T0180998

# Surgical Procedures on the Cirrhotic Patient

Bijan Eghtesad • John Fung
Editors

# Surgical Procedures on the Cirrhotic Patient

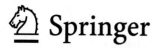 Springer

*Editors*
Bijan Eghtesad
Transplantation Center
Department of General Surgery
Cleveland Clinic
Cleveland, Ohio, USA

John Fung
Department of Surgery
University of Chicago
Chicago, Illinois, USA

ISBN 978-3-319-84896-9      ISBN 978-3-319-52396-5    (eBook)
DOI 10.1007/978-3-319-52396-5

Printed on acid-free paper

This Springer imprint is published by Springer Nature
The registered company is Springer International Publishing AG
The registered company address is: Gewerbestrasse 11, 6330 Cham, Switzerland

# Dedication

*This book is dedicated in memory of Professor Anthony "Tony" Sydney Tavill, who was an extraordinary academic hepatologist and gastroenterologist, but, most of all, a great friend and mentor. Professor Tavill completed his medical training at the University of Manchester and was named Lecturer at the Royal Free Hospital in London before being appointed as Consultant and Clinical Scientist in Middlesex. Professor Tavill emigrated with his family to Cleveland in 1975, where he continued his distinguished career at Metropolitan General Hospital (now known as MetroHealth), then as the Morton Stone Professor of Digestive and Liver Disorders at Mount Sinai Hospital and finally at the Cleveland Clinic Digestive Diseases Institute. He held leadership roles in prestigious professional organizations including President of the American Association for the Study of Liver Diseases (AASLD) and was a regular contributor to and editor of many liver and gastroenterology books and journals. He was Professor Emeritus at Case Western Reserve*

*University for the last 16 years of his career and the recipient of prestigious honors and awards for his teaching and contributions to the study of liver disease and the clinical practice of hepatology. His love of teaching was legendary, and his trainees included two other AASLD presidents: Arthur McCullough and Bruce Bacon. Professor Tavill possessed tremendous social skills and leadership qualities, making him an excellent traveling companion, and often was seen in the company of his beloved wife, Anne Tavill (nee Rayburn), to whom he was married for nearly 57 years. Together they raised 3 children (Leonore, Michael, and Stephanie) and 6 grandchildren. He was a collector of fountain pens and miniature yachts.*

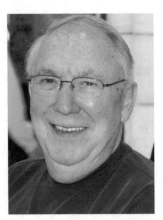

*Kevin D. Mullen*
*Bijan Eghtesad*
*John Fung*

# Foreword

"Cirrhosis", "liver failure", "chronic liver disease" – until recently, mention of these comorbid medical conditions was often cited as a barrier to treatment for patients needing elective or urgent surgery for related or unrelated conditions. However, advances in the understanding of the pathophysiology of liver failure and appreciation of the full spectrum of complications arising from liver disease, as well as treatment for the underlying liver disease and their associated complications, have provided patients afflicted with liver disease, an opportunity for thoughtful preparation and a more realistic understanding of the risks and managing their care after surgery. In this textbook, the co-editors, Bijan Eghtesad and John Fung, both worlds' acknowledged experts in liver surgery and liver transplantation, assemble a veritable "Who's Who" in surgery and liver diseases, to publish a novel, yet extremely important treatise on approaches to optimizing the condition of patients with liver disease and to understand what the procedure specific risks are.

This book is a "must-read" for all surgeons and anesthesiologists, as well as hepatologists and internists that care for these patients before and after their surgery. This will surely become a classic in medical textbooks.

Thomas E. Starzl, MD, PhD

# Preface

Liver disease is a growing public health problem in the United States and around the world. It is estimated that 1 in 10 Americans has some form of liver disease, while estimates of 5–10% of the general population globally have cirrhosis. The prevalence of cirrhosis is likely to be underestimated because of the lack of symptoms in up to one-third of patients with early stages of cirrhosis. Nevertheless, liver disease is the second leading cause of death among digestive diseases, and primary liver cancers now rank as the fastest growing cause of cancer deaths in developed countries. While chronic viral hepatitis accounts for the prevalence of liver disease in developing countries, alcohol and nonalcoholic fatty liver disease account for the growth of liver disease in developed countries.

In this light, surgical practitioners are more than likely to face patients with varying stigmata of chronic liver disease in their practice. The derangements in chronic liver disease may affect multiple physiological systems, including coagulation, circulatory, neurological, renal, and pulmonary manifestations. Patients can be managed with knowledge of those derangements, if the practitioner can recognize the signs and symptoms of chronic liver disease and knows how those derangements impact the organ/tissue that requires surgery and how best to manage such patients prior to, during, and after a surgical procedure. Consultation with a specialist in digestive disorders (gastroenterology) or liver specifically (hepatology), to assist in the management of these patients, should be sought, for those patients with known moderate or greater liver disease and those with newly detected liver disease. Early detection offers an opportunity to treat and stabilize and potentially even reverse chronic liver disease.

We have complied contributions from experts in hepatology and surgical subspecialists to provide evidence-based practices as well as their personal perspectives in the management of patients with chronic liver disease in need of surgery. It is our intention to educate the targeted audience (surgeons, intensivists, hospitalists, and internists) on the risks of surgery, on methods to reduce those risks, and on guidelines on perioperative management. This book is intended to frame the physiologic, pharmacologic, and nutritional disorders in chronic liver disease, as it relates to specific organ systems that are in need of a surgical procedure, as well as to the patient as a whole.

Bijan Eghtesad, MD
John Fung, MD, PhD

# Contents

# Contributors

**Kareem Abu-Elmagd, MD, PhD** Transplant Center, Cleveland Clinic, Cleveland, OH, USA

**Antonios Arvelakis** Recanati/Miller Transplantation Institute, The Mount Sinai Hospital, New York, NY, USA

**Edward C. Benzel, MD** Department of Neurosurgery, Cleveland Clinic, Neurological Institute, Cleveland, OH, USA

**Eren Berber, MD** Cleveland Clinic, Cleveland, OH, USA

**Matthew Blum** Cleveland Clinic, Department of General Surgery, Cleveland, OH, USA

**Jessica E. Bollinger, Pharm D, BCPS** Department of Pharmacy, Cleveland Clinic, Cleveland, OH, USA

**Peter A Caputo, MD** Center for Robotic and Advanced Laparoscopic Surgery, Glickman Urologic Institute, Cleveland Clinic, Cleveland, OH, USA

**Alvin Chan, BS** Medical College of Wisconsin, Milwaukee, WI, USA

**Kenneth D. Chavin, MD, PhD** Department of Surgery, Case Western Reserve University, Cleveland, OH, USA

**Gabriel R. Chedister, MD** Medical University of South Carolina, Charleston, SC, USA

**Christopher P. Coppa, MD** Department of Radiology, Cleveland Clinic, Cleveland, OH, USA

**Guilherme Costa, MD, PhD** Transplant Center, Department of General Surgery, Cleveland Clinic, Cleveland, OH, USA

**Bijan Eghtesad, MD** Transplant Center, Department of General Surgery, Cleveland Clinic, Cleveland, OH, USA

**Haytham Elgharably** Cleveland Clinic Department of Thoracic and Cardiovascular Surgery, Cleveland, OH, USA

**Andrew W. Eller, MD** The Retina Service, UPMC Eye Center, Department of Ophthalmology, University of Pittsburgh School of Medicine, The Eye and Ear Institute, Pittsburgh, PA, USA

**Tommaso Falcone, MD, FRCSC, FACOG** Cleveland Clinic Lerner College of Medicine and Chair Obstetrics, Gynecology and Women's Health Institute, Cleveland, OH, USA

**Sander Florman** Recanati/Miller Transplantation Institute, The Mount Sinai Hospital, New York, NY, USA

**Yuman Fong, MD** Department of Surgery, City of Hope National Medical Center, Duarte, CA, USA

**Masato Fujiki, MD, PhD** Transplant Center, Department of General Surgery, Cleveland Clinic, Cleveland, OH, USA

**Maysoon Gamaleldin, MD** Department of Colorectal Surgery, Digestive Disease Institute, Cleveland Clinic, Cleveland, OH, USA

**Manjushree Gautam, MD, MAS** Department of Internal Medicine, Texas A&M College of Medicine, Bryan, TX, USA
Simmons Transplant Institute, Baylor All Saints Medical Center, Fort Worth, TX, USA

**James Guggenheimer, DDS** Department of Diagnostic Sciences, University of Pittsburgh School of Dental Medicine, Pittsburgh, PA, USA

**Zubaidah Nor Hanipah, MD** Bariatric and Metabolic Institute, M61, Cleveland Clinic, Cleveland, OH, USA

**Ivy N. Haskins, MD** Comprehensive Hernia Center, Digestive Disease and Surgery Institute, Cleveland, OH, USA

**Jeanette Hasse, PhD, RD, LD, FADA, CNSC** Annette C. and Harold C. Simmons Transplant Institute, Baylor University Medical Center, Dallas, TX, USA

**Bahaa Eldeen Senousy Ismail, MD, MSc** Gastroenterology Department, Cleveland Clinic Florida, Weston, FL, USA

**Jihad H. Kaouk, MD, FACS** Center for Robotic and Advanced Laparoscopic Surgery, Glickman Urologic Institute, Cleveland Clinic, Cleveland, OH, USA

**Linden Karas, MD** Bariatric and Metabolic Institute, M61, Cleveland Clinic, Cleveland, OH, USA

**Ajai Khanna, MD, PhD** Transplant Center, Department of General Surgery, Cleveland Clinic, Cleveland, OH, USA

**David J. Kramer, MD, FACP** Aurora Critical Care Service, Aurora Health Care, Milwaukee, WI, USA
University of Wisconsin School of Medicine and Public Health, Madison, USA

**Robert R. Lorenz, MD** Cleveland Clinic Head and Neck Institute, Cleveland, OH, USA

**Haider Mahdi, MD, MPH** Section of Gynecologic Oncology, Cleveland Clinic Lerner College of Medicine, Cleveland, OH, USA

**Kenneth R. McCurry, MD** Cleveland Clinic Department of Thoracic and Cardiovascular Surgery, Cleveland, OH, USA

**Jeffrey P. Mullin, MD, MBA** Department of Neurosurgery, Cleveland Clinic, Neurological Institute, Cleveland, OH, USA

**Jennifer W. Nguyen-Lee, MD** Department of Anesthesiology and Perioperative Medicine, UCLA Health System, Los Angeles, CA, USA

**Jila Noori, MD** The Retina Service, Department of Ophthalmology, University of Pittsburgh Medical Center, Pittsburgh, PA, USA

**Toshihiro Okamoto** Cleveland Clinic Department of Thoracic and Cardiovascular Surgery, Cleveland, OH, USA

**Arun P. Palanisamy, PhD** Department of Surgery, Case Western Reserve University, Cleveland, OH, USA

**Andrew B. Peitzman, MD** Trauma and Surgical Services, Pittsburgh, PA, USA

**Uma Perni, MD, MPH** Section of Maternal-Fetal Medicine, Cleveland Clinic Lerner College of Medicine, Cleveland, OH, USA

**Jeffery L. Ponsky, MD, FACS** Lerner College of Medicine, Department of General Surgery, Digestive Diseases and Surgery Institute, Cleveland Clinic Foundation, Cleveland, OH, USA
Cleveland Clinic Lerner College of Medicine, Digestive Disease and Surgery Institute, Cleveland, OH, USA

**Naftali Presser, MD** Department of General Surgery, Digestive Disease Surgical Institute, Cleveland Clinic Foundation, Cleveland, OH, USA

**Margaret V. Ragni, MD, MPH** Department of Medicine, University of Pittsburgh, Hemophilia Center of Western Pennsylvania, Pittsburgh, PA, USA

**Jorge D. Reyes, MD** Roger K. Giesecke Distinguished Chair, Professor and Chief, Division of Transplant Surgery, Department of Surgery, University of Washington, Director of Transplant Services, Seattle Children's Hopsital, Seattle, WA, USA

**John M. Rivas, MD** Liver Transplant Department, Cleveland Clinic Florida, Weston, FL, USA

**Vinayak S. Rohan, MD** Medical University of South Carolina, Charleston, SC, USA

**Michael J. Rosen, MD FACS** Comprehensive Hernia Center, Digestive Disease and Surgery Institute, Cleveland, OH, USA

**Nelson A. Royall, MD** Cleveland Clinic Foundation, Cleveland, OH, USA

**Samuel Eleazar Ruskin, MD** Department of Radiology, Cleveland Clinic, Cleveland, OH, USA

**Philip R. Schauer, MD** Bariatric and Metabolic Institute, M61, Cleveland Clinic, Cleveland, OH, USA

**Craig D. Seaman, MD, MS** Department of Medicine, University of Pittsburgh, Hemophilia Center of Western Pennsylvania, Pittsburgh, PA, USA

**Ron Shapiro** Recanati/Miller Transplantation Institute, The Mount Sinai Hospital, New York, NY, USA

**Nicholas Smedira, MD** Heart and Vascular Institute, Cleveland Clinic, Cleveland, OH, USA

**Basem Soliman, MD, PhD** Cleveland Clinic Department of General Surgery, Cleveland, OH, USA

**Randolph H. Steadman, MD, MS** Department of Anesthesiology and Perioperative Medicine, UCLA Health System, Los Angeles, CA, USA

**Luca Stocchi, MD, FACS** Department of Colorectal Surgery, Digestive Disease Institute, Cleveland Clinic, Cleveland, OH, USA

**Dennis Tang, MD** Cleveland Clinic Head and Neck Institute, Cleveland, OH, USA

**R. Matthew Walsh, MD** Department of General Surgery, Academic Department of Surgery, Cleveland Clinic Foundation, Cleveland, OH, USA

**Susanne Warner, MD** Department of Surgery, City of Hope National Medical Center, Duarte, CA, USA

**Connor Wathen, BS** Cleveland Clinic Lerner College of Medicine, Cleveland, OH, USA

**Nisar Zaidi, MD** Essentia Health/Duluth Clinic, Duluth, MN, USA

**Ahmad Zeeshan, MD** Heart and Vascular Institute, Cleveland Clinic, Cleveland, OH, USA
Heart and Vascular Institute, Cleveland Clinic Florida, Weston, FL, USA

**Xaralambos B. Zervos, DO, MS** Liver Transplant Department, Cleveland Clinic Florida, Weston, FL, USA

# Chapter 1
# Pathophysiology of Cirrhosis and Portal Hypertension

Bahaa Eldeen Senousy Ismail, John M. Rivas, and Xaralambos B. Zervos

## Introduction

The regenerative capability of the liver is one of the many unique characteristics that distinguish it from the other major organ systems. Its dual blood supply via the portal vein and hepatic artery further delineate the liver from other organs. They provide the rich nourishing environment for the hepatocytes to thrive but also serve as the entry for toxin-mediated inflammation. Insult from either exogenous or endogenous sources that lead to persistent liver injury exemplifies the liver's natural ability to regenerate toward sustained healing. However, prolonged exposure to an inflammatory cascade eventually paves the way for abnormal excessive fibrogenesis, which results in replacement of liver tissue by fibrous bands and regenerative nodules. As this disease progression occurs, the hepatic architecture becomes distorted; rings of collagen bands develop indicating the establishment of cirrhosis. Hepatic vasculature distortion with impairment of hepatic function signals the progression of cirrhosis and subsequent associated decompensation [1].

Although cirrhosis histologically is a process that involves the liver tissue, major systemic manifestations develop due to both impaired function of the hepatocytes and development of portal hypertension. The resulting hormonal and generalized circulatory changes impact other organs, such as the kidney and heart. Patients with cirrhosis undergoing surgery have considerable increased risk for complications compared to the normal population due to impaired hepatic function and altered systemic venous flow dynamics. Understanding the basic concepts of cirrhosis

B.E.S. Ismail, MD, MSc
Gastroenterology Department, Cleveland Clinic Florida, Weston, FL, USA

J.M. Rivas, MD • X.B. Zervos, DO, MS (✉)
Liver Transplant Department, Cleveland Clinic Florida, Weston, FL, USA
e-mail: zervosx@ccf.org

© Springer International Publishing AG 2017
B. Eghtesad, J. Fung (eds.), *Surgical Procedures on the Cirrhotic Patient*,
DOI 10.1007/978-3-319-52396-5_1

1

pathogenesis and development of portal hypertension is essential to clinicians and surgeons tasked to appropriately risk stratify this patient population prior to any invasive procedure.

## Liver Histology

### *Hepatocytes*

Hepatocytes represent 70–80% of the cell mass in the normal liver [2]. They serve multiple functions including synthesis of proteins, cholesterol, bile, hormones, and cytokines, as well as metabolism of carbohydrates [2]. Hepatocytes are the target for most hepatotoxic agents, and although they have the ability to regenerate, cell death may result from either direct insult of the hepatotoxin and/or from the immune response elicited by the affected hepatocytes [3].

The liver architecture consists of rows of hepatocytes arranged in sheets with intervening vascular spaces that make up the hepatic sinusoids. They are lined by fenestrated endothelial cells without a true basement membrane but with a surrounding perisinusoidal space (Space of Disse). The Space of Disse contains a permeable connective tissue [4] known as the extracellular matrix. It predominately consists of collagen and glycoproteins, and in the normal liver this matrix is loose to facilitate exchange of molecules through endothelium fenestrae. This perisinusoidal space also serves as the main site of fibrous tissue deposition in a diseased liver. Hepatic stellate cells, also commonly known as Ito cells, when activated are responsible for the deposition of collagen in this space with persistent liver injury. When the production of fibrous material exceeds degradation thus changing the matrix to dense connective tissue, this change is associated with loss of endothelial fenestration and formation of a dense basement membrane. This process is known as capillarization of the hepatic sinusoids [5] and is a well-described hallmark of liver cirrhosis.

The development of fibrous deposition is a complex process involving interaction between multiple liver cells via a series of enzymes and cytokines [6]. Many liver cells are involved in this progression but the hepatocyte remains central to the process. Hepatocytes stimulate hepatic fibrogenesis through production of matrix metalloproteinases (MMP-2 and MMP-3), while concurrently, there is an imbalance between metalloproteinase and tissue inhibitor of metalloproteinases (TIMP) that are normally secreted by the hepatocytes (TIMP-1 and TIMP-2) [7]. Hepatocytes release multiple inducers of fibrogenesis including transforming growth factor-$\beta 1$ (TGF-$\beta 1$) and reactive oxygen species that induce activation of hepatic stellate cells [8].

Other important nonparenchymal cells involved in fibrogenesis are located mainly around the lining of the hepatic sinusoids. These cells include the sinusoidal endothelial cells, Kupffer cells, and the Hepatic stellate (Ito) cells.

## Liver Sinusoidal Endothelial Cells

These cells differ from other vascular endothelium to allow filtration and exchange of fluids and molecules between blood in hepatic sinusoids and the hepatic parenchyma. The presence of fenestrae and loose surrounding connective tissue allow the passage of pathogens and facilitate the scavenger function of these cells and their ability to present antigen. With excess fibrous tissue deposition, capillarization of endothelial cells occurs interfering with their exchange process ability [9]. They secrete cytokines such as IL-33, which activate stellate cells and contribute in the formation of liver fibrosis [10].

## Kupffer Cells

Part of the reticuloendothelial system, they are the second most abundant cells in the liver after hepatocytes, constituting about 15% of the liver cell mass [11]. They function as the hepatic macrophage lining the sinusoids where they are exposed to toxins and infectious agents. Once exposed to antigens they act as antigen presenting cells. In addition, they have a role in detoxification and tumor surveillance [12]. Following antigen presentation, Kupffer cells produce other cytokines that attract T-cells, which initiate apoptosis of the hepatocytes [13, 14]. In the diseased liver, Kupffer cells contribute to hepatocyte injury through production of reactive oxygen species and lysosomal enzymes that are destructive to the liver. Finally, their role in fibrosis is via the TGF-β1 production that activates stellate cells [15].

## Stellate Cells (Ito Cells)

The hepatic stellate cells (HSCs) are located in the space of Disse around the hepatic sinusoids. They store fat and are the primary site for retinoid storage [16]. Ito cells are considered the key player in fibrogenesis.

Fibrogenesis takes place through activation of HSCs that can be defined as a process of proliferation, transformation into myofibroblasts, followed by migration and formation of large amounts of dense collagen fibers into the extracellular matrix [17]. Activation follows liver injury and is driven by exposure to cytokines such as transforming growth factor TGF-β and platelet-derived growth factor (PDGF) among other gathering stimulants [18].

Stellate cell activation has been commonly divided into two phases: initiation and perpetuation. Initiation is the early step involving alteration in gene expression and receptor changes that make cells responsive to cytokines, while perpetuation indicates a later stage of maintaining activation and ongoing fibrogenesis [19].

Initiation is driven by several mechanisms: (1) Oxidative stress and release of free radicals into the extracellular space [20] resulting from infiltration of inflammatory cells that follow liver injury. A similar process occurs via direct oxidative stress with excess iron presence in disease entities such as hemochromatosis and alcoholic liver disease [21]. (2) Fas-mediated hepatocyte apoptosis and formation of apoptotic fragments initiate activation when engulfed by HSCs. This stimulates upregulation of nicotinamide adenine dinucleotide phosphate (NADPH) oxidase, which further generates oxidative stress [22]. (3) Injury of endothelial cells and release of cellular fibronectin activate HSCs [23]. (4) Platelet injury during inflammation stimulates the most potent HSC activation through PDGF and associated epidermal growth factor (EGF) release [24]. (5) The steatosis present in hepatitis C infection may directly affect HSC activation in addition to the binding of the HCV envelope protein (E2) with surface CD81 on the HSC surface. This has been shown to increase the expression of MMP-2 [25]. During the process of activation there is loss of the HSC perinuclear retinoid droplets thought to play a role in activation through interaction with nuclear retinoid receptors [26].

After activation, the number of HSCs in the injured liver tissue is increased, which occurs due to both proliferation and migration. There are several identified HSC mitogens involved in this process, but the most prominent is PDGF that induces proliferation through intracellular calcium signaling. The PDFG receptor upregulation correlates with liver tissue damage [27]. Additionally, PDGF serves as a HSC chemotaxic agent, stimulating migration of HSCs to areas of injured liver tissue [28]. Other mitogens for HSCs are endothelin and insulin-like growth factor 1 (IGF-1) [29]. The notable structural change in activated HSCs is the increase in intracellular actin fibrils that increases cell contractility. This is stimulated by endothelin-1 and decreased by nitric oxide, an agent that significantly decreases in the setting of cirrhosis [30]. Activated HSCs are found in large numbers in the collagenous bands found in cirrhosis. Alteration in portal blood flow occurs via remodeling of the sinusoid as these bands shorten leading to the overall morphology of the cirrhotic liver.

Once activation occurs, there is a positive feedback loop that maintains this process to allow for the second stage of perpetuation. This occurs through interaction between HSCs and certain extracellular matrix components that have biologic activity directing cell differentiation, proliferation, chemotaxis, fibrogenesis as collagen VI, fibronectin, and the noncollagenous glycoprotein laminin-1 [31]. The net result of HSC activation is fibrogenesis. This is mediated by different cytokines but the most identified is TGF-β1 and others are summarized in Table 1.1.

In addition to cytokines, there has been a growing interest in the role of micro RNA (miRNA), which are noncoding RNA segments that act as posttranscriptional regulators of many other genes. The miRNA can be divided into profibrogenic and antifibrogenic [6] (Table 1.2). Both animal and human studies show a significant role in hepatic fibrogenesis and a potential target for therapy.

As the deposition of excess collagen occurs, matrix degradation ensues through MMP. However, in the case of chronic liver injury, matrix production occurs at a higher rate than degradation resulting in turn over, matrix remodeling, and formation of the acellular dense collagen rich matrix [52]. Moreover, there is a process of

**Table 1.1** Multiple cytokines are involved in hepatic stellate cells activation and in the process of fibrogenesis

| Cytokine | Source | Role in fibrogenesis |
|---|---|---|
| TGF-β1 | Main source is HSCs (autocrine loop). Other source: KCs, Liver sinusoidal endothelial cells, and hepatocytes [32] | Smad3 signaling to activate HSCs [33] |
| | | Expression of the matrix-producing genes |
| | | Promoting TIMP |
| | | Downregulates MMPs |
| | | Induces apoptosis of hepatocytes [34] |
| TNF-α | Main source is macrophage and monocyte; other sources HSCs, and KCs [35] | Induces synthesis of extracellular matrix by HSCs |
| | | Inhibits HSCs apoptosis (downregulation of p53) [36] |
| PDGF (mostly PDGF-B and PDGF-D) | KCs [6] | Proliferation of HSCs (through mitogen-activated protein kinase (MAPK) and protein kinase (PK)B/Akt pathways [37] |
| Interferon | Leukocytes [6] | *IFN-α*: antiapoptotic effect on activated HSCs [38] |
| | | *IFN-γ*: [38, 39] |
| | | Inhibiting HSC activation through TGFβ1 pathways |
| | | Proapoptotic effect on HSCs by downregulating heat-shock protein 70 |
| | | Decreases production of α-smooth muscle actin and collagen |
| Profibrogenic IL | T lymphocytes, KC, in addition to endothelial cells | *IL1*: HSCs activation and stimulate production of MMP and TIMP-1 [40] |
| | | *IL-17*: particularly in hepatitis B, upregulation of TNF-α, TGF-β1, and collagen 1α [41] |
| Leptin | Adipose cells | Upregulates collagen expression in HSCs [42] |

*TGF-β1* transforming growth factor beta, *TNF-α* tumor necrosis factor alpha, *PDGF* platelet-derived growth factor, *KCs* kupffer cells, *TIMP* tissue inhibitor of metalloproteinases, *MMPs* matrix metalloproteinases, *HSCs* hepatic stellate cells, *IFN* interferon, *IL* interleukin

**Table 1.2** Profibrogenic and antifibrogenic miRNAs

| Profibrogenic miRNA | Antifibrogenic miRNAs |
|---|---|
| *miR-214-5p*: increase expression of fibrosis-related genes (such as MMP-2, MMP-9, α-SMA, and TGF-β1) [43]<br>*miR-181b and miR-221/222* : promote HSC proliferation by regulating p27 gene and the cell cycle [44, 45]<br>*miR-155*: increase TNF-α production in response to gut-derived lipopolysaccharide in alcoholic hepatitis [46, 47]<br>In addition to others that are upregulated in response to TGF-β as miR-571 [48] | *miRNA-150 and miRNA-194*: inhibit HSC activation through downregulation of c-myb [49]<br>*miR-21*: inhibits HSC activation through downregulation of TGF-β expression [50]<br>*miR- 133a*: decreases expression of collagens and is inhibited by TGF-β in the setting of chronic hepatitis [51] |

*TGF-β1* transforming growth factor beta, *MMP* matrix metallopeptidase, *α-SMA* α-smooth muscle actin, *HSC* hepatic stellate cell matrix stabilization, leading to accumulation of elastic fibers and covalent cross-linking of collagen. This progression enables the matrix to be more resistant to enzymatic degradation and is driven by enzymes such as lysyl oxidase, a potential target for inhibition of fibrogenesis [53].

## Outcome of Activated Stellate Cells

Changes in activated HSCs, for example, increase the expression of nerve growth factor receptor (NGFR) and make them more susceptible to apoptosis [54]. However, even with such changes, there are other factors associated with ongoing liver tissue injury that inhibit HSC apoptosis and the net result is prolonged life of activated cells. This is mediated by factors, such as the antiapoptotic activity of TIMP-1; which was shown to inhibit MMP-2 activity, and blocks apoptosis [55]. Other agents as TNF-$\alpha$ and IGF-I inhibit HSC apoptosis through interaction with NF-$\kappa$B and phosphatidylinositol-3 kinase (PI3-K) pathways, respectively [54, 56]. Also as mentioned earlier, some components of the fibrotic matrix (i.e., collagen VI) can stimulate activated HSC survival [57]. Resolution of injury is associated with stimulation of apoptosis that was inhibited by the abovementioned mechanisms. Reversal of HSCs to quiescent form occurs after resolution of inflammation and contributes to decreased number of activated cells [58]. In the case of unresolved liver injury, for example, with untreated chronic hepatitis C infection, HSC activation continues, along with active fibrogenesis, eventually resulting in liver cirrhosis.

Macrophages play a critical regulatory role in wound healing and in the resolution of fibrogenesis. They can stimulate liver regeneration and scar resolution through production of fibrinolytic agents such as MMP 13 [59]. Found within areas of fibrosis, scar-associated macrophages (SAMs) have been identified as potential targets of therapy to reverse fibrosis [60, 61].

## Definition and Classification of Portal Hypertension

Portal hypertension is defined as the rise in portal pressure above the normal hepatic venous pressure of 1–5 mmHg. The key physiologic feature of portal hypertension is an increase in resistance to portal blood flow. Portal hypertension can be broadly classified into three types: (1) prehepatic, (2) intrahepatic, (3) posthepatic depending on the site of where the resistance develops. Prehepatic portal hypertension involves any obstruction along the portal vein. Intrahepatic portal hypertension in turn can be further subclassified into three subcategories, including (i) presinusoidal (e.g., schistosomiasis, granuloma, congenital fibrosis), (ii) sinusoidal (e.g., cirrhosis), and (iii) postsinusoidal (e.g., sinusoidal obstruction syndrome). In turn, posthepatic portal hypertension involves inferior vena cava obstruction (e.g., Budd–Chiari syndrome) or heart disease (e.g., constrictive pericarditis) [62]. The underlying pathophysiology and the consequences of portal hypertension vary according to the etiology and the location of increased resistance. The focus of this section is portal hypertension at the level of the hepatic sinusoids in the setting of end-stage liver disease [63].

## Intrahepatic Changes

### Increased Intrahepatic Resistance

Multiple factors contribute to the increase in vascular resistance within the liver. Decreased intrahepatic vasodilators (nitric oxide, NO) and an increase in vasoconstrictors (cyclooxygenase-1, COX-1) appear to be the main drivers of intrahepatic vasoconstriction. Decrease in NO results from a combination of lower concentrations of the NO producing enzyme, endothelial synthase, as well as, NO depletion via formation of peroxynitrite in the setting of chronic bacterial endotoxemia [64]. This increase in vasoconstriction occurs as a result of increased activity of COX-1, which in turn causes an upregulation of thromboxane A2 production, leading to intrahepatic vasoconstriction. Other additional upregulated intrahepatic vasoconstrictors, include endothelin-1, angiotensin-II, and norepinephrine [65]. To a lesser extent, activated stellate cells, which are present in the perisinusoidal space, also play an important role in intrahepatic resistance, as a result of endothelin-1 stimulation [66].

### Intrahepatic Angiogenesis

Increased numbers of blood vessels are observed in the cirrhotic fibrotic septa and in the surrounding regenerative nodules. Activated stellate cells stimulate endothelial cells through the release of certain factors, such as, vascular endothelial growth factor (VEGF) and angiopoietin [67, 68]. In theory, the formation of these new blood vessels is expected to decrease hepatic vascular resistance. However, the opposite occurs because these new vessels are abnormal, leading to irregular flow patterns, known as splitting (or intussusceptive) angiogenesis [69].

### Intrahepatic Microthrombosis

Part of the hypercoagulable state associated with cirrhosis is the formation of microthrombi in intrahepatic vasculature. These microthrombi propagate in the progression of fibrosis and the increase in intrahepatic vascular resistance contributing to portal hypertension [70]. This can be seen when examining the histology of liver explants. Obliterative lesions and intimal fibrosis – suggestive of healed microthrombi – were present in hepatic and portal venules and associated with regions of confluent fibrosis and cirrhotic nodules (focal parenchymal extinction theory) [71].

This may have clinical application shown through significantly delayed decompensation in cirrhotic patients treated with a 12-month course of enoxaparin [72]. In summary, increased intrahepatic resistance occurs secondary to both structural and dynamic changes. Structural changes in the cirrhotic nodule can be seen by the presence of impaired blood flow, fibrous septa, angiogenesis, and microthrombi. Dynamic changes occur secondary to intrahepatic cytokine-induced vasoconstriction and stellate cell contraction.

## Extrahepatic Changes

### *Extrahepatic Arteriolar Vasodilation*

In the setting of cirrhosis, vasodilation is noted in both splanchnic and systemic circulations that significantly contribute to the development of portal hypertension. Similar to the intrahepatic environment, NO is the most potent vasodilator molecule. An increase in portal pressure when sensed by endothelial cells leads to stimulation of endothelial NO synthase, resulting in an increase NO production [73]. Other vasodilator molecules that have been identified to participate in extrahepatic arteriolar vasodilation, include carbon monoxide, prostacyclin, and endocannabinoids [65]. In addition to increased levels of potent vasodilator molecules, there is also a decreased production of potent vasoconstrictor molecules, such as bradykinin [65].

Aside from the disequilibrium between said vasodilators and vasoconstrictors, structural changes such as (1) decreased vascular sympathetic tone as a result of atrophy of sympathetic nerve [74] and (2) thinning of mesenteric arteries may also contribute to splanchnic vasodilation [75].

The net result of splanchnic and systemic vasodilation is the relative decrease in the effective blood volume and systemic vascular filling. This eventually causes stimulation of compensatory mechanism, such as release of antidiuretic hormone and activation of the renin–angiotensin–aldosterone system. This, in turn, leads to both sodium and water retention and increase in blood volume. In accordance to Ohm's law, such a compensatory mechanism leads to an increase in portal pressure that is proportionate to both flow resistance and portal inflow [76]. The latter is increased by both splanchnic vasodilation and the increased blood volume seen mentioned earlier (Fig. 1.1).

### *Collateral Blood Vessel Formation*

This occurs primarily through opening of preexisting blood vessels. Increased circulating vascular endothelial growth factor and placental growth factor play a major role leading to significant angiogenesis [73, 77, 78].

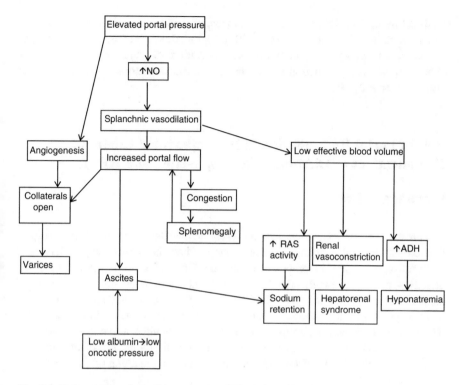

**Fig. 1.1** Pathogenesis of portal hypertension (*NO* nitric oxide, *RAS* renin–angiotensin system, ADH *antidiuretic hormone*)

## Splenomegaly and Increased Spleen Stiffness

Splenomegaly is a common sign of portal hypertension. It initially occurs as a result of congestion of the spleen's red pulp in the setting of decreased low venous drainage from the spleen into the now higher portal pressure system. However, as the spleen enlarges its elasticity decreases and stiffness increases, thus creating higher resistance in the portal system [79]. Additionally, the sheer blood volume acquired reservoirs in the now larger spleen, leading to an overall increase in portal blood flow. Given that the portal system is a fixed circuit, the increasing amount of volume overwhelms the system leading to drainage through alternate routes (e.g., varices) [80].

## *Role of Bacterial Translocation*

In cirrhosis there is an increase in bacterial translocation and lipopolysaccharides endotoxemia, as a result of increased (1) intestinal bacterial overgrowth, (2) increased intestinal permeability [81, 82], (3) decreased endotoxin clearance by malfunctioning Kupffer cells and hepatocytes, as well as, low circulating albumin, which has an endotoxin-binding effect [83]. Endotoxins also cause increases in NO production, hepatocyte inflammation via activation of tumor necrosis factor-α (TNF-α) [84], and production of intrahepatic vasoconstrictors, endothelin-1, and thromboxane A2 [85].

## Role of Portal Hypertension in Development of Common Complications of Cirrhosis (Varices, Ascites, and HRS)

### *Esophageal Varices*

The presence of esophageal varices represent an elevated portal pressure gradient. Dilated submucosal esophageal veins enlarge when the periesophageal tributary drain through become incompetent communicating veins. As the portal pressure increases, more blood is diverted into the submucosa in an attempt to decompress the portal circulation. The loose submucosal connective tissue and the negative intra thoracic pressure allow further expansion and increase in size of the varices [86, 87]. Increased neovascularization in splanchnic organs plays a role in formation of portal collaterals including varices, shown in animal studies to be mediated by VEGF. When VGEF and PDGF are inhibited, there is a reduction of collateral vein formation [88, 89].

One of the most serious complications of cirrhosis is when esophageal wall tension is exceeded and rupture of the varices occurs leading to bleeding. This increased tension is best described by Laplace's law $[Q \times (nl/ \prod r^4)] \times r/w$, where $Q$ refers to blood flow per unit of time, $r$ and $l$ are radius and length of the blood vessel, and $w$ is wall thickness. The longer and larger the varices with higher flow rate within a thin wall the more likely for spontaneous rupture and bleeding to occur [90].

### Gastric and Ectopic Varices

Gastric varices develop via the same principle and are identified based on their anatomical relationship to esophageal varices and location in the stomach. Gastroesophageal varices when in continuity with the esophagus are classified into two types: type 1 (GOV 1) found along the lesser curvature, whereas type 2 (GOV 2) run along the greater curvature toward the fundus of the stomach. Larger varices are commonly found in GOV 1 than in GOV 2. This is likely due to their relationship to the left gastric vein [91].

Isolated gastric varices do not communicate with the esophagus and are also classified into two types: type 1 (IGV 1) are seen as a cluster of isolated varices in the fundus where type 2 (IGV 2) are isolated varices seen in other parts of the stomach. Splenic vein thrombosis is often associated with presence of IGV1 where portal vein thrombosis is associated with IGV2 [92].

Other ectopic varices can be seen at sites of previous surgery where there is a cross relationship between portal circulation (gastrointestinal tract) and systemic circulation (abdominal wall). Patients with portal hypertension undergoing bowel surgery and stoma formation are susceptible to peristomal varice formation [93].

## Portal Hypertensive Gastropathy

The presence of portal hypertensive gastropathy (PHG) is a highly prevalent complication of portal hypertension which manifests as chronic versus overt blood loss. The severity correlates with the progression of liver disease and presence of other signs of portal hypertension such as large esophageal varices [94]. How PHG develops is not fully understood; however, available evidence suggests that portal hypertension increases congestion of capillaries and venules in the gastric submucosa [95], leading to mucosal microcirculation abnormalities causing hypoxia and dysregulation of local cytokines which impair healing and increase risk of bleeding [96]. Patients who suffer from PHG-associated chronic blood loss may requiring repeat blood transfusion and thus considered for decompression with shunt surgery or transjugular intrahepatic portosystemic shunt [97].

It is clinically important to understand how the pathogenesis of PHG differs from gastric antral vascular ectasia (GAVE-watermelon stomach). GAVE is not directly related to the degree of portal hypertension and may be seen in other disease processes like chronic gastritis. Patients with GAVE have an increased concentration of locally acting vasodilator substances (mainly gastrin and prostaglandin E) along with altered antral motility, hence, the histologic appearance of mucosal capillary dilation along with fibrin thrombi and fibromuscular hyperplasia [98]. As the pathophysiology implies, GAVE does not respond to reduction of portal pressure with shunting or beta-blocker therapy [99].

## Ascites, Refractory Ascites and Hepatorenal Syndrome

The most acceptable theory currently on how cirrhotic ascites develops is the forward theory [100]. The presence of sinusoidal portal hypertension results in splanchnic arterial vasodilation leading to a forward increase in filtration across splanchnic capillaries and lymphatics. As decompensation worsens, filtration increases beyond the capability of the lymphatic system to complement return to the circulation [101] This effective intravascular reduction activates the renin–angiotensin–aldosterone system stimulating sodium and water retention in an attempt to compensate for underfilling by increasing blood volume. However, because of the increased filtration and the low plasma oncotic pressure, continuous leakage into the peritoneal cavity occurs leading to more ascites [102]. In more advanced cirrhosis, renal vasoconstriction develops along with enhanced sodium reabsorption in the renal tubule.

This leads to very low urinary excretion of sodium and development of refractory ascites and eventually hepatorenal syndrome [103].

## Diagnosis and Measurement of Portal Hypertension

The diagnosis of portal hypertension is portrayed in patients who have a history of cirrhosis with clinical signs of ascites, varices, or low platelet count. Imaging findings suggestive of portal hypertension are not sensitive or specific to the diagnosis [104]. The presence of splenomegaly, dilated portal vein with reversed flow, recanulized umbilical vein or other intra-abdominal collaterals is relative markers for but do not quantify the degree of portal hypertension.

The measuring of portal pressure is indicated to confirm diagnosis and help determine etiology and/or stratify the risk of complications. Hepatic venous pressure gradient (HVPG) is the method preferred to measure portal hypertension. Performed by interventional radiology, a 6 or 7 French balloon catheter is inserted through the right internal jugular vein and then placed into the hepatic vein to measure the free hepatic pressure. HVPG is an approximate measure of the gradient between the systemic circulation (represented by the free hepatic pressure-FHVP) and portal pressure (represented by the wedge hepatic pressure-WHVP), HVPG = WHVP − FHVP. The wedge hepatic pressure is measured after inflating the balloon. A difference of 6 mmHg or more is consistent with portal hypertension with a gradient > 10–12 mmHg required for clinically significant portal hypertension and development of complications such as ascites and varices [105].

It is important to note that although there is direct measurement of hepatic vein pressure, the portal vein pressure is an indirect method, as wedge hepatic venous pressure is performed with the catheter still in the end tributary of the hepatic vein. This is a limitation of this technique in cases of postsinusoidal induced portal hypertension, as the gradient will remain normal and will not reflect the actual portal hypertension. An alternative method that is more accurate but more invasive is to directly pass the catheter to the portal venous system through a transhepatic catheter. A new technique using the endoscopic guidance of ultrasound (EUS) has been described in animal models with adequate correlation with the conventional interventional radiology method [106].

One noninvasive way to predict HPVG is transient elastography that showed adequate correlation for detecting clinically significant portal hypertension. However, there was significant variability in the correlating elastography cutoff value; ranging from 13.6 to 34.9 kPa, probably due to variability in the etiology of the underlying liver disease in the different studies [107]. There are several limitations of transient elastography that impact its accuracy detecting liver fibrosis and eventually predicting the portal pressure. The presence of ascites, increased abdominal wall thickness, conditions with increased liver edema such as passive congestion, acute hepatitis, cholestasis, or the technically difficult patient with narrow rib space [108]. Promising results are available on the value of magnetic resonance elastography in predicting the HPVG [109, 110] and if validated through further studies it can provide higher technical success rate and better accuracy compared to transient elastography as magnetic resonance elastography scans the entire liver rather than a limited segment.

# References

1. Schuppan D, Afdhal NH. Liver cirrhosis. Lancet. 2008;371:838–51.
2. Ramadori G, Moriconi F, Malik I, Dudas J. Physiology and pathophysiology of liver inflammation, damage and repair. J Physiol Pharmacol. 2008;59:107–17.
3. Wallace K, Burt AD, Wright MC. Liver fibrosis. Biochem J. 2008;411:1–18.
4. Park YN, Yang CP, Fernandez GJ, Cubukcu O, Thung SN, Theise ND. Neoangiogenesis and sinusoidal "capillarization" in dysplastic nodules of the liver. Am J Surg Pathol. 1998;22:656–62.
5. Xu B, Broome U, Uzunel M, Nava S, Ge X, Kumagai-Braesch M, et al. Capillarization of hepatic sinusoid by liver endothelial cell-reactive autoantibodies in patients with cirrhosis and chronic hepatitis. Am J Pathol. 2003;163:1275–89.
6. Zhou WC, Zhang QB, Qiao L. Pathogenesis of liver cirrhosis. World J Gastroenterol. Baishideng Publishing Group Inc. 2014;20:7312–24.
7. Del Carmen Garcíade León M, Montfort I, Tello Montes E, López Vancell R, Olivos García A, González Canto A, et al. Hepatocyte production of modulators of extracellular liver matrix in normal and cirrhotic rat liver. Exp Mol Pathol. 2006;80:97–108.
8. Ali MA, Koura BA, el Mashad N, Zaghloul MH. The Bcl-2 and TGF-beta1 levels in patients with chronic hepatitis C, liver cirrhosis and hepatocellular carcinoma. Egyptian J Immunol. 2004;11:83–90.
9. Yokomori H, Oda M, Yoshimura K, Hibi T. Recent advances in liver sinusoidal endothelial ultrastructure and fine structure immunocytochemistry. Micron. 2012;43:129–34.
10. Marvie P, Lisbonne M, L'helgoualc'h A, Rauch M, Turlin B, Preisser L, et al. Interleukin-33 overexpression is associated with liver fibrosis in mice and humans. J Cell Mol Med. 2010;14:1726–39.
11. Bouwens L, Baekeland M, De ZR, Wisse E. Quantitation, tissue distribution and proliferation kinetics of Kupffer cells in normal rat liver. Hepatology. 1986;6:718–22.
12. Kolios G, Valatas V, Kouroumalis E. Role of Kupffer cells in the pathogenesis of liver disease. World J Gastroenterol. 2006;12:7413–20.
13. Fausto N, Laird AD, Webber EM. Role of growth regeneration factors and cytokines in hepatic. FASEB J. 1995;9:1527–36.
14. MacPhee PJ, Schmidt EE, Groom AC. Evidence for Kupffer cell migration along liver sinusoids, from high-resolution in vivo microscopy. Am J Physiol. 1992;263:G17–23.
15. Bayón LG, Izquierdo MA, Sirovich I, Van Rooijen N, Beelen RHJ, Meijer S. Role of Kupffer cells in arresting circulating tumor cells and controlling metastatic growth in the liver. Hepatology. 1996;23:1224–31.
16. Elsharkawy AM, Oakley F, Mann DA. The role and regulation of hepatic stellate cell apoptosis in reversal of liver fibrosis. Apoptosis. 2005;10:927–39.
17. Safadi R, Friedman SL. Hepatic fibrosis-role of hepatic stellate cell activation. Med Gen Med. 2002;4:27.
18. Gressner AM, Weiskirchen R. Modern pathogenetic concepts of liver fibrosis suggest stellate cells and TGF-beta as major players and therapeutic targets. J Cell Mol Med. 2006;10:76–99.
19. Rockey DC, Friedman SL. Hepatic fibrosis and cirrhosis. Zakim and Boyer's hepatology, 6th edn. Elsevier Saunders, Philadelphia. 2012:64-85.2012:64–85.

20. Bataller R, Schwabe RF, Choi YH, Yang L, Paik YH, Lindquist J, et al. NADPH oxidase signal transduces angiotensin II in hepatic stellate cells and is critical in hepatic fibrosis. J Clin Invest. 2003;112:1383–94.
21. Fletcher LM, Powell LW. Hemochromatosis and alcoholic liver disease. Alcohol. 2003;30:131–6.
22. Canbay A, Taimr P, Torok N, Higuchi H, Friedman S, Gores GJ. Apoptotic body engulfment by a human stellate cell line is profibrogenic. Lab Invest. 2003;83:655–63.
23. Yoshiji H, Kuriyama S, Yoshii J, Ikenaka Y, Noguchi R, Hicklin DJ, et al. Vascular endothelial growth factor and receptor interaction is a prerequisite for murine hepatic fibrogenesis. Gut. 2003;52:1347–54.
24. Pinzani M, Milani S, Herbst H, DeFranco R, Grappone C, Gentilini A, et al. Expression of platelet-derived growth factor and its receptors in normal human liver and during active hepatic fibrogenesis. Am J Pathol. 1996;148:785–800.
25. Mazzocca A, Sciammetta SC, Carloni V, Cosmi L, Annunziato F, Harada T, et al. Binding of hepatitis C virus envelope protein E2 to CD81 up-regulates matrix metalloproteinase-2 in human hepatic stellate cells. J Biol Chem. 2005;280:11329–39.
26. Ohata M, Lin M, Satre M, Tsukamoto H. Diminished retinoic acid signaling in hepatic stellate cells in cholestatic liver fibrosis. Am J Physiol. 1997;272:G589–96.
27. Eng FJ, Friedman SL, Fibrogenesis I. New insights into hepatic stellate cell activation: the simple becomes complex. Am J Physiol Gastrointest Liver Physiol. 2000;279:G7–11.
28. Kinnman N, Hultcrantz R, Barbu V, Rey C, Wendum D, Poupon R, et al. PDGF-mediated chemoattraction of hepatic stellate cells by bile duct segments in cholestatic liver injury. Lab Invest. 2000;80:697–707.
29. Mann DA, Smart DE. Transcriptional regulation of hepatic stellate cell activation. Gut. 2002;50:891–6.
30. Rockey D. The cellular pathogenesis of portal hypertension: Stellate cell contractility, endothelin, and nitric oxide. Hepatology. 1997;25:2–5.
31. Schuppan D, Ruehl M, Somasundaram R, Hahn EG. Matrix as a modulator of hepatic fibrogenesis. Semin Liver Dis. 2001;21:351–72.
32. Wells RG, Kruglov E, Dranoff JA. Autocrine release of TGF-beta by portal fibroblasts regulates cell growth. FEBS Lett. 2004;559:107–10.
33. Leu JI, Crissey MAS, Taub R. Massive hepatic apoptosis associated with TGF- β 1 activation after Fas ligand treatment of IGF binding protein-1 – deficient mice. J Clin Invest. 2003;111:129–39.
34. Liu X, Hu H, Yin JQ. Therapeutic strategies against TGF-β signaling pathway in hepatic fibrosis. Liver Int. 2006;26:8–22.
35. Crespo J, Rivero M, Fábrega E, Cayón A, Amado JA, García-Unzeta MT, et al. Plasma leptin and TNF-alpha levels in chronic hepatitis C patients and their relationship to hepatic fibrosis. Dig Dis Sci. 2002;47:1604–10.
36. Gressner AM, Weiskirchen R, Breitkopf K, Dooley S. Roles of TGF-beta in hepatic fibrosis. Front Biosci. 2002;7:d793–807.
37. Czochra P, Klopcic B, Meyer E, Herkel J, Garcia-Lazaro JF, Thieringer F, et al. Liver fibrosis induced by hepatic overexpression of PDGF-B in transgenic mice. J Hepatol. 2006;45:419–28.
38. Saile B, Eisenbach C, Dudas J, El-Armouche H, Ramadori G. Interferon-gamma acts pro-apoptotic on hepatic stellate cells (HSC) and abrogates the antiapoptotic effect of interferon-alpha by an HSP70-dependant pathway. Eur J Cell Biol. 2004;83:469–76.
39. Baroni GS, D'Ambrosio L, Curto P, Casini A, Mancini R, Jezequel AM, et al. Interferon gamma decreases hepatic stellate cell activation and extracellular matrix deposition in rat liver fibrosis. Hepatology. 1996;23:1189–99.
40. Gieling RG, Wallace K, Han Y-P. Interleukin-1 participates in the progression from liver injury to fibrosis. Am J Physiol Gastrointest Liver Physiol. 2009;296:G1324–31.

41. Du W-J, Zhen J-H, Zeng Z-Q, Zheng Z-M, Xu Y, Qin L-Y, et al. Expression of interleukin-17 associated with disease progression and liver fibrosis with hepatitis B virus infection: IL-17 in HBV infection. Diagn Pathol. 2013;8:40.
42. Aleffi S, Petrai I, Bertolani C, Parola M, Colombatto S, Novo E, et al. Upregulation of proin-flammatory and proangiogenic cytokines by leptin in human hepatic stellate cells. Hepatology. 2005;42:1339–48.
43. Iizuka M, Ogawa T, Enomoto M, Motoyama H, Yoshizato K, Ikeda K, et al. Induction of microRNA-214-5p in human and rodent liver fibrosis. Fibrogenesis Tissue Repair. 2012;5:12.
44. Roderburg C, Mollnow T, Bongaerts B, Elfimova N, Cardenas DV, Berger K, et al. Micro-RNA profiling in human serum reveals compartment-specific roles of miR-571 and miR-652 in liver cirrhosis. PLoS One. 2012;7:e32999.
45. Bala S, Marcos M, Kodys K, Csak T, Catalano D, Mandrekar P, et al. Up-regulation of microRNA-155 in macrophages contributes to increased tumor necrosis factor {alpha} (TNF{alpha}) production via increased mRNA half-life in alcoholic liver disease. J Biol Chem. 2011;286:1436–44.
46. Wang B, Li W, Guo K, Xiao Y, Wang Y, Fan J. MiR-181b Promotes hepatic stellate cells proliferation by targeting p27 and is elevated in the serum of cirrhosis patients. Biochem Biophys Res Commun. 2012;421:4–8.
47. Ogawa T, Enomoto M, Fujii H, Sekiya Y, Yoshizato K, Ikeda K, et al. MicroRNA-221/222 upregulation indicates the activation of stellate cells and the progression of liver fibrosis. Gut. 2012;61:1600–9.
48. Baltimore D, Boldin MP, O'Connell RM, Rao DS, Taganov KD. MicroRNAs: new regulators of immune cell development and function. Nat Immunol. 2008;9:839–45.
49. Noetel A, Kwiecinski M, Elfimova N, Huang J, Odenthal M. MicroRNA are central players in anti- and profibrotic gene regulation during liver fibrosis. Front Physiol. 2012;3:49.
50. Venugopal SK, Jiang J, Kim T-H, Li Y, Wang S-S, Torok NJ, et al. Liver fibrosis causes down-regulation of miRNA-150 and miRNA-194 in hepatic stellate cells, and their overexpression causes decreased stellate cell activation. Am J Physiol Gastrointest Liver Physiol. 2010;298:G101–6.
51. Roderburg C, Luedde M, Vargas Cardenas D, Vucur M, Mollnow T, Zimmermann HW, et al. miR-133a mediates TGF-β-dependent derepression of collagen synthesis in hepatic stellate cells during liver fibrosis. J Hepatol. 2013;58:736–42.
52. Calabro SR, Maczurek AE, Morgan AJ, Tu T, Wen VW, Yee C, et al. Hepatocyte produced matrix metalloproteinases are regulated by CD147 in liver fibrogenesis. PLoS One. 2014;9:e90571.
53. Barry-Hamilton V, Spangler R, Marshall D, McCauley S, Rodriguez HM, Oyasu M, et al. Allosteric inhibition of lysyl oxidase-like-2 impedes the development of a pathologic micro-environment. Nat Med. 2010;16:1009–17.
54. Oakley F, Trim N, Constandinou CM, Ye W, Gray AM, Frantz G, et al. Hepatocytes express nerve growth factor during liver injury. Am J Pathol. 2003;163:1849–58.
55. Preaux AM, D'Ortho MP, Bralet MP, Laperche Y, Mavier P. Apoptosis of human hepatic myofibroblasts promotes activation of matrix metalloproteinase-2. Hepatology. 2002;36:615–22.
56. Lang A, Schoonhoven R, Tuvia S, Brenner DA, Rippe RA. Nuclear factor kappaB in prolif-eration, activation, and apoptosis in rat hepatic stellate cells. J Hepatol. 2000;33:49–58.
57. Issa R, Williams E, Trim N, Kendall T, Arthur MJ, Reichen J, et al. Apoptosis of hepatic stel-late cells: involvement in resolution of biliary fibrosis and regulation by soluble growth fac-tors. Gut. 2001;48:548–57.
58. Sohara N, Znoyko I, Levy MT, Trojanowska M, Reuben A. Reversal of activation of human myofibroblast-like cells by culture on a basement membrane-like substrate. J Hepatol. 2002;37:214–21.

59. Fallowfield JA, Mizuno M, Kendall TJ, Constandinou CM, Benyon RC, Duffield JS, et al. Scar-associated macrophages are a major source of hepatic matrix metalloproteinase-13 and facilitate the resolution of murine hepatic fibrosis. J Immunol. 2007;178:5288–95.
60. Duffield JS, Forbes SJ, Constandinou CM, Clay S, Partolina M, Vuthoori S, et al. Selective depletion of macrophages reveals distinct, opposing roles during liver injury and repair. J Clin Invest. 2005;115:56–65.
61. Tsuchiya A, Forbes SJ. Macrophage Therapy for Liver Fibrosis and Regeneration. In Gene Therapy and Cell Therapy Through the Liver 2016 (pp. 15-23). Springer Japan.
62. Berzigotti A, Seijo S, Reverter E, Bosch J. Assessing portal hypertension in liver diseases. Expert Rev Gastroenterol Hepatol. 2013;7:141–55.
63. García-Pagán JC, Gracia-Sancho J, Bosch J. Functional aspects on the pathophysiology of portal hypertension in cirrhosis. J Hepatol. 2012;57:458–61.
64. Radi R. Peroxynitrite, a stealthy biological oxidant. J Biol Chem. 2013;288:26464–72.
65. Morales-Ruiz M, Rodríguez-Vita J, Jiménez W, Ribera J. Pathophysiology of portal hypertension. Pan Vascular Med Second Ed. 2015;18:3631–65.
66. Rockey DC, Weisiger RA. Endothelin induced contractility of stellate cells from normal and cirrhotic rat liver: implications for regulation of portal pressure and resistance. Hepatology. 1996;24:233–40.
67. Taura K, De Minicis S, Seki E, Hatano E, Iwaisako K, Osterreicher CH, et al. Hepatic stellate cells secrete angiopoietin 1 that induces angiogenesis in liver fibrosis. Gastroenterology. 2008;135:1729–38.
68. Novo E, Cannito S, Zamara E, di Bonzo LV, Caligiuri A, Cravanzola C, et al. Proangiogenic cytokines as hypoxia-dependent factors stimulating migration of human hepatic stellate cells. Am J Pathol. 2007;170:1942–53.
69. Dill MT, Rothweiler S, Djonov V, Hlushchuk R, Tornillo L, Terracciano L, et al. Disruption of Notch1 induces vascular remodeling, intussusceptive angiogenesis, and angiosarcomas in livers of mice. Gastroenterology. Elsevier. 2012;142:967–77. e2
70. Simonetto DA, Yin YH, Yin M, de Assuncao TM, Kwon JH, Hilscher M, et al. Chronic passive venous congestion drives hepatic fibrogenesis via sinusoidal thrombosis and mechanical forces. Hepatology. 2015;61:648–59.
71. Wanless IR, Wong F, Blendis LM, Greig P, Heathcote EJ, Levy G. Hepatic and portal vein thrombosis in cirrhosis: possible role in development of parenchymal extinction and portal hypertension. Hepatology. 1995;21:1238–47.
72. Villa E, Zecchini R, Marietta M, Bernabucci V, Lei B, Vukotic R, et al. Enoxaparin prevents portal vein thrombosis (PVT) and decompensation in advanced cirrhotic patients: final report of a prospective randomized controlled study. Hepatology. 2011;54:418A–9A.
73. Abraldes JG, Iwakiri Y, Loureiro-Silva M, Haq O, Sessa WC, Groszmann RJ. Mild increases in portal pressure upregulate vascular endothelial growth factor and endothelial nitric oxide synthase in the intestinal microcirculatory bed, leading to a hyperdynamic state. Am J Physiol Gastrointest Liver Physiol. 2006;290:G980–7.
74. Ezkurdia N, Coll M, Raurell I, Rodriguez S, Cuenca S, Gonzalez A, et al. Blockage of the afferent sensitive pathway prevents sympathetic atrophy and hemodynamic alterations in rat portal hypertension. Liver Int. 2012;32:1295–305.
75. Iwakiri Y. Endothelial dysfunction in the regulation of cirrhosis and portal hypertension. Liver Int. 2012;32:199–213.
76. Sass DA, Chopra KB. Portal hypertension and variceal hemorrhage. Med Clin North Am. 2009;93:837–53.
77. Sieber CC, Sumanovski LT, Stumm M, van der Kooij M, Battegay E. In vivo angiogenesis in normal and portal hypertensive rats: role of basic fibroblast growth factor and nitric oxide. J Hepatol. 2001;34:644–50.
78. Van SC, Ribera J, Geerts A, Pauta M, Tugues S, Casteleyn C, et al. Inhibition of placental growth factor activity reduces the severity of fibrosis, inflammation, and portal hypertension in cirrhotic mice. Hepatology. 2011;53:1629–40.

79. Takuma Y, Nouso K, Morimoto Y, Tomokuni J, Sahara A, Toshikuni N, et al. Measurement of spleen stiffness by acoustic radiation force impulse imaging identifies cirrhotic patients with esophageal varices. Gastroenterology. 2013;144:92–101. e2

80. Voros D, Mallas E, Antoniou A, Kafantari E, Kokoris SI, Smyrniotis B, et al. Splenomegaly and left sided portal hypertension. Ann Gastroenterol. 2005;18:341–5.

81. Ilan Y. Leaky gut and the liver: a role for bacterial translocation in nonalcoholic steatohepatitis. World J Gastroenterol. 2012;18:2609–18.

82. Fukui H. Gut-liver axis in liver cirrhosis: how to manage leaky gut and endotoxemia. World J Hepatol. 2015;7:425–42.

83. Messingham KAN, Faunce DE, Kovacs EJ. Alcohol, injury, and cellular immunity. Alcohol. Elsevier. 2002;28:137–49.

84. Tang Y, Forsyth CB, Keshavarzian A. The role of miRNAs in alcohol-induced endotoxemia, dysfunction of mucosal immunity, and gut leakiness. Alcohol Clin Exp Res. 2014;38:2331–4.

85. Miller AM, Masrorpour M, Klaus C, Zhang JX. LPS exacerbates endothelin-1 induced activation of cytosolic phospholipase A2 and thromboxane A2 production from Kupffer cells of the prefibrotic rat liver. J Hepatol. 2007;46:276–85.

86. Bosch J, Groszmann RJ, Shah VH. Evolution in the understanding of the pathophysiological basis of portal hypertension: how changes in paradigm are leading to successful new treatments. J Hepatol. 2015;62:S121–30.

87. Rigau J, Bosch J, Bordas JM, Navasa M, Mastai R, Kravetz D, et al. Endoscopic measurement of variceal pressure in cirrhosis: correlation with portal pressure and variceal hemorrhage. Gastroenterology. Wiley. 1989;96:873–80.

88. Fernandez M, Vizzutti F, Garcia-Pagan JC, Rodes J, Bosch J. Anti-VEGF receptor-2 monoclonal antibody prevents portal-systemic collateral vessel formation in portal hypertensive mice. Gastroenterology. 2004;126:886–94.

89. Fernandez M, Mejias M, Garcia-Pras E, Mendez R, Garcia-Pagan JC, Bosch J. Reversal of portal hypertension and hyperdynamic splanchnic circulation by combined vascular endothelial growth factor and platelet-derived growth factor blockade in rats. Hepatology. 2007;46:1208–17.

90. Escorsell A, Bordas JM, Feu F, Garcia-Pagan JC, Gines A, Bosch J, et al. Endoscopic assessment of variceal volume and wall tension in cirrhotic patients: effects of pharmacological therapy. Gastroenterology. 1997;113:1640–6.

91. Garcia-Pagán JC, Barrufet M, Cardenas A, Escorsell A. Management of gastric varices. Clin Gastroenterol Hepatol. 2013;12:1–11.

92. Ryan BM, Stockbrugger RW, Ryan JM. A Pathophysiologic, gastroenterologic, and radiologic approach to the management of gastric varices. Gastroenterology. 2004;126:1175–89.

93. Helmy A, Al Kahtani K, Al FM. Updates in the pathogenesis, diagnosis and management of ectopic varices. Hepatol Int. 2008;2:322–34.

94. Cubillas R, Rockey DC. Portal hypertensive gastropathy: a review. Liver Int. 2010;30:1094–102.

95. Gupta R, Sawant P, Parameshwar RV, Lele VR, Kulhalli PM, Mahajani SS. Gastric mucosal blood flow and hepatic perfusion index in patients with portal hypertension gastropathy. J Gastroenterol Hepatol. 1998;13:921–6.

96. Perini RF, Camara PRS, Ferraz JGP. Pathogenesis of portal hypertensive gastropathy: translating basic research into clinical practice. Nat Clin Pract Gastroenterol Hepatol. 2009;6:150–8.

97. Mezawa S, Homma H, Ohta H, Masuko E, Doi T, Miyanishi K, et al. Effect of transjugular intrahepatic portosystemic shunt formation on portal hypertensive gastropathy and gastric circulation. Am J Gastroenterol. 2001;96:1155–9.

98. Patwardhan VR, Cardenas A. Review article: the management of portal hypertensive gastropathy and gastric antral vascular ectasia in cirrhosis. Aliment Pharmacol Ther. 2014;40:354–62.

99. Kamath PS, Lacerda M, Ahlquist DA, McKusick MA, Andrews JC, Nagorney DA. Gastric mucosal responses to intrahepatic portosystemic shunting in patients with cirrhosis. Gastroenterology. 2000;118:905–11.
100. Senousy BE, Draganov PV. Evaluation and management of patients with refractory ascites. World J Gastroenterol. 2009;15:67–80.
101. Cardenas A, Bataller R, Arroyo V. Mechanisms of ascites formation. Clin Liver Dis. 2000;4:447–65.
102. Arroyo V, Bosch J, Gaya-Beltran J, Kravetz D, Estrada L, Rivera F, et al. Plasma renin activity and urinary sodium excretion as prognostic indicators in nonazotemic cirrhosis with ascites. Ann Intern Med. 1981;94:198–201.
103. Arroyo V, Guevara M, Ginès P. Hepatorenal syndrome in cirrhosis: pathogenesis and treatment. Gastroenterology. 2002;122:1658–76.
104. Kim MY, Jeong WK, Baik SK. Invasive and non-invasive diagnosis of cirrhosis and portal hypertension. World J Gastroenterol. 2014;20:4300–15.
105. Groszmann RJ, Wongcharatrawee S. The hepatic venous pressure gradient: anything worth doing should be done right. Hepatology. 2004;39:280–2.
106. Huang JY, Samarasena JB, Tsujino T, Chang KJ. EUS-guided portal pressure gradient measurement with a novel 25-gauge needle device versus standard transjugular approach: a comparison animal study. Gastrointest Endosc. Elsevier. 2016;84:358–62.
107. Castera L, Pinzani M, Bosch J. Non invasive evaluation of portal hypertension using transient elastography. J Hepatol. 2012;56:696–703.
108. Castera L, Foucher J, Bernard PH. Pitfalls of liver stiffness measurement: a 5-years prospective study of 13,369 examinations. Hepatology. 2010;51:828–35.
109. Guo J, Büning C, Schott E, Kröncke T, Braun J, Sack I, et al. In vivo abdominal magnetic resonance elastography for the assessment of portal hypertension before and after transjugular intrahepatic portosystemic shunt implantation. Invest Radiol. 2015;00:1.
110. Ronot M, Lambert S, Elkrief L, Doblas S, Rautou PE, Castera L, et al. Assessment of portal hypertension and high-risk oesophageal varices with liver and spleen three-dimensional multifrequency MR elastography in liver cirrhosis. Eur Radiol. 2014;24:1394–402.

# Chapter 2
# Coagulopathy in Cirrhosis

Craig D. Seaman and Margaret V. Ragni

## Introduction

Coagulopathy in cirrhosis can be difficult to manage. This chapter will provide a concise, but detailed, overview of the role of the normal and abnormal liver in hemostasis and introduce the concept of rebalanced hemostasis in chronic liver disease. Hepatic production of pro- and antihemostatic proteins in normal and altered hepatic function will be described. Laboratory testing will be discussed, including the effects of chronic liver disease on their interpretation. Finally, bleeding and thrombotic complications, and recommended therapy, will be reviewed.

## Physiology of Normal Hemostasis

Appreciating the coagulation abnormalities that occur in liver dysfunction requires a basic understanding of the physiology of normal hemostasis. The process of hemostasis is initiated at the site of injured blood vessels where von Willebrand factor (VWF) binds to subendothelial collagen. Subsequent binding of platelets to VWF results in platelet activation and aggregation. This process is termed primary hemostasis [1]. Concurrently, tissue factor (TF) is released from the endothelium of the damaged vasculature. TF binds to circulating activated factor VII (FVIIa) forming the intrinsic tenase complex, which converts factor X to factor Xa (FXa). FXa proteolytically cleaves a small amount of prothrombin to thrombin. The minimal amount of thrombin generated amplifies the coagulation cascade by activating

C.D. Seaman, MD, MS • M.V. Ragni, MD, MPH (✉)
Department of Medicine, University of Pittsburgh, Hemophilia Center of Western
Pennsylvania, 3636 Blvd of the Allies, Pittsburgh, PA 15213, USA
e-mail: seaman@upmc.edu; ragni@pitt.edu

© Springer International Publishing AG 2017
B. Eghtesad, J. Fung (eds.), *Surgical Procedures on the Cirrhotic Patient*,
DOI 10.1007/978-3-319-52396-5_2

19

factors VIII (FVIIIa), IX (FIXa), and XI (FXIa), among others. FXIa generates FIXa, which complexes with FVIIIa to form the extrinsic tenase complex. This complex produces large amounts of FXa, which generates enough thrombin to convert fibrinogen to fibrin. Polymerized fibrin monomers are cross-linked by factor XIIIa. This process is referred to as secondary hemostasis and involves a complex interplay among the abovementioned coagulation factors, activated platelets, membrane phospholipids, and calcium for stable clot formation [2].

Unchecked activation of the coagulation cascade may lead to unintended clot formation; therefore, anticoagulant proteins function to ensure that clot formation is limited to sites of vascular injury. The major components of the anticoagulant system are protein C, protein S, antithrombin III (ATIII), and tissue factor pathway inhibitor (TFPI). Protein C, following activation by thrombin bound thrombomodulin, along with protein S – a protein C cofactor, inactivates factors Va and VIIIa [3]. ATIII inactivates factors IXa, Xa, XIa, and XIIa. TFPI limits thrombin generation by inhibiting the TF-FVIIa-FXa complex [4].

Another important component of hemostasis is fibrinolysis. Eventually, fibrinolysis is necessary to prevent excess clot formation. The chief components of the fibrinolytic system are plasmin, tissue plasminogen activator (TPA), alpha-2-antiplasmin, and plasminogen activator inhibitor (PAI). Fibrin-bound plasminogen is converted to plasmin by TPA. Plasmin digests fibrin releasing fibrin degradation products. Regulation of this process is necessary to prevent excess clot breakdown and hemorrhage. Alpha-2-antiplasmin and PAI function in this role and inhibit plasmin and TPA, respectively [5].

## Hemostasis in Liver Disease

The liver plays an integral role in hemostasis. Hepatocytes are responsible for the synthesis of the majority of procoagulant, anticoagulant, and fibrinolytic proteins. Liver dysfunction disrupts this process altering the normal hemostatic balance. Historically, liver disease was felt to represent a bleeding diathesis as suggested by the presence of thrombocytopenia and prolongation of the prothrombin time (PT) and activation partial thromboplastin time (aPTT) on routine laboratory tests. More recently, an increasing amount of evidence supports a model of rebalanced hemostasis where concomitant prohemostatic and antihemostatic changes lead to a rebalanced hemostatic system [6–8].

The hemostatic changes that occur in chronic liver disease can be divided into those affecting primary hemostasis (platelet activation), secondary hemostasis (thrombin generation), and fibrinolysis (Table 2.1). Reduced hepatic synthesis of thrombopoietin causes thrombocytopenia and a bleeding tendency. Furthermore, splenic sequestration of platelets in portal hypertension-induced splenomegaly contributes to thrombocytopenia. Alternatively, increased levels of von Willebrand factor, in response to endothelial dysfunction, and decreased production of ADAMTS-13, a VWF cleaving protease, promote platelet adhesion, and hemostasis [9]. Secondary hemostasis is affected by deficiencies of the following procoagulants produced by

**Table 2.1** Alterations in hemostasis in chronic liver disease

| Phase of hemostasis | Promote hemostasis | Impair hemostasis |
| --- | --- | --- |
| Primary hemostasis (platelet activation) | Increased VWF Decreased ADAMTS-13 | Thrombocytopenia |
| Secondary hemostasis (thrombin generation) | Decreased protein C and S Decreased antithrombin III Increased factor VIII | Decreased factors II, V, VII, IX, X, and XI Decreased fibrinogen Dysfibrinogenemia |
| Fibrinolysis | Decreased plasminogen Increased PAI | Increased tPA Decreased alpha 2-antiplasmian Decreased factor XIII Decreased TAFI |

*VWF* von Willebrand antigen, *ADAMTS-13* a disintegrin and metalloprotease with thrombospondin type 1 motif 13, *PAI* plasminogen activator inhibitor, *tPA* tissue plasminogen activator, *TAFI* thrombin-activatable fibrinolysis inhibitor

the liver: fibrinogen and factors II, V, VII, IX, X, and XI. Additionally, dysfibrinogemia occurs, which promotes bleeding. There is a concurrent decrease in natural anticoagulants, protein C, protein S, and antithrombin III, due to reduced hepatic production, and a marked increase in factor VIII, secondary to endothelial dysfunction. These changes act as drivers of hemostasis [10]. Fibrinolysis is affected in a similar fashion. Decreased plasminogen and elevated PAI promote clot resolution, while increased TPA and reduced alpha-2-antiplasmin inhibit clot breakdown [8].

While the concept of rebalanced hemostasis argues against a hypocoagulable state long believed to be present in chronic liver disease, this balance is far more unstable in comparison to healthy individuals. Multiple factors, such as infection or renal disease, may precipitate bleeding or thrombosis by altering the hemostatic balance in either direction [6].

## Clinical Features of Coagulopathy in Liver Disease

One of the most common, and feared, bleeding complications in liver disease is bleeding esophageal varices; however, variceal bleeding is largely related to local vascular abnormalities, including vessel radius, thickness, and pressure, rather than hemostatic disturbances. Vessel pressure is predominantly dictated by splanchnic blood pressure, which is often increased due to hypervolemia, a common problem in liver disease [11]. Other features of bleeding in liver dysfunction include ecchymosis, epistaxis, oral mucosal bleeding, and gastrointestinal bleeding. Further, bleeding can be precipitated by invasive procedures.

Previously, it was assumed liver disease provided protection against thrombosis given the prolonged PT on routine laboratory tests. This now appears to be incorrect. The rate of deep venous thrombosis and pulmonary embolism is anywhere between 0.5 and 8.1% [12]. A more common complication is portal venous thrombosis (PVT), which has a reported prevalence of 11–36% [13]. Portal venous stasis appears to be the major change in liver disease contributing to the increased risk for PVT [14]. Hypercoagulability (i.e., increased FVIII, decreased protein C, etc.) likely plays a role in clotting when the hemostatic balance is tipped in the favor of thrombosis. The prevention and treatment bleeding and thrombotic complications in chronic liver disease will be discussed later.

## Coagulation Tests in Liver Disease

No one test can accurately predict the risk of bleeding in liver disease (Table 2.2). Two of the most commonly used tests are the PT and aPTT, which measure the time to formation of a fibrin clot. While inexpensive and widely available, both gauge just one aspect of coagulation and are not predictive of bleeding in chronic liver disease [15]. Similarly, obtaining a platelet count is another common test to evaluate bleeding risk. A platelet count less than 50,000/µL confers an increased risk of bleeding with invasive procedures in liver disease; however, higher platelet counts

**Table 2.2** Diagnostic tests to measure hemostasis in chronic liver disease

| Name of test | Comments |
| --- | --- |
| Platelet count | Widely available, timely results, and inexpensive |
| | Predicts risk of bleeding only at extreme levels |
| | Does not indicate platelet function |
| PT/INR | Widely available, timely results, and inexpensive |
| | Correlates with severity of liver disease but does not predict risk of bleeding in chronic liver disease |
| | Measures narrow aspect of procoagulant system |
| | High interlaboratory variability |
| aPTT | Widely available, timely results, and inexpensive |
| | Often normal in chronic liver disease |
| | Measures narrow aspect of procoagulant system |
| Coagulation factor activity | Does not correlate with risk of bleeding or thrombosis |
| | Not widely available |
| | High interlaboratory variability |
| Fibrinogen | Acute phase reactant |
| | Does not correlate with risk of bleeding in chronic liver disease |
| Thromboelastography | Global measure of hemostasis that can detect multiple perturbations in coagulation |
| | Rapid results |
| | Requires expertise in interpretation |
| | Not validated for predicting risk of bleeding or thrombosis in nonsurgical patients |
| Endogenous thrombin potential | Better representation of pro- and anticoagulant balance |
| | Not validated |
| | Experimental |

do not appear to predict bleeding risk [16]. Various other less commonly used laboratory tests are employed. Fibrinogen is a measure of the fibrinolytic system and decreased levels are indicative of fibrinolysis; however, fibrinogen is not correlated with bleeding risk in liver disease [16].

A major disadvantage of the above tests is their inability to assess more than a single aspect of the hemostatic system, which is less than ideal in chronic liver disease, a disorder with multiple perturbations of hemostasis. Global tests of hemostasis, such as thromboelastography (TEG), are methods of measuring whole-blood coagulation. TEG is often used perioperatively by surgeons and anesthesiologists. Given the numerous abnormalities present in liver disease, many acting in opposition to one another, tests such as TEG, may provide a more accurate assessment of bleeding risk. Indeed, TEG has been shown to be useful in detecting coagulopathy in liver disease [17]. Another global measure of hemostasis, the thrombin generation assay measures thrombin production and may be beneficial when evaluating coagulopathy in liver dysfunction. Thrombin generation is often normal or increased in liver disease, which highlights the concept of rebalanced hemostasis previously mentioned [18]. Thrombin generation assays are still experimental and may provide a more accurate measure of bleeding and thrombotic risk in chronic liver disease but further study is needed.

## Management of Bleeding in Liver Disease

A variety of options are available for the treatment and prevention of bleeding in chronic liver disease (Table 2.3). Prevention of bleeding is a concern in certain high-risk patients and prior to invasive procedures.

**Table 2.3** Treatment options for chronic liver disease related coagulopathy

| Type of product | Comment |
| --- | --- |
| Red blood cells | Transfusions should be administered to maintain minimally acceptable hemoglobin threshold depending on the clinical situation |
| Platelets | Reserved for severe thrombocytopenia or platelet count less than 50,000/μL with active bleeding |
| Fresh frozen plasma | Reserved for active bleeding |
| | Large volume (20–40 mL/kg) necessary for correction of coagulation factor deficiencies and may result in volume overload |
| | Not recommend for bleeding prevention prior to invasive procedures |
| Cryoprecipitate | Reserved for active bleeding with hypofibrinogenemia |
| Transexamic acid | Administered in patients with hypofibrinogenemia |
| Desmopressin | May improve platelet function but no data regarding efficacy in chronic liver disease |
| Prothrombin complex concentrates and recombinant factor VIIa | Reserved for severe and/or refractory bleeding |
| | Risk of thrombosis |
| | Expensive |
| | Limited data regarding efficacy in chronic liver disease |

One of the most commonly encountered bleeding complications experienced in liver disease is esophageal variceal bleeding. As previously mentioned, the etiology of variceal bleeding is related to local vascular abnormalities, such as splanchnic blood pressure, rather than abnormalities of hemostasis. Thus, treatment is not necessarily directed at correcting hemostatic abnormalities; however, as is the case with all potentially life-threatening bleeding events, volume resuscitation with red blood cells is critical. The goal hemoglobin concentration is 7–8 mg/dL [19]. It is important to avoid excessive transfusion since excess volume can increase splanchic portal pressure and further exacerbate bleeding. The key treatment modality in acute variceal bleeding is endoscopic variceal banding or ligation. While not the mainstay of treatment, correction of hemostatic defects is frequently attempted prior to invasive procedures, such as endoscopic therapy, to prevent worsened bleeding. Other potential bleeding complications that may arise in chronic liver disease include portal hypertensive gastropathy or gastric vascular ectasia-related bleeding and bleeding associated with invasive procedures. Commonly performed invasive procedures in liver dysfunction include percutaneous or transjugular liver biopsy, abdominal paracentesis, and accessing vascular sites (i.e., central venous catheter placement), among others.

Various blood products and hemostatic agents are administered for the treatment and prevention of bleeding in liver disease. Red blood transfusions to replace blood loss have already been discussed. The others are aimed at improving underlying hemostatic defects. Fresh frozen plasma (FFP) contains both pro- and anticoagulation factors and can be administered to replace deficiencies of either. FFP is most commonly administered to correct a prolonged PT. The efficacy of FFP to prevent bleeding has never been demonstrated [20]. Moreover, the volume of FFP necessary to correct coagulation factor deficiencies is large – 20–40 mL/kg – and complete correction is seldom accomplished [21, 22]. Potential adverse effects include pulmonary edema and increased portal venous blood pressure, among others. Therefore, in chronic liver disease, FFP is not recommend for the prevention of bleeding in patients with a prolonged PT prior to invasive procedures, and its use in actively bleeding patients is questionable. Platelet transfusions are often administered for thrombocytopenia. Adequate thrombin production occurs with a platelet count greater than 50,000/µL. Transfusion to obtain this value is warranted in active bleeding and should be considered for prophylaxis prior to invasive procedures [23–25]. In some instances, it may be difficult to achieve a platelet count of 50,000/µL or greater due to splenic sequestration of platelets in portal hypertension-induced splenomegaly, often present in liver disease. Cryoprecipitate, which contains fibrinogen and coagulation factors V and VIII, should be administered in bleeding patients with hypofibrinogenemia until fibrinogen levels normalize [26]. Its use as a prophylactic agent to prevent hemorrhage is not well studied. Similarly, when hyperfibrinolysis is a concern, antifibrinolytic agents, such as tranexamic acid, may be used. Last, recombinant factor VIIa (rFVIIa) and prothrombin complex concentrates (PCC) represent low-volume prohemostatic alternatives to FFP. Recombinant FVIIa has not been shown to be beneficial in bleeding esophageal varices or with prophylactic use prior to liver transplantation [27]. Therefore, routine use is not recommended except during very high-risk procedures, such as intracranial pressure monitor placement and rescue therapy for refractory, life-threatening bleeding. There are limited data regarding the use of PCCs in similar situations, so it cannot be recommended for routine use either. Adverse effects of both therapies include thrombogenicity, high expense, and need for frequent therapy.

## Management of Thrombosis in Liver Disease

Although liver disease was formerly believed to represent a bleeding diathesis, thus providing protection from thrombotic events, it is now known that this is not true. The precarious nature of the pendulum in rebalanced hemostasis in chronic liver disease can swing in the direction of bleeding or clotting. Despite the presence of thrombocytopenia and an elevated INR, termed autoanticoagulation, a misnomer, deep venous thrombosis (DVT) and pulmonary embolism (PE) do occur and affected patients should receive anticoagulation.

Deciding which anticoagulant to recommend can be difficult in chronic liver disease. Often, the INR is already elevated due to reduced hepatic synthesis of coagulation factors. Therefore, the addition of oral vitamin K antagonists (VKA) is problematic because it is challenging to determine if the INR value is due to liver disease or related to VKA use and it may not be possible to determine the INR range that represents therapeutic anticoagulation. Furthermore, the interlaboratory variability in INR is unacceptably high [28]. A more appropriate choice of therapy may be low molecular weight heparin (LMWH) since it does not require INR monitoring, although it presents potential difficulties too. LMWH functions by enhancing ATIII activity, which is often reduced in liver disease. This may result in unpredictable efficacy and necessitate anti-Xa level monitoring to ensure therapeutic dosing; however, anti-Xa levels may not be completely reliable. Despite subtherapeutic anti-Xa levels, thrombin generation assays have shown reduced thrombin generation in patients with chronic liver disease indicative of an increased responsiveness to LMWH in liver disease [29]. Limited data are available on the use of direct oral anticoagulants to treat venous thromboembolism in chronic liver disease; therefore, their efficacy and safety are uncertain for now and cannot be recommended.

PVT is the most common thrombotic complication experienced in chronic liver disease and is more often related to portal venous stasis rather than hypercoagulability. Clinical data from randomized clinical trials regarding the optimal treatment of PVT in cirrhosis are lacking; thus, the American Association for the Study of Liver Disease neither recommends for or against anticoagulation. Despite this shortcoming, there are a limited number of nonrandomized clinical studies demonstrating the efficacy and safety of VKA and LMWH. The goal of anticoagulation in PVT is recanalization of the obstructed blood vessel and decreasing the risk of extension to the superior mesenteric vein (SMV) to prevent intestinal ischemia and reduce portal hypertension. Exactly who should receive treatment is uncertain. Generally, anticoagulation is recommended for liver transplantation candidates since PVT is associated with decreased survival in patients undergoing liver transplantation. Patients not eligible for liver transplantation should receive anticoagulation on an individualized basis. The presence of PVT extension into the SMV or a coexisting thrombophilia usually warrants anticoagulation [30]. Successful recanalization occurs anywhere from one-third to nearly one-half of the time in patients receiving LMWH and VKA, respectively [31]. Initiation of anticoagulation within 6 months of PVT diagnosis is associated with a higher rate of recanalization [32]. Importantly, since bleeding in liver disease is most commonly related to portal hypertension, esophageal varices should be treated prior to beginning anticoagulation. Patients with prior variceal bleeding, large varices, and no history of bleeding, or small varices and a high risk of bleeding should undergo endoscopic therapy or begin treatment with a nonselective beta blocker [33]. The optimal duration of anticoagulation in PVT and cirrhosis is uncertain. Most studies treated the subjects for 6 months. If complete recanalization is not present at 6 months, a more prolonged duration of anticoagulation may still result in successful resolution of thrombosis [34]. Given the high rate of recurrent PVT following anticoagulation cessation, a longer duration of therapy to prevent recurrent thrombosis may be warranted in liver transplantation candidates and individuals with underlying thrombophilia. Other therapeutic options for PVT include thrombolysis and transjugular intrahepatic portosystemic shunt (TIPS). Limited evidence is available regarding the use of thrombolysis in PVT, but it may be advantageous in intestinal ischemia or anticoagulation failure. A considerable more amount of evidence is available for the use of TIPS in PVT, and it may serve a role in failure or contraindication of anticoagulation [35].

Several studies have shown the risk of VTE in hospitalized patients with chronic liver disease is no lower than hospitalized noncirrhotic patients, and in fact, may be greater [36–38]. Despite the risk of thrombosis in chronic liver disease, patients often do not receive thromboprophylaxis during hospitalization [39, 40]. This is likely related to a fear of bleeding and the inappropriate assumption that a prolonged INR in liver disease is protective against clotting. While not specifically addressed in the most recent consensus guidelines, accumulating data are leading to an increasing amount of evidence to support thromboprophylaxis in hospitalized patients with chronic liver disease [41].

# References

1. Gale AJ. Current understanding of hemostasis. Toxicol Pathol. 2011;39:273–80.
2. Versteef HH, Heemskerk JWM, Levi M, et al. New fundamentals in hemostasis. Physiol Rev. 2013;3:1327–58.
3. Esmon CT. The protein C pathway. Chest. 2003;124:26S–32S.
4. Bajaj MS, Birktoft JJ, Steer SA, et al. Structure and biology of tissue factor pathway inhibitor. Thromb Haemost. 2001;86:959–72.
5. Chapin JC, Hajjar KA. Fibrinolysis and the control of blood coagulation. Blood Rev. 2015;29:17–24.

6. Lisman T, Porte RJ. Rebalanced hemostasis in patients with liver disease: evidence and clinical consequences. Blood. 2009;116:878–85.
7. Lisman T, Caldwell SH, Burroughs AK, et al. Hemostasis and thrombosis in patients with liver disease: the ups and downs. J Hepatol. 2010;53:362–7. x
8. Tripodi A, Mannucci PM. The coagulopathy of chronic liver disease. N Engl J Med. 2011;365:147–56.
9. Mannucci PM, Canciani MT, Forza I, et al. Changes in health and diseases of the metalloprotease that cleaves von Willebrand factor. Blood. 2001;98:2730–5.
10. Tripodi A, Primignani M, Chantarangkul V, et al. An imbalance of pro- vs anti-coagulation factors in plasma from patients with cirrhosis. Gastroenterology. 2009;137:2105–11.
11. Dell'era A, Bosch J. The relevance of portal pressure and other risk factors in acute gastro-esophageal variceal bleeding. Aliment Pharmacol Ther. 2004;20:8–15.
12. Aggarwal A, Puri K, Lianpunsakul S. Deep vein thrombosis and pulmonary embolism in cirrhotic patients: systematic review. World J Gastroenterol. 2014;20:5737–45.
13. Wanless IR, Wong F, Blendis LM, et al. Hepatic and portal vein thrombosis in cirrhosis: a possible role in development of parenchymal extinction and portal hypertension. Hepatology. 1995;21:1238–47.
14. Amitrano L, Guardascione MA, Ames PR. Coagulation abnormalities in cirrhotic patients with portal vein thrombosis. Clin Lab. 2007;53:583–9.
15. Tripodi A, Caldwell SH, Hoffman M, et al. Review article: the prothrombin time test as a measure of bleeding risk and prognosis in liver disease. Aliment Pharmacol Ther. 2007;26:141–8.
16. Northup PG, Caldwell SH. Coagulation in liver disease: a guide for the clinician. Clin Gastroenterol Hepatol. 2013;11:1064–74.
17. Tripodi A, Primignani M, Chantarangkul V, et al. The coagulopathy of cirrhosis assessed by thromboelastometry and its correlation with conventional coagulation parameters. Thromb Res. 2009;124:132–6.
18. Tripodi A, Salerno F, Chantarangkul V, et al. Evidence of normal thrombin generation in cirrhosis despite abnormal conventional coagulation tests. Hepatology. 2005;41:553–8.
19. Villanueva C, Colomo A, Bosch A, et al. Transfusion strategies for acute upper gastrointestinal bleeding. N Engl J Med. 2013;368:11–21.
20. Segal JB, Dzik WH. Paucity of studies to support that abnormal coagulation test results predict bleeding in the setting of invasive procedures: an evidence-based review. Transfusion. 2005;45:1413–25.
21. Holland LL, Brooks JP. Toward rational fresh frozen plasma transfusion: the effect of plasma transfusion on coagulation test results. Am J Clin Pathol. 2006;126:133–9.
22. Youssef WI, Salazar F, Dasarathy S, et al. Role of fresh frozen plasma infusion in correction of coagulopathy of chronic liver disease: a dual phase study. Am J Gastroenterol. 2003;98:1391–4.
23. Tripodi A, Primignani M, Chantarangkul V, et al. Thrombin generation in patients with cirrhosis: the role of platelets. Hepatology. 2006;44:440–5.
24. Violo F, Basili S, Raparelli V, et al. Patients with liver cirrhosis suffer from primary hemostatic defects? Factor or fiction? J Hepatol. 2011;55:1415–27.
25. Rockey DC, Caldwell SH, Goodman ZD, et al. Liver biopsy. Hepatology. 2009;49:1017–44.
26. Amarapurkar PD, Amarapurkar DN. Management of coagulopathy in patients with decompensated liver cirrhosis. Int J Hepatol. 2011;11:1–5.
27. Lodge JP, Jonas S, Jones RM, et al. Efficacy and safety of perioperative dose of recombinant factor VIIa in liver transplantation. Liver Transpl. 2005;11:973–9.
28. Trotter JF, Olson J, Lefkowitz J, et al. Changes in international normalized ratio (INR) and model for end stage liver disease (MELD) based on selection of clinical laboratory. Am J Transplant. 2007;7:1624–8.
29. Bechmann LP, Sichau M, Wichert M, et al. Low-molecular-weight-heparin in patients with advanced cirrhosis. Liver Int. 2011;31:75–82.

30. Vall DC, Rautou PE. The coagulation system in patients with end stage liver disease. Liver Int. 2015;35:139–44.
31. Huard G, Bissonnette J, Bilodeau M. Optimal management of portal vein thrombosis in patients with liver cirrhosis: a review. Curr Hepatol Rep. 2015;14:203–11.
32. Senzolo M, Sartori TM, Rossetto V, et al. Prospective evaluation of anticoagulation and transjugular intrahepatic portosystemic shunt for the management of portal vein thrombosis in cirrhosis. Liver Int. 2012;32:919–27.
33. Garcia-Tsao G, Sanyal AJ, Grace ND, et al. Prevention and management of gastroesophageal varices and variceal hemorrhage in cirrhosis. Hepatology. 2007;46:922–38.
34. Amitrano L, Guardascione MA, Menchise A, et al. Safety and efficacy of anticoagulation therapy with low molecular weight heparin for portal vein thrombosis in patients with liver cirrhosis. J Clin Gastroenterol. 2010;44:448–51.
35. Qi X, Han G, Fan D. Management of portal vein thrombosis in liver cirrhosis. Nature. 2014;11:435–46.
36. Gulley D, Teal E, Suvannasankha A, et al. Deep vein thrombosis and pulmonary embolism in cirrhosis patients. Dig Dis Sci. 2008;53:3012–7.
37. Sogaard KK, Horvath-Puho E, Gronbaek H, et al. Risk of venous thromboembolism in patients with liver disease: a nationwide population-based case-control study. Am J Gastroenterol. 2009;104:96–101.
38. Ali M, Ananthakrishnan AN, McGibley EL, et al. Deep vein thrombosis and pulmonary embolism in hospitalized patients with cirrhosis: a nationwide analysis. Dig Dis Sci. 2011;56:2152–9.
39. Northup PG, McMahon MM, Ruhl AP, et al. Coagulopathy does not fully protect hospitalized cirrhosis patients from peripheral venous thromboembolism. Am J Gastroenterol. 2006;101:1524–8.
40. Runyon BA. Introduction to the revised American Association for the Study of Liver Diseases Practice Guideline management of adult patients with ascites due to cirrhosis. Hepatology. 2013;57:1651–3.
41. Kahn SR, Lim W, Dunn AS, et al. Prevention of VTE in nonsurgical patients: antithrombotic therapy and prevention of thrombosis, 9th ed: American college of chest physicians evidence-based clinical practice guidelines. Chest. 2012;141:195–226.

# Chapter 3
# The Impact of Liver Disease on Drug Metabolism

Jessica E. Bollinger

## Abbreviations

| | |
|---|---|
| ACE | Angiotensin converting enzyme |
| AUC | Area under the concentration-time curve |
| $CL_H$ | Hepatic clearance |
| $CL_{int}$ | Intrinsic clearance |
| $CL_p$ | Total plasma clearance |
| $C_{max}$ | Maximum serum concentration |
| CYP | Cytochrome P450 |
| $E_H$ | Hepatic extraction ratio |
| FDA | Food and Drug Administration |
| fu | Fraction of unbound drug in blood |
| GFR | Glomerular filtration rate |
| IV | Intravenous |
| NAPQI | N-acetyl-p-benzoquinone imine |
| $Q_H$ | Hepatic blood flow |

Any drug that is introduced to the body must be eliminated by either metabolism or excretion via the urine, bile, or feces. The liver is the primary site of drug metabolism. End stage liver disease, or liver cirrhosis, can alter drug pharmacokinetics significantly – mainly through decreased clearance, which may lead to drug accumulation and increased risk of adverse drug reactions. In addition to being the primary site of drug metabolism, variables that contribute to drug pharmacokinetics such as liver blood flow, plasma protein binding, intrinsic clearance, and biliary excretion can change with the progression of hepatic disease. Difficulty lies within

J.E. Bollinger, Pharm D, BCPS
Department of Pharmacy, Cleveland Clinic, Cleveland, OH, USA
e-mail: bollinj@ccf.org

© Springer International Publishing AG 2017
B. Eghtesad, J. Fung (eds.), *Surgical Procedures on the Cirrhotic Patient*,
DOI 10.1007/978-3-319-52396-5_3

the fact that there are no direct biomarkers that represent the rate or extent of drug metabolism. Unlike renal dysfunction, where a glomerular filtration rate (GFR) can be calculated to estimate renal function, there is no test to predict the effect of hepatic dysfunction on drug metabolism. Patients with liver cirrhosis are a unique population in which dosage adjustment is troublesome but necessary to achieve therapeutic efficacy and avoid serious adverse drug reactions.

## Hepatic Drug Clearance

Hepatic clearance ($CL_H$) is defined as the volume of blood from which a drug is irreversibly removed by the liver per unit of time and is represented by the following equation where $Q_H$ represents hepatic blood flow and $E_H$ represents the hepatic extraction ratio of the drug:

$$CL_H = Q_H \times E_H$$

Because $E_H$ depends on liver blood flow, the intrinsic clearance (enzymatic metabolism) of unbound drug ($CL_{int}$), and the fraction of unbound drug in blood (fu), the following expanded equation is used:

$$CL_H = Q_H \times ((fu \times CL_{int})/(Q_H + fu \times CL_{int}))$$

Drugs can be categorized according to the hepatic extraction ratio into three categories: highly extracted drugs ($E_H > 0.7$), drugs of intermediate extraction ($E_H$ 0.3–0.7), and drugs of low extraction ($E_H < 0.3$). Drugs with a high hepatic extraction ratio are highly lipid-soluble molecules whose clearance depends primarily on blood flow. For a drug with high hepatic extraction ratio, the hepatic clearance is independent of the unbound fraction in the blood. For a drug with intermediate hepatic extraction, the hepatic clearance depends on liver blood flow, the unbound fraction, and intrinsic clearance of unbound drug. For a drug with low hepatic extraction, the hepatic clearance depends on the unbound fraction in the blood. Poorly extracted drugs are influenced by both changes in plasma protein binding and enzymatic activity, which makes predicting effects of liver disease challenging. This is particularly important considering an increase in volume of distribution is found with drugs bound to albumin in patients with cirrhosis. Decreased synthesis of albumin and other plasma proteins occurs as liver function declines. The resultant fall in albumin is responsible for a decreased plasma binding of a drug, which leads to the increase in volume of distribution and an associated increase in clearance for a drug of low extraction [1].

## Drug Metabolism

Hepatocytes, which make up >90% of the cells in the liver, carry out most drug metabolism. Drugs are subjected to one or multiple enzymatic pathways that metabolize through Phase I reactions (oxidation, reduction, hydrolysis) or Phase II reactions (glucuronidation, sulfation, acetylation, methylation). Phase I enzymes lead to the introduction of functional groups such as –OH, –COOH, –SH, –O–, or –NH2, and typically cause inactivation of the drug. The cytochrome P450 (CYP450) family of enzymes carry out the majority of phase I metabolism of drugs. CYP3A is the predominant subfamily, which is responsible for the metabolism of approximately 50% of drugs commonly used. Occasionally, metabolism results in activation of a drug. Inactive drugs that undergo metabolism (usually via hydrolysis) to an active compound are called prodrugs. Phase II enzymes facilitate the elimination of drugs and the inactivation of toxic metabolites produced by oxidation. Phase II reactions produce a metabolite with improved water solubility, a change that facilitates the elimination of the drug from the tissue, normally via efflux pumps [2].

## Pharmacokinetic Alterations in Cirrhosis

Chronic liver diseases without cirrhosis usually result in minimal changes to drug pharmacokinetics. Disease states such as chronic active hepatitis and liver cancer are not associated with significantly impaired hepatic elimination unless cirrhosis is present [3]. Patients with cirrhosis show a decrease in liver mass and hepatic enzyme activity, a reduction in liver blood flow, and portosystemic shunting. As such, the extent of oral bioavailability of drugs with a high first-pass metabolism increases due to the reduction of intrinsic clearance and the existence of portosystemic shunting. Drugs with a high first-pass metabolism such as morphine, meperidine, verapamil, metoprolol, labetalol, carvedilol, or midazolam may double their bioavailability in cirrhosis [4]. In contrast, the oral administration of prodrugs is associated with increased inactive drug concentrations and decreased active metabolite levels. CYP450 activity may be increased or decreased, depending on the stage of progression of hepatic dysfunction. Phase II reactions do not appear to be altered in most liver diseases and only decrease when liver mass is significantly reduced [5].

In 2008, Frye and colleagues proposed a "sequential progressive model of hepatic dysfunction." This concept reveals specific CYP450 enzyme families are affected at different stages of liver disease. In the study, the authors used a validated cocktail of four drugs (caffeine, mephenytoin, debrisoquine, and chlorzoxazone) to determine the effect of liver disease on these enzymes. They found that in early stages of liver disease, the enzyme activity of CYP2C19 would be reduced, while the activity of CYP1A2, CYP2D6, and CYP2E1 will be retained. At an intermediate stage of liver disease, the activity of CYP2C19 and CYP1A2 will exhibit reduced clearance while CYP2D6 and CYP2E1 will be normal. In advanced end-stage liver disease all of the aforementioned enzymes will have decreased activity [6].

## Prodrug Metabolism

The successful use of a prodrug relies on its conversion to the active form, usually in the liver. The angiotensin converting enzyme (ACE) inhibitors are an example of a common group of prodrugs that require conversion to an active metabolite. Most

ACE inhibitors are prodrugs because the active drug has poor oral absorption, whereas their ester prodrugs are readily absorbed. Conversion of enalapril, cilazapril, quinalapril, and perindopril to their respective active metabolite is decreased in cirrhosis, reflecting impaired hydrolysis. However, with the exception of cilazapril, this seems to be of no clinical significance because ACE inhibition and the antihypertensive effect of these drugs are not altered in cirrhosis. This is likely due to the fact that reduced clearance of the active metabolite may make up for decreased conversion of the prodrug to the active form [3, 7].

## Liver Function Assessment and Dosage Adjustment

Chronic liver disease follows a gradual progression, and theoretically, a correlation should exist between changes in pharmacokinetics of drugs, especially intrinsic clearance (metabolism) and appropriate measure of hepatic function. Attempts to establish such relationships have been generally unsuccessful. This failure probably arises because, unlike drug excretion, there are numerous pathways of drug metabolism, each affected to a different degree in hepatic disorders. The contribution of each pathway to total drug elimination also varies with the drug. Drug metabolism is often decreased in severe cirrhosis, signified by the combination of a low albumin (<2.8 g/dL), an elevated INR (>2.2), refractory ascites, and the presence of Grade III or IV hepatic encephalopathy, which would warrant reducing the dose and monitoring the patient for adverse reactions. One needs to consider if an extensively metabolized drug is truly needed or if an alternative is available. Conversely, drug dosage adjustment is typically not warranted unless cirrhosis is present [1]. Currently, the Child-Pugh score (Table 3.1) is the most widely used tool (also recommended by the Food and Drug Administration [FDA]) to guide a prescriber by the functional capacity of the liver [8]. Originally designed to stratify perioperative risk in patients with cirrhosis, the Child-Pugh score has been shown to correlate with survival and the development of complications of cirrhosis. This classification scheme is useful in following an individual patient's disease course and may offer some guidance for dose adjustment. However, unlike in renal disease, where estimates of GFR correlate with kinetic parameters of drug elimination such as renal clearance, the Child-Pugh score lacks the sensitivity to measure the specific ability of the liver to metabolize

**Table 3.1** Child-Pugh classification and scoring of the severity of liver disease

| Clinical/biochemical indicator | 1 point | 2 points | 3 points |
|---|---|---|---|
| Serum bilirubin (mg/dL) | <2 | 2–3 | >3 |
| Serum albumin (g/dL) | >3.5 | 2.8–3.5 | <2.8 |
| Prothrombin time (s > control) | <4 | 4–6 | >6 |
| Encephalopathy (grade) | None | 1 or 2 | 3 or 4 |
| Ascites | Absent | Slight | Moderate |

Points are summed, and the total score is classified according to severity as follows: 5–6 points = group A (mild), 7–9 points = group B (moderate), 10–15 points = group C (severe)

individual drugs. According to a recent survey, there are few medications with prescribing information that outlines specific recommendations for dosage adjustment based on hepatic function as determined by Child-Pugh [9].

A static model to predict the relative change of drug exposure in cirrhotic patients has been developed. Although further evaluation of the model needs to be made, the Child-Pugh based tool may help clinicians in adjusting drug dose regimens in this problematic patient population. The model is based on ratios of the altered drug area under the concentration-time curve (AUC*) in a typical cirrhotic patient to the AUC measured in a typical healthy subject, predicted as a function of the Child-Pugh classes A, B, or C. A web-based version can be found at www.ddi-predictor.org [10].

## Drug-Drug Interactions

Patients with cirrhosis have many risk factors that may predispose them to drug-drug interactions and subsequent adverse drug reactions [11]. The magnitude of drug-drug interactions is expected to vary with the severity of liver impairment, however, there are very few studies documenting the impact of drug interactions on drug exposure in patients with cirrhosis. A limited amount of data suggests minimally decreased irreversible CYP3A enzyme inhibition and significantly increased free fraction (from decreased plasma protein binding) in patients with liver disease [12]. Cirrhosis also results in blood shunting around hepatocytes which may reduce drug delivery to metabolizing enzymes. In addition to alterations in drug metabolism through the CYP system, these patients are often times prescribed multiple medications to manage complications of their cirrhosis which would only increase their odds for a drug-drug interaction. A sound knowledge of the principles of dose adjustment in cirrhosis and an awareness of the most important potential drug-drug interactions of the therapeutic agents used to treat the complications of liver disease in this population is essential.

## Recommendations for Select Medications in Surgical Patients

### *Analgesics*

Acetaminophen is commonly recommended as a first-line analgesic due to its overall tolerability. However, the use of acetaminophen in patients with liver dysfunction is often avoided due to the established relationship between acetaminophen overdose and hepatotoxicity. Acetaminophen is primarily metabolized in the liver by three separate pathways: conjugation with glucuronide, conjugation with sulfate, and oxidation via the cytochrome P450 enzyme pathway, primarily CYP2E1, to form a reactive and hepatotoxic metabolite N-acetyl-*p*-benzoquinone imine (NAPQI). With therapeutic doses, NAPQI undergoes rapid conjugation with glutathione. Acetaminophen metabolites are mainly excreted in the urine.

In acute or chronic overdose, the glucuronidation and sulfation pathways become saturated. When this occurs, more of the toxic metabolite NAPQI is formed by CYP450-mediated N-hydroxylation. When glutathione stores are depleted with increased exposure to acetaminophen, NAPQI accumulates resulting in liver damage [13].

Pharmacokinetic studies in patients with severe liver disease have shown an increase in half-life, an increase in the AUC, and decreased plasma clearance [14–16]. With an increased acetaminophen exposure, patients are at higher risk of overdose and subsequent toxicity. Acetaminophen is contraindicated in patients with severe hepatic impairment or severe active liver disease and should be used with caution by limiting the total daily dose to no more than 2 g/day in patients with mild to moderate hepatic impairment or active liver disease.

## Opioid Analgesics

The metabolism of oxycodone depends on oxidation by CYP3A4 and CYP2D6, which transform oxycodone to noroxycodone and the active metabolite oxymorphone. An impairment in oxycodone metabolism might occur as a result of decreased liver blood flow and/or decreased liver metabolism. Data from a study involving 12 patients with hepatic impairment following a single dose of controlled release oxycodone 20 mg, the oxycodone AUC was increased by 90% and the half-life was prolonged by 2 h. Oxymorphone AUC values were lowered by 50%. These data suggest that oral oxycodone should be initiated at lower doses in patients with hepatic impairment and/or the dosing interval should be increased in patients with severe liver cirrhosis [17].

Morphine undergoes first-pass metabolism after oral administration and is approximately 30–40% bioavailable. It is also a moderate to highly extracted drug with a hepatic extraction ratio of ~0.7. Decreased total clearance is mostly due to a decrease in liver blood flow and a small decrease in intrinsic clearance. Several studies have shown impairment in the metabolism of morphine in patients with liver disease. In a study by Mazoit et al., morphine's half-life doubled (201 vs. 111 min) and the clearance decreased by 37% in patients with cirrhosis (hypoalbuminemia, hyperbilirubinemia, and prolonged prothrombin time) as compared to normal subjects after a single dose of intravenous morphine was given [18]. The authors recommend that the dosing interval of morphine may need to be increased by 1.5–2 times in patients with cirrhosis to avoid accumulation and untoward effects. A study by Hasselström et al. reiterates that the metabolism of morphine is impaired significantly in patients with severe cirrhosis (Child-Pugh B or C). In addition to finding an increased half-life (4.2 vs. 1.7 h) and decreased clearance (11.4 vs. 28.0 ml/min/kg), the investigators found the oral bioavailability of morphine in patients with hepatic impairment is likely to be increased (100% vs. 47%) due to decreased first-pass metabolism [19]. These studies suggest that if morphine is given intravenously to patients with cirrhosis, the dosing interval should be increased. For oral administration, a consideration should be made to decrease the dose in addition to increasing the dosing interval.

Hydromorphone is a semisynthetic opioid that also undergoes first-pass metabolism, resulting in low (~24%) bioavailability. Hydromorphone is extensively metabolized via glucuronidation in the liver, with greater than 95% of the dose metabolized to hydromorphone-3-glucuronide along with minor amounts of 6-hydroxy reduction metabolites. After oral administration of hydromorphone at a single 4 mg dose, $C_{max}$ and AUC were increased fourfold in patients with moderate (Child-Pugh B) hepatic impairment compared with subjects with normal hepatic function [20]. This increase in overall bioavailability was likely a consequence of reduced first-pass metabolism. The half-life of the drug in patients with hepatic impairment was the same as that in controls. The authors concluded that a reduction of hydromorphone dose is necessary in patients with moderate liver disease. The pharmacokinetics of hydromorphone in patients with severe hepatic impairment have not been studied. A further increase in $C_{max}$ and AUC of hydromorphone in this group is expected. As such, the starting dose should be even more conservative.

## Antiemetics

The pharmacokinetics of metoclopramide were studied in eight patients with severe alcoholic cirrhosis (Child-Pugh class C) as compared to eight healthy volunteers [21]. A single 20 mg dose of intravenous (IV) and oral metoclopramide was given. A 50% reduction in clearance ($0.34 \pm 0.09$ vs. $0.16 \pm 0.07$ L/kg/h, $p < 0.05$) was observed following both routes of drug administration. The authors concluded the adverse effects of metoclopramide observed in marked hepatic impairment are likely to be due to accumulation of the drug as a result of lowered clearance. A 50% dose reduction should be recommended in patients with cirrhosis. Considering that 20% of metoclopramide is also excreted unchanged in the urine, metoclopramide is best avoided if severe hepatic impairment is accompanied by severe renal dysfunction.

Ondansetron is well absorbed from the gastrointestinal tract and undergoes some first-pass metabolism. Mean bioavailability is approximately 60% and ondansetron is extensively metabolized in humans. In vitro metabolism studies have shown that ondansetron is a substrate for CYP450 enzymes, including CYP1A2, CYP2D6, and CYP3A4 (predominant). In patients with hepatic impairment, clearance is reduced twofold (28.3 L/h. vs. 14.7 L/h) and the mean half-life is increased to 14.3 h compared with 5.7 h in healthy individuals. Specifically, in patients with severe hepatic impairment (Child-Pugh C), half-life is increased to 20 h. In these patients, a total daily dose of 8 mg should not be exceeded [22].

A subsequent study analyzed 19 patients with varying degrees of hepatic impairment from chronic liver disease and compared them to six healthy volunteers after a single intravenous dose of ondansetron (8 mg) [23]. The patients with mild to moderate hepatic impairment had similar pharmacokinetic changes: decreased total plasma clearance ($CL_p$ 211–299 vs. 478 ml/min), increase in area under the curve (AUC 446–633 vs. 279 ng/L/h), and a longer half-life ($t_{1/2}$ 9.1–9.2 vs. 3.6 h). The changes were even more apparent in patients with severe hepatic impairment ($CL_p$ 96 mL/min, AUC 1383 ng/L/h, $t_{1/2}$ 20.6 h).

## Antimicrobials

Cirrhosis has multiple effects on the pharmacokinetic parameters of many antimicrobials. Appropriate antibiotic therapy selection and individualized dosing can contribute to optimal clinical outcomes while decreasing the risk of side effects. When individualizing dosing regimens, one should consider the indication, the site and severity of infection, and the duration of therapy. For example, shorter courses of therapy (<7 days), may not require dose adjustments. In general, dose adjustments should be considered in the setting of decompensated cirrhosis for antibiotics that undergo phase I metabolism, have high protein binding, or are associated with high rates of hepatotoxicity [24]. A review of commonly used antimicrobials in surgical patients that undergo hepatic metabolism is included below.

The majority of penicillins are eliminated renally, with a minor component of biliary excretion. The exception to this rule is nafcillin, which is primarily hepatically metabolized. One study that analyzed the effects of cirrhosis and biliary obstruction demonstrated that the plasma clearance of nafcillin was significantly decreased in patients with hepatic dysfunction (nearly twofold). In patients with cirrhosis, nafcillin excretion in the urine was significantly increased from about 30–50% of the administered dose, suggesting that renal disease superimposed on hepatic disease could further decrease nafcillin clearance [25].

Fluoroquinolones demonstrate low protein binding and a combination of hepatic and renal clearance. Levofloxacin in largely excreted by the kidneys and undergoes minimal hepatic metabolism. Ciprofloxacin is excreted by a combination of renal and hepatic metabolism. Moxifloxacin undergoes the most extensive metabolism in the liver where approximately half of a dose is changed to inactive metabolites. One study that evaluated the pharmacokinetics of moxifloxacin in patients with liver insufficiency found no significant differences in pharmacokinetic parameters as compared to healthy controls [26]. Therefore, fluoroquinolone dosage adjustment is not likely to be necessary in patients with cirrhosis.

Macrolides that are primarily metabolized by the liver include erythromycin and azithromycin. Clarithromcyin undergoes both hepatic and renal clearance. Studies have demonstrated prolonged half-life, decreased clearance, and increased concentration of free erythromycin in patients with cirrhosis [27, 28]. Dose adjustment and cautious use are recommended in light of erythromycin's adverse effect profile and potential for drug interactions via the CYP3A4 enzymes.

Metronidazole is metabolized by the liver to several metabolites, including an active hydroxyl metabolite, which maintains 30–65% activity of the primary compound. Studies in patients with cirrhosis have shown a prolonged half-life, decreased total plasma clearance, and an increased AUC [29, 30]. Due to these pharmacokinetic changes, a 50% dose reduction of metronidazole is recommended in patients with severe hepatic impairment (Child-Pugh C).


## Proton Pump Inhibitors

Patients with impaired hepatic function usually require gastric acid suppression therapy but are at increased risk for adverse drug reactions and may require dosage adjustments. Lansoprazole, omeprazole, and pantoprazole all have similar bioavailability (85%, 60%, and 77%, respectively). They are completely metabolized by CYP2C19 and exhibit high plasma protein binding (>95%).

The pharmacokinetics of lansoprazole after a single oral dose of 30 mg were studied in 18 healthy volunteers and 24 patients with hepatic failure (8 hepatitis, 16 with cirrhosis) [31]. The patients with cirrhosis showed a decreased clearance (0.04–0.07 vs. 0.26 L/h/kg), higher AUC (10.7–11.7 vs. 2.67 µg·h/mL), and longer half-life (6.1–7.2 vs. 1.4 h) of lansoprazole when compared with healthy patients. It is recommended that a lansoprazole dosage of 30 mg/day should not be exceeded in patients with liver dysfunction.

Cirrhosis causes marked changes in the pharmacokinetics of omeprazole. In patients with chronic hepatic disease, the bioavailability increased to approximately 100% compared approximately 50% in young healthy volunteers, reflecting decreased first-pass effect, and the plasma half-life of the drug increased to nearly 3 h compared with the half-life in healthy patients of 0.5–1 h. Plasma clearance decreased to 70 mL/min, compared with a value of 500–600 mL/min in normal subjects. Dose reduction in patients with hepatic dysfunction should be considered [32].

In patients with moderate to severe hepatic impairment (Child-Pugh B and C), maximum pantoprazole concentrations increased only slightly relative to healthy subjects. Although serum half-life values increased from 3.5 to 7–9 h and AUC values increased by five- to sevenfold in moderate to severe cirrhosis, these increases were no greater than those observed in CYP2C19 poor metabolizers, where no dosage adjustment is necessary. These pharmacokinetic changes in hepatic-impaired patients result in minimal drug accumulation following once-daily, multiple-dose administration. No dosage adjustment is needed in patients with mild to severe hepatic impairment [33].


## Conclusions

The pharmacokinetics of many types of drugs metabolized by the liver are changed in patients with cirrhosis. Liver disease can affect drug clearance by reducing drug-metabolizing capacity, reducing the synthesis of plasma proteins, and altering liver blood flow. These pharmacokinetic modifications can vary based on the chemical characteristics of the drug and the severity of liver disease. Delineating the impact these changes have on drug metabolism is quite difficult because at present, there is no single satisfactory test that gives a quantitative measure of liver function. Safe and effective drug use in patients with liver disease requires an awareness of the possibility of interactions between changes in hepatic function and pharmacodynamics. In patients with cirrhosis, dosage reduction and/or dosage interval modification should be considered, particularly those with severe liver disease (Child-Pugh C).

# References

1. Rowland M, Tozer TN. Clinical pharmacokinetics: concepts and applications. 4th ed. Baltimore: Lippincott Williams & Wilkins; 2011.
2. Brunton LL, Chabner BA, Knollman BC. Goodman & Gilman's: the pharmacological basis of therapeutics. 12th ed. New York: McGraw-Hill; 2011.
3. Morgan DJ, McLean AJ. Clinical pharmacokinetic and pharmacodynamic considerations in patients with liver disease – an update. Clin Pharmacokinet. 1995;29(5):370–91.
4. Pena MA, Horga JF, Zapater P. Variations of pharmacokinetics of drugs in patients with cirrhosis. Expert Rev Clin Pharmacol. 2016;9(3):441–58.
5. Verbeeck RK. Pharmacokinetics and dosage adjustment in patients with hepatic dysfunction. Eur J Clin Pharmacol. 2008;64(12):1147–61.
6. Frye RF, Zgheib NK, Matzke GR, Chaves-Gnecco D, Rabinovitz M, Shaikh O, et al. Liver disease selectively modulates cytochrome P450-mediated metabolism. Clin Pharmcol Ther. 2006;80(3):235–45.
7. Rodighiero V. Effects of liver disease of pharmacokinetics. Clin Pharmacokinet. 1999;37(5):399–491.
8. Pugh RN, Murray-Lyon IM, Dawson JL, Pietroni MC, Williams R. Transection of the oesophagus for bleeding oesophageal varices. Br J Surg. 1973;60(8):646–9.
9. Spray JW, Willett K, Chase D, Sindelar R, Connelly S. Dosage adjustment for hepatic dysfunction based on Child-Pugh scores. Am J Health Syst Pharm. 2007;64(7):690. 692-3
10. Steelandt J, Jean-Bart E, Goutelle S, Tod M. A prediction model of drug exposure in cirrhotic patients according to Child-Pugh classification. Clin Pharmacokinet. 2015 Dec;54(12):1245–58.
11. Franz CC, Egger S, Born C, Rätz Bravo AE. Krähenbühl. Potential drug-drug interactions and adverse drug reactions in patients with liver cirrhosis. Eur J Clin Pharmacol. 2012;68(2):179–88.
12. Orlando R, De Martin S, Pegoraro P, Quintieri L, Palatini P. Irreversible CYP3A inhibition accompanied by plasma protein-binding displacement: a comparative analysis in subjects with normal and impaired liver function. Clin Pharmacol Ther. 2009;85(3):319–26.
13. Schilling A, Corey R, Leonard M, Eghtesad B. Acetaminophen: old drug, new warnings. Cleve Clin J Med. 2010;77(1):19–27.
14. Andreasen PB, Hutters L. Paracetamol (acetaminophen) clearance in patients with cirrhosis of the liver. Acta Med Scand Suppl. 1979;624:99–105.
15. Arnman R, Olsson R. Elimination of paracetamol in chronic liver disease. Acta Hepatogastroenterol. 1978;25(4):283–6.
16. Forrest JA, Adriaenssens P, Finlayson ND, Prescott LF. Paracetamol metabolism in chronic liver disease. Eur J Clin Pharmacol. 1979;15(6):427–31.
17. Kaiko RF. Pharmacokinetics and pharmacodynamics of controlled-release opioids. Acta Anaesthesiol Scand. 1997;41(1):166–74.

18. Mazoit J-X, Sandouk P, Zetlaoui P, Scherrmann J-M. Pharmacokinetics of unchanged morphine in normal and cirrhotic subjects. Anesth Analg. 1987;66(4):293–8.
19. Hasselström J, Eriksson S, Persson A, Rane A, Svensson JO, Säwe J. The metabolism and bioavailability of morphine in patients with severe cirrhosis. Br J Clin Pharmacol. 1990;29(3):289–97.
20. Durnin C, Hind ID, Ghani SP, Yates DB, Molz KH. Pharmacokinetics of oral immediate-release hydromorphone in subjects with moderate hepatic impairment. Proc West Pharmacol Soc. 2001;44:83–4.
21. Magueur E, Hagege H, Attali P, Singlas E, Etienne JP, Taburet AM. Pharmacokinetics of metoclopramide in patients with liver cirrhosis. Br J Clin Pharmacol. 1991;31(2):185–7.
22. Figg WD, Dukes GE, Pritchard JF, Hermann DJ, Lesesne HR, Carson SW, et al. Pharmacokinetics of ondansetron in patients with hepatic insufficiency. J Clin Pharmacol. 1996;36(3):206–15.
23. Blake JC, Palmer JL, Minton NA, Burroughs AK. The pharmacokinetics of intravenous ondansetron in patients with hepatic impairment. Br J Clin Pharmacol. 1993;35(4):441–3.
24. Halilovic J, Heintz BH. Antibiotic dosing in cirrhosis. Am J Health Syst Pharm. 2014;71(19):1621–34.
25. Marshall 2nd JP, Salt WB, Elam RO, Wilkinson GR, Schenker S. Disposition of nafcillin in patients with cirrhosis and extrahepatic biliary obstruction. Gastroenterology. 1977;73(6):1388–92.
26. Barth J, Jäger D, Mundkowski R, Drewelow B, Welte T, Burkhardt O. Single- and multiple-dose pharmacokinetics of intravenous moxifloxacin in patients with severe hepatic impairment. J Antimicrob Chemother. 2008;62(3):575–8.
27. Kroboth PD, Brown A, Lyon JA, Kroboth FJ, Juhl RP. Pharmacokinetics of single-dose erythromycin in normal and alcoholic liver disease subjects. Antimicrob Agents Chemother. 1982;21(1):135–40.
28. Hall KW, Nightingale CH, Gibaldi M, Nelson E, Bates TR, DiSanto AR. Pharmacokinetics of erythromycin in normal and alcoholic liver disease subjects. J Clin Pharmacol. 1982;22(7):321–5.
29. Lau AH, Evans R, Chang CW, Seligsohn R. Pharmacokinetics of metronidazole in patients with alcoholic liver disease. Antimicrob Agents Chemother. 1987;31(11):1662–4.
30. Muscara MN, Pedrazzoli Jr J, Miranda EL, Ferraz JG, Hofstätter E, Leite G, et al. Plasma hydroxy-metronidazole/metronidazole ratio in patients with liver disease and in healthy volunteers. Br J Clin Pharmacol. 1995;40(5):477–80.
31. Delhotal-Landes B, Flouvat B, Duchier J, Molinie P, Dellatolas F, Lemaire M. Pharmacokinetics of lansoprazole in patients with renal or liver disease of varying severity. Eur J Clin Pharmacol. 1993;45(4):367–71.
32. Andersson T, Olsson R, Regårdh C-G, Skånberg I. Pharmacokinetics of [14C]omeprazole in patients with liver cirrhosis. Clin Pharmacokinet. 1993;24(1):71–8.
33. Ferron GM, Preston RA, Noveck RJ, Pockros P, Mayer P, Getsy J, et al. Pharmacokinetics of pantoprazole in patients with moderate and severe hepatic dysfunction. Clin Ther. 2001;23(8):1180–92.

# Chapter 4
# Imaging in Cirrhotic Patients Undergoing Surgical Procedures

Christopher P. Coppa and Samuel Eleazar Ruskin

## Abbreviations

| | |
|---|---|
| CT | Computed tomography |
| IMV | Inferior mesenteric vein |
| IVC | Inferior vena cava |
| MR (or MRI) | Magnetic resonance (or magnetic resonance imaging) |
| MRE | Magnetic resonance elastography |
| SVC | Superior vena cava |
| TIPS | Transjugular intrahepatic portosystemic shunt |
| US | Ultrasound |

## Introduction

Preoperative imaging plays an important role in cirrhotic patients undergoing surgery. The imaging may make an initial diagnosis of cirrhosis in a patient with no known history of liver disease and demonstrate findings of advanced liver disease, such as ascites, splenomegaly, and portosystemic collateral pathways. In both scenarios, the identification of cirrhosis and complications is important in the preoperative setting, since cirrhotic patients have increased risk of surgical complications [1]. In this chapter, we will discuss the imaging findings used to make the radiographic

C.P. Coppa, MD (✉) • S.E. Ruskin, MD
Department of Radiology, Cleveland Clinic,
Cleveland, OH, USA
e-mail: coppac@ccf.org; ruskins@ccf.org

© Springer International Publishing AG 2017
B. Eghtesad, J. Fung (eds.), *Surgical Procedures on the Cirrhotic Patient*,
DOI 10.1007/978-3-319-52396-5_4

41

diagnosis of cirrhosis. Extrahepatic manifestations of cirrhosis will also be reviewed with an emphasis on portal hypertension and portosystemic collaterals. Further, the clinical implication of some of these findings will be touched upon.

## Radiographic Diagnosis of Cirrhosis

While the diagnosis of cirrhosis is traditionally based on clinical and histologic findings, it is often suggested at imaging [2]. Many imaging findings of cirrhosis have been described and most commonly involve cirrhosis-induced changes in hepatic morphology that can be detected with computed tomography (CT), magnetic resonance (MR) imaging, or ultrasound (US) [3]. While these features are specific, they lack sensitivity [4]. Some modalities potentially offer diagnostic information not afforded by others.

Changes in liver morphology include contour nodularity and classic lobar findings, including atrophy of the right lobe and medial segment of the left lobe, and hypertrophy of the caudate and the lateral segment of the left lobe [5].

Generalized widening of the interlobar fissures is another feature of cirrhosis. Examples of such widening include the "expanded gallbladder fossa" sign, which is 98% specific (but only 68% sensitive) for the diagnosis of cirrhosis and is manifested by a widened, fat-filled pericholecystic space, most commonly on the basis of anterior and medial segment liver atrophy [3, 5]. Enlargement of the hilar periportal space is a similar example [5, 6] and this space is considered widened when the distance between the anterior wall of the right portal vein and the posterior edge of the medial segment of the left hepatic lobe is greater than 10 mm (Fig. 4.1).

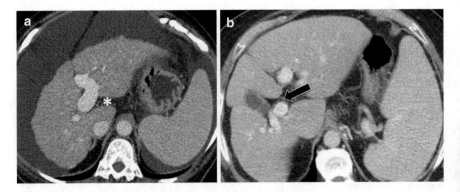

**Fig. 4.1** Spectrum of morphologic changes in the cirrhotic liver. (**a**) Nodular liver contour and fissural widening, in this case the fissure for the ligamentum venosum (*). Ascites is also present. (**b**) Classic lobar findings of cirrhosis, including atrophy of the *right* lobe and medial segment of the *left* lobe, and hypertrophy of the caudate and the lateral segment of the *left* lobe. There is also widening of the hilar periportal space (*arrow*)

Additionally, the ratio of caudate lobe width to right lobe width can also be used to assist in the diagnosis of cirrhosis. As the caudate lobe enlarges and the right lobe becomes atrophic, this ratio increases and several researches have used this ratio as a quantifiable measure of cirrhosis [2, 7].

Confluent hepatic fibrosis can also be seen as wedge-shaped areas along the periphery of the liver, classically in segments IV, V, or VIII, with associated capsular retraction and delayed enhancement on contrast enhanced CT and MRI [5, 8].

In a few instances, the etiology of cirrhosis can be suggested by the imaging findings. The classic example is primary sclerosing cholangitis-induced cirrhosis, which is manifested by atrophy of the peripheral hepatic segments, and mass-like caudate enlargement, as well as multifocal regions of intrahepatic ductal prominence created by irregular bile ducts stricture (Fig. 4.2) [5].

Of note, there are several entities that induce morphologic changes in the liver that resemble cirrhosis radiographically but are not cirrhosis histologically. Examples would include "pseudocirrhosis," which is the name given to the scarred and fibrotic appearance of the liver that occasionally occurs after treating hepatic metastases with chemotherapy, and the "atrophy-hypertrophy complex," which refers to the changes in hepatic morphology induced by portal vein thrombosis and cavernous transformation in patients *without* cirrhosis (Fig. 4.3). Therefore, it is important to keep these potential mimickers of cirrhosis in mind when evaluating any liver with altered morphology [9, 10].

In addition to the anatomic/morphologic information described thus far, MRI provides additional diagnostic information in the evaluation of cirrhosis. For example, MRI has improved contrast resolution and is superior to CT and US in the visualization of cirrhotic nodules and intervening bands of fibrosis (Fig. 4.4). It can also be used to assess and quantify fat and iron deposition [2, 11].

MR elastography (MRE) is a relatively new MR imaging technique that can quantify liver stiffness by analyzing propagation of mechanical waves through the liver parenchyma. These stiffness measurements are used as a marker for liver fibrosis, that is, liver stiffness measured by elastography increases with increased stages

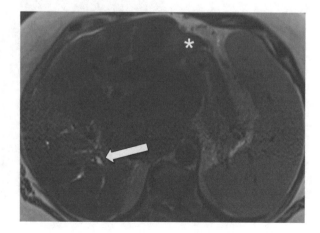

**Fig. 4.2** Primary sclerosing cholangitis-related cirrhosis. Mass-like caudate enlargement and central regeneration, lateral segment atrophy (*) and multiple mildly dilated *right* lobe intrahepatic bile ducts (*arrow*) created by irregular ductal strictures (Note the splenomegaly due to portal hypertension)

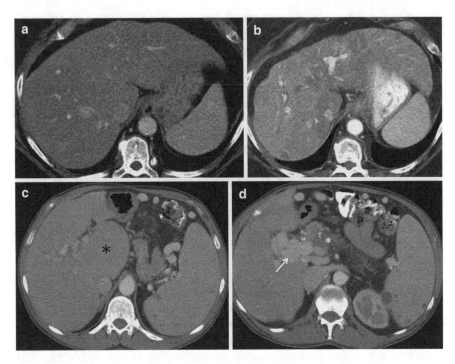

**Fig. 4.3** Mimickers of cirrhosis. Pseudocirrhosis in a woman with breast cancer metastatic to liver before (**a**) and after chemotherapy (**b**) The nodular liver contour on the later image (**b**) developed in a 9-month timeframe and is a treatment affect unrelated to cirrhosis. Atrophy-hypertrophy complex (**c, d**) in a *noncirrhotic* patient with hypercoagulable state. The caudate lobe (*) and *right* lobe are enlarged and the *left* lobe is atrophic (a different pattern than what is classically observed in cirrhosis). The portal vein is thrombosed (*) and there is cavernous transformation, evidenced by numerous tortuous collaterals in the porta hepatis (*arrow*). While cirrhosis is often the cause of these venous changes, it was not the etiology in this case

**Fig. 4.4** MRI in cirrhosis. Dark lines throughout the liver in a somewhat lace-like pattern are created by bands of fibrosis surrounding regenerative nodules in a patient with primary biliary cirrhosis. The superior contrast resolution of MRI enables visualization of cirrhotic nodules, which are not routinely apparent on CT

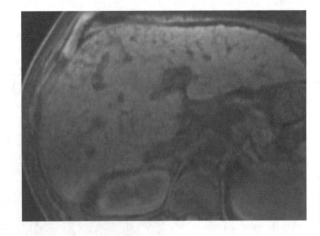

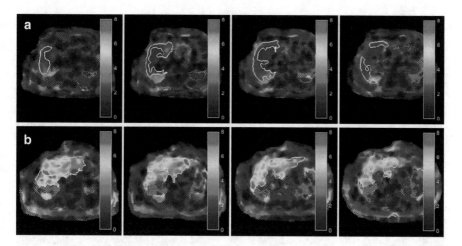

**Fig. 4.5** MR elastography (Courtesy of Dr. Ajit Goenka, Mayo Clinic). (**a**) MR elastogram images demonstrate normal liver stiffness (<2.5 kPa). (**b**) MR elastogram images demonstrate significantly elevated liver stiffness, which was consistent with patient's known biopsy-proven stage 3–4 liver fibrosis

of fibrosis (Fig. 4.5) [4]. MRE is emerging as a reliable and noninvasive alternative to biopsy for grading liver fibrosis [12].

In addition to assessing for parenchymal and morphologic changes of cirrhosis with grayscale US, Doppler ultrasound has proven to be a valuable tool in the cirrhotic population. Most commonly, it is used to detect alterations in portal venous flow. While normal portal flow is hepatopetal (or directed towards the liver), cirrhosis and portal hypertension can result in slower portal venous flow, hepatofugal (or retrograde) flow (Fig. 4.6), or absent flow due to stagnation or thrombosis.

Altered hepatic venous and hepatic arterial flow can also be detected in the setting of cirrhosis. For example, altered hepatic vein waveforms can be seen in up to 50% of patients with cirrhosis and may correlate with the severity of the disease. Usually this manifests as a monophasic, or flat, hepatic vein flow pattern since the stiff or fibrotic liver does not permit transmission of cardiac pulsation, which is responsible for the tri-phasic waveform in normal individuals. The hepatic arteries may show increased caliber and flow to compensate for the relatively decreased portal flow that develops in the setting of cirrhosis and portal hypertension [13–15].

Additionally, Doppler interrogation is the study of choice for initial and follow-up evaluation of transjugular intrahepatic portosystemic shunts (TIPS) [14–16].

US elastography is an additional sonographic tool used as a noninvasive technique for quantifying liver fibrosis, sometimes in lieu of liver biopsy. Although specific details are beyond the scope of this discussion, elastography attempts to correlate liver stiffness with the different pathologic stages of liver fibrosis in patients with chronic hepatitis, similar to MRE [17].

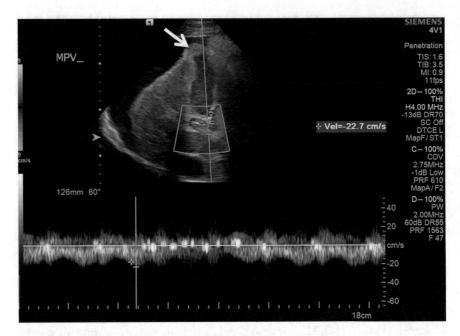

**Fig. 4.6** Ultrasound in cirrhosis. Doppler evaluation of the main portal vein demonstrates hepatofugal flow. The *blue* color within the vein indicates flow away from the ultrasound transducer and away from the liver; the corresponding spectral venous waveform is below the baseline, also consistent with retrograde flow. Incidentally, note the nodular liver contour, the perihepatic ascites, and the gallbladder wall thickening (*arrow*), commonly present in the setting of cirrhosis and portal hypertension

## Extrahepatic Imaging Manifestations

### Portal Hypertension and Portosystemic Collaterals

Portal hypertension is the major clinical manifestation of cirrhosis. In addition to being a major risk factor for postoperative mortality [18], portal hypertension is as associated with increased incidence of intraoperative complications, especially in abdominal surgery, largely related to bleeding. This is especially true in patients with prior abdominal surgery and adhesions [19]. Not unexpectedly, extreme care must be taken during surgical procedures when handling varices as they have thin walls and high pressure, which can result in massive bleeding if injured [1]. As such, collateral venous pathways should be described on preoperative imaging studies.

Interestingly, some advocate the placement of a TIPS in cirrhotic patients with portal hypertension before abdominal surgery in order to reduce the likelihood of intraoperative bleeding. However, there is currently insufficient evidence to support the routine use of TIPS preoperatively [20, 21].

Classically, collateral pathways are believed to develop due to passive opening of preexisting portosystemic channels or anastomoses in the setting of increased portal pressure. More recently some research suggests that portosystemic circulation may also be due to endothelial growth factor–induced angiogenesis [22].

While conventional angiography was historically the procedure of choice for detection of varices [23], CT and MRI are less intrusive alternatives now commonly used in the delineation of portosystemic collaterals that develop secondary to portal hypertension.

As described previously, Doppler ultrasound is an additional technique to evaluate portal hypertension, especially in situations where contrast enhanced CT and MRI are contraindicated (e.g., acute kidney injury). Ultrasound features of portal hypertension include increased diameter of the main portal vein, hepatofugal portal vein flow, and identification of collateral vessels.

As portal hypertension progresses, there is gradual slowdown in the portal vein velocity secondary to elevated intrahepatic resistance. As reversal of portal venous flow progresses, splanchnic blood is shunted via portosystemic collateral vessels to the systemic circulation [24]. For simplicity, collateral vessels can be subdivided into those that drain into the superior vena cava (SVC) and those that drain into the inferior vena cava (IVC).

Collaterals draining into the SVC include:

- Left gastric (or coronary) vein
- Posterior and short gastric veins
- Esophageal and paraesophageal varices

Collaterals draining to the IVC include:

- Gastrorenal and splenorenal shunts
- Paraumbilical vein and abdominal wall veins (including caput medusae)
- Retroperitoneal shunts
- Mesenteric varices (e.g., rectal varices) [22, 25]

The left gastric (coronary) vein is the most commonly visible varix in portal hypertension and is considered abnormal and indicative of portal hypertension when it measures larger than 5–6 mm in diameter. It originates from the splenic vein or portal vein and courses between the medial wall of the stomach and posterior surface of the left hepatic lobe. As may be expected, left gastric varices are often associated with esophageal and/or paraesophageal varices (Fig. 4.7) [26].

Short gastric veins are normal veins that drain the gastric fundus and left side of the greater curvature and empty into the splenic vein. With portal hypertension, they form gastric varices, mostly near the fundus. The posterior gastric vein represents a potential venous drainage system between the left and short gastric veins and can connect to the SVC via esophageal varices or the IVC via the left renal vein [22].

Esophageal varices refer to those within the wall of the lower esophagus, while paraesophageal varices refer to those outside the wall (Fig. 4.8). These varices are mostly supplied by the left gastric vein, which splits into the anterior branch supplying esophageal varices, and posterior branch supplying paraesophageal varices. Along with gastric varices, these are the most common portosystemic pathways detected on cross-sectional imaging. Esophageal varices are clinically important, as they are the most common cause of upper gastrointestinal bleeding. Although

**Fig. 4.7** Varix of the *left* gastric (coronary) vein. Dilated coronary vein (*arrows*) courses between the stomach and *left* hepatic lobe. There are associated (para) esophageal varices more cranially

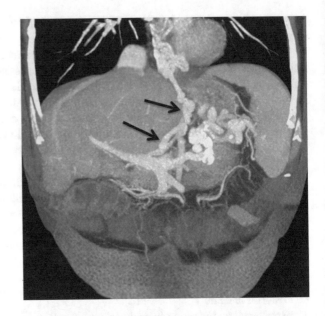

**Fig. 4.8** Paraesophageal varices. Multiple tortuous veins surround the distal esophagus secondary to portal hypertension. Splenomegaly is also present

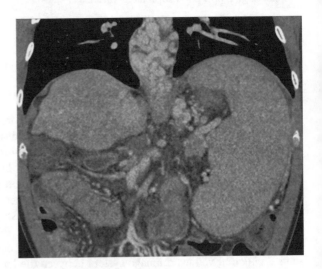

endoscopy is important for diagnosis and often treatment of esophageal and gastric varices, CT and MR better depict the extent of collateralization [26].

Gastrorenal shunts form between the gastric and perigastric varices and drain into the left renal vein via the left inferior phrenic vein and adrenal vein. Splenorenal shunts can be separated into direct and indirect shunts. A direct splenorenal shunt is a direct communication between the splenic vein and left renal vein (Fig. 4.9). These can be large shunts that take a circuitous path and can cause significant enlargement of the left renal vein. Indirect splenorenal shunts represent communication of the splenic vein and left renal vein via the short and posterior gastric veins [22].

**Fig. 4.9** Spontaneous splenorenal shunt. A prominent venous collateral (*) extends between the splenic vein (*S*) and the *left* renal vein (*R*), which is segmentally dilated to the level of the IVC

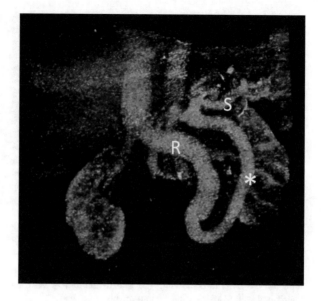

The paraumbilical veins are small veins within the ligamentum teres and falcifom ligament, adjacent to the closed off umbilical vein. Although it was initially postulated that the umbilical vein recanalizes, Lafortune et al. demonstrated that in fact the *para*umbilical veins collateralize with the SVC (via the superior epigastric or internal thoracic veins) or with the IVC (via the inferior epigastric and external iliac veins) in the setting of portal hypertension [27]. Although a recanalized paraumbilical vein increases the predisposition to hepatic encephalopathy, it also tends to correlate with smaller esophageal and gastric varices, therefore, indicating a decreased risk for significant variceal gastrointestinal bleeding [28].

Sometimes the paraumbilical veins connect with subcutaneous abdominal wall veins creating the "caput medusae" pattern (Fig. 4.10) [29, 22]. Such abdominal wall collaterals are a potential source of bleeding during laparoscopic surgeries and their presence (discovered on physical examination or with imaging) will prompt surgeons to modify umbilical trocar placement [30].

Retroperitoneal shunts are one of the most common collateral pathways in portal hypertension and develop from mesenteric veins draining into the renal veins or directly in to the IVC via the veins of Retzius. Although not associated with gastrointestinal bleeding, they can rarely rupture into the retroperitoneum causing massive blood loss [22, 29].

Mesenteric collateral vessels usually appear as dilated and tortuous branches of the superior and/or inferior mesenteric veins within the mesenteric fat. Due to the complex collateral pathways of the mesenteric vessels, there are a wide variety of potential mesenteric varices [26]. Mesenteric-gonadal varices represent anastomoses between the ileocolic veins and the right gonadal vein, or rarely the inferior mesenteric vein (IMV) and the left gonadal vein. Rectal varices are secondary to retrograde flow of blood from the IMV into the rectal veins (Fig. 4.11), which then drain into the IVC via the internal iliac and pudendal veins. Rectal varices have been

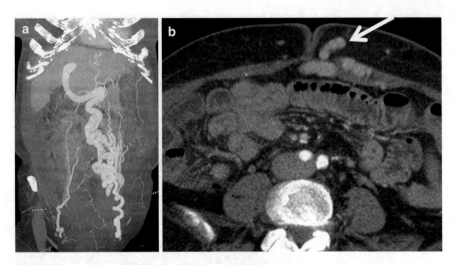

**Fig. 4.10** Recanalized paraumbilical vein. (**a**) Large recanalized paraumbilical vein collateralizes with the *left* external iliac vein. (**b**) The paraumbilical vein also connects with subcutaneous abdominal wall veins creating a caput medusae (*arrow*)

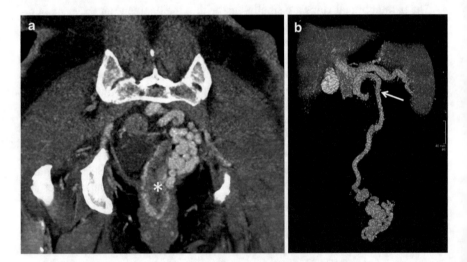

**Fig. 4.11** Rectal varices. (**a**) Multiple tortuous venous collaterals surround the rectum (*). (**b**) Volume rendered image demonstrates the communication between the rectal varices and the inferior mesenteric vein (*arrow*). Incidentally, gallstones are present

reported in 10–20% of patients with cirrhosis and cause bleeding in up to 5% of cases. Distinguishing between anorectal varices and hemorrhoids is of great importance to avoid surgical procedures that can result in massive hemorrhage [31].

Collateralization can occur in the setting of prior abdominal surgery. For example, patients with portal hypertension and prior stoma formation (e.g., ileostomy and colostomy) may develop stomal varices, which result from the communication created between high-pressure mesenteric veins and low-pressure abdominal wall veins [22, 32]. Another example is the jejunoileal varices that collateralize to the abdominal wall through postoperative adhesions [22, 33].

## Cavernous Transformation

In addition to portosystemic collaterals that can develop in the setting of portal hypertension, slow portal venous flow or thrombosis can result in cavernous transformation of the portal vein. CT findings include a tangle of veins with a beaded appearance in the porta hepatitis, and often the absence of a normal-appearing portal vein (Fig. 4.3d) [26].

## Splenomegaly

In the United States, splenomegaly is most commonly caused by portal hypertension. Splenomegaly is easily detected by CT (Figs. 4.2 and 4.9), MRI, or US. In addition to generalized splenic enlargement due to backpressure and reversal of flow from the portal venous system into the splenic vein, hemosiderin is sometimes deposited within the spleen (approximately 10% of patients with portal hypertension). On MR imaging, such deposits appear as multiple tiny foci of decreased signal intensity called Gamna-Gandy bodies and can demonstrate susceptibility artifact due to iron deposition (Fig. 4.12) [34]. Platelet sequestration in the setting splenomegaly can result in thrombocytopenia, which poses a bleeding risk operatively and postoperatively [35].

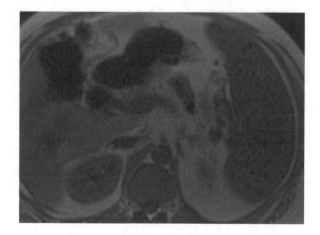

**Fig. 4.12** Gamna-Gandy bodies. Multiple punctate dark spots, known as Gamna-Gandy bodies, are present in the spleen and result from hemosiderin deposition in about 10% of patients with portal hypertension

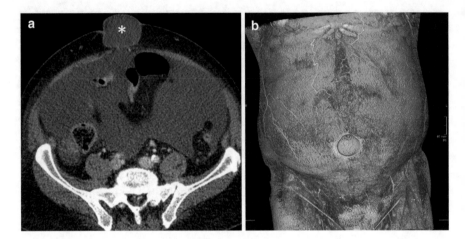

**Fig. 4.13** Umbilical hernia and ascites. (**a**) A large volume of ascites throughout the peritoneal cavity also extends into a moderate-sized umbilical hernia (*). (**b**) Volume rendered image of the same patient illustrates the degree of abdominal distention before therapeutic paracentesis

## Ascites

The etiology of ascites (Fig. 4.13) in cirrhosis is multifactorial, but portal hypertension is certainly a contributing factor. The development of ascites in cirrhotic patients is not inconsequential, since ascites is associated with 50% mortality over 2 years [36]. In cirrhotic patients being considered for surgery, the presence of ascites is associated with worse outcomes, including increased incidence of infection and renal failure [18, 21]. Further ascites can aggravate pulmonary function [20] and impair wound healing [1]. As such, cirrhotic patients being considered for surgery should undergo ultrasound to assess for ascites, assuming other current, preoperative imaging (e.g., CT or MR) is not available. Depending on the volume of fluid, preoperative paracentesis, diuresis, and/or sodium restriction may be warranted. If ascites is refractory to medical management, TIPS may be used to control ascites in eligible patients [1, 21].

## Abdominal Wall Hernia

Cirrhotic patients are at a greater risk for developing umbilical, inguinal, and incisional hernias compared to the general population. This is secondary to abdominal distention from ascites and atrophy of the abdominal wall musculature (Fig. 4.13) [1, 18].

# Cholelithiasis

Cholelithiasis occurs about two times more frequently in cirrhotic patients than in the general population (Fig. 4.11) [19]. While gallstones are easily identified with ultrasound, the sonographic diagnosis of acute cholecystitis can be difficult in the setting of cirrhosis. Gallbladder wall thickening is often observed in cirrhotic patients (Fig. 4.6), probably due to portal hypertension and hypoproteinemia [25]. Gallstones, pericholecystic fluid, and right upper quadrant pain can also be present. As such, the potential overlap in the imaging appearance of acute calculous cholecystitis and asymptomatic cholelithiasis with cirrhosis can create a diagnostic dilemma [37].

While many Child-Pugh A and B cirrhotic patients with acute calculous cholecystitis can be managed with laparoscopic cholecystectomy, surgery is usually not performed in Child-Pugh C patients due to the prohibitive death rate [19]. In the high-risk group, alternative treatments are recommended including antibiotics and percutaneous drainage [1, 38]. Percutaneous cholecystostomy is considered equally safe in cirrhotic patients and other high-risk patients (e.g., patients with heart failure, end-stage renal disease) and is used as temporizing measure until more definitive surgical procedures can be performed (e.g., cholecystectomy or liver transplant) [39].

# Bowel Wall Thickening

Bowel wall thickening in cirrhotic patients is usually the result of submucosal edema related to portal hypertension and/or hypoalbuminemia. The ascending colon (Fig. 4.14) and jejunum are the most commonly affected bowel segments [25, 40]. Such bowel wall thickening can mimic pathologic processes such as ischemia and infection, but further evaluation is not warranted unless clinically indicated.

# Hydrothorax

Hepatic hydrothorax is defined as a pleural effusion of greater than 500 ml in a patient with cirrhosis but no evidence of cardiopulmonary disease. It likely relates to leakage of ascites through a diaphragmatic defect with a pressure gradient moving fluid from the peritoneal cavity into the pleural space (Fig. 4.15). It is most often right sided (85%), but may be left sided, or rarely bilateral. CT can demonstrate a focal defect in the diaphragm as well as the pleural effusion with or without ascites [41]. In a cirrhotic patient with a pleural effusion, scintigraphic imaging can be used

**Fig. 4.14** Colonic wall
thickening. Wall thickening
of the ascending colon
(*arrows*) results from
submucosal edema in the
setting of portal
hypertension

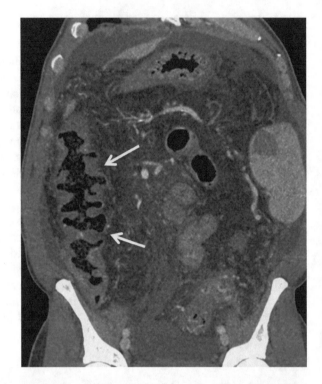

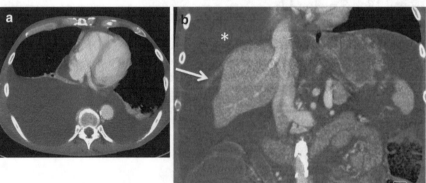

**Fig. 4.15** Hepatic hydrothorax. (**a**) There is a moderate-sized *right* pleural effusion and a small
*left* pleural effusion in a patient with cirrhosis and no cardiopulmonary disease. (**b**) Coronal image
of the same patient shows ascites and a *right* pleural effusion (\*) with an intervening slip of diaphragm (*arrow*), without a visible diaphragmatic defect

to prove the presence of hepatic hydrothorax. Technetium-99 m sulfur colloid is
injected into the peritoneal cavity and serial imaging of the thorax is performed to
detect radiotracer activity above the diaphragm, the presence of which confirms a
hepatic hydrothorax [42].

# References

1. Im GY, Lubezky N, Facciuto ME, Schiano TD. Surgery in patients with portal hypertension: a preoperative checklist and strategies for attenuating risk. Clin Liver Dis. 2014;18:477–505.
2. Awaya H, Mitchell DG, Kamishima T, Holland G, Ito K, Matsumoto T. Cirrhosis; modified caudate-right lobe ratio. Radiology. 2002;224:769–74.
3. Ito K, Mitchell DG, Gabata T, Hussain SM. Expanded gallbladder fossa: simple MR imaging sign of cirrhosis. Radiology. 1999;211:723–6.
4. Faria SC, Ganesan K, Mwangi I, Shiehmorteza M, Vamonte B, Mazhar S, et al. MR imaging of liver fibrosis: current state of the art. Radiographics. 2009;29:1615–35.
5. Brancatelli G, Federle MP, Ambrosini R, Lagalla R, Carriero A, Midiri M, et al. Cirrhosis: CT and MR imaging evaluation. Eur J Radiol. 2007;61(1):57–69.
6. Tan KC. Enlargement of the hilar periportal space. Radiology. 2008;248:699–700.
7. Harbin WP, Robert NJ, Ferrucci JJ. Diagnosis of cirrhosis based on regional changes in hepatic morphology: a radiological and pathological analysis. Radiology. 1980;135:273–83.
8. Valls C, Andía E, Roca Y, Cos M, Figueras J. CT in hepatic cirrhosis and chronic hepatitis. Semin Ultrasound CT MR. 2002;23(1):37–61.
9. Gupta AA, Kim DC, Krinsky GA, Lee VS. CT and MRI of cirrhosis and its mimics. Am J Roentgenol. 2004;183(6):1595–601.
10. Vilgrain V, Condat B, Bureau C, Hakime A, Plessier A, Cazals-Hatem D, et al. Atrophy-hypertrophy complex in patients with cavernous transformation of the portal vein: CT evaluation. Radiology. 2006;241(1):149–55.
11. Hussain SM, Reinhold C, Mitchell DG. Cirrhosis and lesion characterization at MR imaging. Radiographics. 2009;29:1637–52.
12. Mariappan YK, Glaser KJ, Ehman RL. Magnetic resonance elastography: a review. Clin Anat. 2010;23(5):497–511.
13. Nicolau C, Bianchi L, Vilana R. Gray-scale ultrasound in hepatic cirrhosis and chronic hepatitis: diagnosis, screening and intervention. Semin Ultrasound CT MR. 2002; 23(1):3–18.
14. Goyal N, Jain N, Rachapalli V, Cochlin DL, Robinson M. Non-invasive evaluation of liver cirrhosis using ultrasound. Clin Radiol. 2009;64(11):1056–66.
15. Martínez-Noguera A, Montserrat E, Torrubia S, Villalba J. Doppler in hepatic cirrhosis and chronic hepatitis. Semin Ultrasound CT MR. 2002;23(1):19–36.
16. McNaughton DA, Abu-Yousef MA. Doppler US of the liver made simple. Radiographics. 2011;31:161–88.
17. Barr RG, Ferraioli G, Palmeri ML, Goodman ZD, Garcia-Tsao G, Rubin J, et al. Elastography assessment of liver fibrosis: society of radiologists in ultrasound consensus conference statement. Radiology. 2015;276(3):845–61.
18. Sabbagh C, Fuks D, Regimbeau JM. Non-hepatic gastrointestinal surgery in patients with cirrhosis. J Visc Surg. 2014;151(3):203–11.
19. Bhangui P, Laurent A, Amathieu R, Azoulay D. Assessement of risk for non-hepatic surgery in cirrhotic patients. J Hepatol. 2012;57(4):874–84.
20. Lopez-Delgado JC, Ballus J, Esteve F, Betancur-Zambrano NL, Corral-Velez V, Mañez R, et al. Outcomes of abdominal surgery in patients with liver cirrhosis. World J Gastroenterol. 2016;22(9):2657–67.
21. Rai R, Nagral S, Nagral A. Surgery in a patient with liver disease. J Clin Exp Hepatol. 2012;2(3):238–46.
22. Moubarak E, Bouvier A, Boursier J, Lebigot J, Ridereau-Zins C, Thouveny F, et al. Portosystemic collateral vessels in liver cirrhosis: a three-dimensional MDCT pictorial review. Abdom Imaging. 2012;37(5):746–66.
23. Cho KC, Patel YD, Wachsberg RH, Seeff J. Varices in portal hypertension: evaluation with CT. Radiographics. 1995;15:609–22.

24. Wachsberg RH, Bahramipour P, Sofocleous CT, Barone A. Hepatofugal flow in the portal venous system: pathophysiology, imaging findings and diagnostic pitfalls. Radiographics. 2002;22(1):123–40.
25. Sangster GP, Previgliano CH, Nader M, Chwoschtschinsky E, Heldmann MG. MDCT imaging findings of liver cirrhosis: spectrum of hepatic and extrahepatic abdominal complications. HPB Surg. 2013;2013:1–12.
26. Kang HK, Jeong YY, Choi JH, Choi S, Chung TW, Seo JJ, et al. Three-dimensional multi-detector row CT portal venography in the evaluation of portosystemic collateral vessels in liver cirrhosis. Radiographics. 2002;22(5):1053–61.
27. Lafortune M, Constantin A, Breton G, Légaré AG, Lavoie P. The recanalized umbilical vein in portal hypertension: a Myth. Am J Roentgenol. 1985;144(3):549–53.
28. Gupta D, Chawla YK, Dhiman RK, Suri S, Dilawari JB. Clinical significance of patent para-umbilical vein in patients with liver cirrhosis. Dig Dis Sci. 2000;45(9):1861–4.
29. Kim MJ, Mitchell DG, Ito K. Portosystemic collaterals of the upper abdomen: review of anatomy and demonstration on MR imaging. Abdom Imaging. 2000;25(5):462–70.
30. Evans SRT. Surgical pitfalls: prevention and management. Philadelphia: Saunders-Elsevier; 2009.
31. Hosking SW, Smart HL, Johnson AG, Triger DR. Anorectal varices, haemorrhoids, and portal hypertension. Lancet. 1989;1(8634):349–52.
32. Fucini C, Wolff BG, Dozois RR. Bleeding from peristomal varices: perspectives on prevention and treatment. Dis Colon Rectum. 1991;34(12):1073–8.
33. Lebrec D, Benhamou JP. Ectopic varices in portal hypertension. Clin Gastroenterol. 1985;14(1):105–21.
34. Elsayes KM, Narra VR, Mukundan G, Lewis Jr JS, Menias CO, Heiken JP. MR imaging of the spleen: spectrum of abnormalities. Radiographics. 2005;25(4):967–82.
35. Hayashi H, Beppu T, Shirabe K, Maehara Y, Baba H. Management of thrombocytopenia due to liver cirrhosis: a review. World J Gastroenterol. 2014;20(10):2595–605.
36. Moore KP, Aithal GP. Guidelines on the management of ascites in cirrhosis. Gut. 2006;55(Suppl 6):vi1–12.
37. Sohail S, Shaheen R, Khatri ZA. Calculous cholecystitis and hepatic cirrhosis as sonographic co-confounders for gallbladder evaluation. J Coll Physicians Surg Pak. 2006;16(11):693–5.
38. Currò G, Iapichino G, Melita G, Lorenzini C, Cucinotta E. Laparoscopic cholecystectomy in child-pugh class C cirrhotic patients. JSLS. 2005;9(3):311–5.
39. Jayadevan R, Garg M, Schiano T, Divino CM. Is cholecystostomy a safe procedure in patients with cirrhosis. Am Surg. 2014;80(11):1169–71.
40. Ormsby EL, Duffield C, Ostovar-Sirjani F, McGahan JP, Troppmann C. Colonoscopy findings in end-stage liver disease patients with incidental CT colonic wall thickening. Am J Roentgenol. 2007;189(5):1112–7.
41. Kim YK, Kim Y, Shim SS. Thoracic complications of liver cirrhosis: radiologic findings. Radiographics. 2009;29(3):825–37.
42. Bhattacharya A, Mittal BR, Biswas T, Dhiman RK, Singh B, Jindal SK, et al. Radioisotope scintigraphy in the diagnosis of hepatic hydrothorax. J Gastroenterol Hepatol. 2001; 16(3):317–21.

# Chapter 5

# Anesthesia for Surgical Procedures in Cirrhotic Patients Other than Liver Transplantation: Management, Concerns, and Pitfalls

Randolph H. Steadman and Jennifer W. Nguyen-Lee

## Introduction

In 2010, 101,000 patients were admitted with chronic liver disease and cirrhosis as their primary diagnosis. These patients were predominately male (62%) with chronic alcoholic cirrhosis (52.5%) [1]. Chronic liver disease represents the 12th leading cause of mortality nationwide in the USA [2]. Because of improved treatments and extended life expectancies, the percentage of patients with chronic end-stage liver disease (ESLD) undergoing procedures is increasing. Patients with cirrhosis are at relatively increased risk of biliary obstruction requiring cholecystectomy, and ascites predisposes patients to inguinal and ventral hernias requiring repair.

In a review of the Nationwide Inpatient Sample, 22,569 patients with cirrhosis underwent cholecystectomies, colectomies, abdominal aortic repair, and coronary artery bypass grafting between 1998 and 2005. Of these surgeries, cholecystectomy was the most frequently performed operation on cirrhotic patients (63%) followed by colectomies (26%). As expected, mortality, hospital length of stay, and cost are significantly increased in patients with ESLD and increased further in patients with portal hypertension. Even after adjusting for risk factors and comorbid diseases, patients with compensated cirrhosis undergoing elective surgery have a 3.4–8 times increased risk of mortality depending on the type of surgery [3]. In another study of 733 patients with the diagnosis of cirrhosis, who had surgery between 1980 and

R.H. Steadman, MD, MS (✉) • J.W. Nguyen-Lee, MD
Department of Anesthesiology and Perioperative Medicine, UCLA Health System, Los Angeles, CA, USA
e-mail: Rsteadman@mednet.ucla.edu

© Springer International Publishing AG 2017
B. Eghtesad, J. Fung (eds.), *Surgical Procedures on the Cirrhotic Patient*,
DOI 10.1007/978-3-319-52396-5_5

1991, the 30-day postsurgical mortality was 11.6% and the complication rate was 30.1%. Postoperative pneumonia was the most frequent complication [4]. Therefore, a detailed evaluation of preoperative risk and potential risk reduction strategies is prudent in patients with known liver disease.


## Perioperative Risk Associated with Liver Disease

Prior to surgery, the etiology, duration, and severity of hepatic dysfunction should be determined including history of complications related to portal hypertension, including encephalopathy, ascites, gastrointestinal bleeding, and renal dysfunction. Routine laboratory assessment includes evaluation of hemoglobin, electrolytes, and coagulation (INR, fibrinogen and platelets). In patients with fever, leukocytosis, or acute deterioration, infection should be considered as well as a diagnostic paracentesis to rule out spontaneous bacterial peritonitis.

Based on a retrospective, small case series from the 1960s and 1970s, acute hepatitis confers a prohibitive risk for elective surgery. In a series of 36 patients with undiagnosed hepatitis who underwent laparotomy for diagnosis nearly one-third died and the majority suffered complications i.e. bacterial peritonitis, wound dehiscence, and hepatic failure. All patients with acute hepatitis, either viral or alcohol related, died [5]. When prudent, elective surgery should be postponed in patients with acute hepatitis [6, 7].

A number of studies have investigated the risk of surgery in patients with cirrhosis [8–11]. Each of the studies identified various components of the Child-Turcotte-Pugh score as important prognostic factors for perioperative mortality. In studies conducted over multiple decades, the modified Child score performed similarly in predicting early postoperative mortality: 10% in Child A, 17–30% in Child B, and 60–80% in Child C [10–12]. In comparison, the 3-month mortality for hospitalized patients not undergoing surgery was 4%, 14%, and 51%, respectively, for Child A, B, and C [11].

The MELD score is a useful predictor of 90-day waitlist mortality in liver transplant candidates [13], as well as shows a predictive value of perioperative mortality in cirrhotic patients. In a single-center study of 140 surgical procedures, the $c$-statistic for the MELD score's ability to predict 30-day mortality was 0.72. A $c$-statistic of 0.7 and higher is considered useful. Each MELD point to 20 equated to an additional 1% mortality and each point over 20 equated to an additional 2% mortality. A MELD score between 25 and 30 was associated with a 30-day mortality of 50% [14]. A larger study of 772 cirrhotics found similar results: a MELD score of 25 had a 30-day mortality of 50% [15]. Besides MELD score, other important predictors of perioperative mortality were age (>70 years = 3 MELD points) and coexisting diseases (ASA physical status > 4 = 5.5 MELD points). Common perioperative complications include liver failure, postoperative bleeding, infection, and renal failure. Teh et al. concluded that patients with a MELD score less than 11 have low postoperative mortality, and elective surgery can be considered relatively

**Table 5.1**  Cardiopulmonary Syndromes Related to Portal Hypertension

| Diagnosis | Screening method | Perioperative consequences |
|---|---|---|
| Cirrhotic cardiomyopathy (CCM) | Echocardiography assessment of LV diastolic function | Congestive heart failure[a] |
| Hepatopulmonary syndrome (HPS) | Room air hypoxemia ($PaO_2$ <70 mmHg) in the absence of other causes; confirmed by bubble echo | Although hypoxemia is typically responsive to supplemental oxygen, HPS is associated with increased infectious risk and perioperative mortality during liver transplantation[b] |
| Portopulmonary hypertension (POPH) | Echocardiographic estimate of RVSP; confirmed by right heart catheterization | Moderate to severe POPH associated with right heart failure and perioperative mortality during liver transplantation[c] |

*LV* left ventricle, *RVSP* right ventricle systolic pressure
[a]Ruiz-del-Arbol L, et al. World J Gastroenterol 2015; 21(41): 11502–21; Zardi EM, et al. J Am Coll Cardiol 2010; 56(7): 539–49
[b]Gupta S, et al. Am J Transpl 2010; 10(2): 354
[c]Ramsay M, et al. Curr Opin Anaesthesiol 2010; 23(2): 145–50

safe, preferably at institutions with a liver transplant center. In patients with a MELD score $\geq$ 20, the high mortality contraindicates elective procedures until after liver transplantation. If surgery is unable to be postponed or the patient has an intermediate MELD score (between 12 and 19), then liver transplant work-up should be underway prior to elective surgery in case the need for urgent postoperative transplantation arises. An online calculator of postoperative mortality risk in patients with cirrhosis can be found online at http://www.mayocinic.org/meld/mayomodel9.html.

Nearly every organ system is affected by liver disease. Specific cardiopulmonary consequences related to portal hypertension include cirrhotic cardiomyopathy (CCM), hepatopulmonary syndrome (HPS), and portopulmonary hypertension (POPH). Patients with even mild cirrhosis should be screened for these conditions if undergoing extensive surgery. The screening methods and the perioperative consequences of these conditions can impact perioperative outcomes (see Table 5.1) [16, 17].

Medical management to optimize cirrhotic patients undergoing surgery should be directed toward treating active infection, optimizing central blood volume and renal status while minimizing ascites and improving encephalopathy. However, there is little evidence to support specific goal-directed targets for preoperative care in any of these areas. In particular, preoperative INR correction has little support. Evidence suggests that transfusion of plasma in the absence of bleeding increases central blood volume and worsens portal hypertension, which can lead to an increased risk of variceal bleeding [18]. Recent reviews argue against prophylactic plasma administration [19]. In an observational study of over 1200 patients with preoperative INR > 1.5 undergoing noncardiac surgery, 11% received preoperative plasma transfusion. Despite this, WHO grade 3 bleeding occurred in 53% of those receiving plasma compared to 32% in those who did not (OR 2.35, 95% CI 1.65–3.36) [20]. Standard doses of plasma rarely correct the coagulopathy of cirrhosis and, by worsening portal hypertension, can be harmful [21]. The INR has been recognized as an inadequate indicator of preoperative bleeding risk since PT/INR values depend upon the levels of procoagulants (factors I, II, V, VII and X) without accounting for low levels of endogenous anticoagulant factors. Due to elevated levels of endothelial-derived factor VIII and low levels of protein C, chronic liver disease patients often generate normal or high levels of thrombin [22]. Chronic liver disease patients are often in a delicate balance between inadequate hemostasis and excessive coagulation [23]. With bleeding, fibrinogen levels should be maintained >150–200 mg/dL with transfusion of cryoprecipitate or if available, human fibrinogen concentrate [19].

Perioperative risk depends more on the operative site and the degree of liver impairment than the anesthetic technique [24]. In a retrospective study of 733 cirrhotic patients, mortality was associated with the Child score (ascites, elevated creatinine), male gender, cryptogenic cirrhosis (vs. other etiologies), preoperative infection, higher ASA physical status, and surgery on the respiratory system. One-year mortality in patients with six risk factors was over 80%; mortality with two risk factors was 30% [4].

In addition to optimizing medical management, minimizing surgical risk should be considered. Gallstones are twice as common in cirrhotic patients as in patients without cirrhosis [8]. Laparoscopic surgery is safe in patients with Child A and B cirrhosis [25]. However, Child C patients may benefit from percutaneous drainage of the gallbladder over cholecystectomy [26]. In a series of over 4200 laparoscopic cholecystectomies, cirrhotics ($n = 226$) had a mortality of approximately 1/100, compared to 1/2000 without [27]. Preoperative decompression of portal hypertension by TIPS may improve outcomes in patients with severe portal hypertension [28].

## Intraoperative Management

### Monitoring and Vascular Access

In addition to standard noninvasive monitors, arterial pressure monitoring should be considered for patients with ESLD. The decision is based on preoperative hypotension due to vasodilatation, anticipated blood loss, the need for intraoperative laboratory studies, coexisting disease, and age. The usefulness of CVP monitoring to predict fluid responsiveness is debatable [29]. Many have abandoned CVP monitoring in the setting of liver resection [30–32]. In our practice, we do not place a central venous catheter exclusively for CVP monitoring. Pulmonary artery catheterization is used for patients with known or suspected pulmonary artery hypertension and/or low cardiac ejection fraction. Transesophageal echocardiography (TEE) is a sensitive monitor for the assessment of preload, contractility (including regional wall motion), ejection fraction, static and dynamic valvular abnormalities, emboli, and pericardial fluid. In a small series of patients with esophageal varices, TEE universally aided in diagnosis and was not associated with bleeding complications, although transgastric views were avoided to minimize esophageal manipulation [33]. Other authors have confirmed the safety of TEE in this population [34, 35].

## Coagulation Management

Viscoelastic coagulation testing using thromboelastography or thromboelastometry may be a useful guide, more accurately reflecting the overall effects of altered levels of endogenous pro- and anticoagulant factors [36]. Abnormalities in platelet number and function are in part compensated for by increased levels of von Willebrand factor (VWF), a platelet adhesive protein, and by decreased levels of ADAMTS13, the VWF cleaving protease. Thrombin generation is preserved with platelet counts exceeding $50 \times 10^9$ / L, making this value a practical target in the setting of active bleeding [37].

## Anesthetic Technique: Neuraxial Versus General Anesthesia

The effect of neuraxial or epidural anesthesia on hepatic blood flow appears related to alterations of systemic blood pressure [38, 39]. Standard contraindications to neuraxial blockade should be considered and weighed against the benefits on a case-by-case basis. Many patients with advanced hepatic disease may not be candidates for neuraxial techniques due to coagulopathy and/or thrombocytopenia. Nerve blockade may be appropriate even when neuraxial blockade is contraindicated. The transversus abdominal plane (TAP) block has been used successfully for abdominal surgery, including hepatobiliary procedures [40, 41]. However, the efficacy has been questioned and reported complications include abdominal wall hematoma.

## Volatile Anesthetics

Volatile anesthetics decrease hepatic blood flow to varying degrees. Commonly used agents, isoflurane and sevoflurane, have less significant effects on hepatic blood flow than halothane [42]. Desflurane appears to more substantially decrease hepatic blood flow at one MAC, causing a 30% reduction [43]. At higher anesthetic concentrations, isoflurane causes a dose-dependent reduction in hepatic blood flow not seen with sevoflurane. In animal studies, both sevoflurane and isoflurane maintain the hepatic arterial buffer response, which increases hepatic arterial blood flow in the presence of reductions of portal blood flow [44, 45].

Concerns exist regarding the production of reactive intermediates during the metabolism of inhaled anesthetics. There is little evidence, however, to suggest that volatile anesthetics besides halothane are responsible for hepatic complications. Most volatile anesthetics undergo metabolism that yields reactive trifluoroacetylated (TFA) intermediates. These intermediates bind to hepatic proteins, producing an immunologic reaction leading to liver injury. The incidence of liver injury correlates to the extent to which inhaled anesthetics undergo this oxidative metabolism (halothane 20%, isoflurane 0.2%, desflurane 0.02%). Notably, sevoflurane metabolism does not result in TFA intermediates [46].

## Nitrous Oxide

Nitrous oxide administration has not been shown to cause hepatocellular injury in the absence of hepatic hypoxemia [47]. Due to sympathomimetic effects, nitrous oxide can decrease hepatic blood flow, and inhibition of methionine synthase can occur after even brief exposures. However, the clinical significance of these effects is unclear [48].

## Intravenous Anesthetics

Intravenous anesthetics and sedatives including propofol, etomidate, and midazolam do not appear to alter hepatic function when given for short durations. The effects of IV anesthetics after prolonged infusions in patients with advanced liver disease are not well studied. Propofol infusion syndrome (lactic acidosis, lipemia, rhabdomyolysis, hyperkalemia, and myocardial failure) has resulted in patient deaths [49]. Liver dysfunction resulting in altered lipid metabolism may predispose to cirrhotics to propofol infusion syndrome [50]. Patients on prolonged propofol infusions should be monitored for progressive lactic acidosis and escalating vasopressor requirements.

There is no evidence that opioids have an effect on hepatic function independent of hepatic blood flow. All opioids increase sphincter of Oddi pressure. Some authors have suggested that morphine causes spasm in the sphincter of Oddi, but a review failed to show a differential effect, concluding that morphine may be preferred over meperidine for the treatment of patients with acute pancreatitis due to less risk of seizures [51].

## Pharmacokinetic and Pharmacodynamic Alterations

Decreased hepatocellular mass and portocaval shunts lead to reduced metabolism of drugs that rely on hepatic metabolism. Factors that affect hepatic clearance include blood flow to the liver, the fraction of the drug unbound to plasma proteins, and intrinsic clearance. Drugs with low extraction ratios < 0.3, have restrictive hepatic clearance. Clearance of drugs in this class is affected by protein binding, the induction or inhibition of hepatic enzymes, age, and hepatic pathology, but clearance is not significantly affected by hepatic blood flow. Drugs with high extraction ratios (> 0.7) undergo extensive first-pass metabolism, which alters their bioavailability after oral administration. Drugs with high extraction ratios are significantly affected by alteration in hepatic blood flow, which can occur with hemodynamic changes or hepatic inflow clamping during liver resection.

Benzodiazepines have a low extraction ratio and the elimination half-life can be prolonged (diazepam $t_{1/2} = 43$ h). Studies have shown conflicting effects of cirrhosis on the metabolism of midazolam, possibly due to changes in protein binding [52, 53]. As hepatic protein synthesis declines, the drug fraction bound to protein decreases. While the pharmacokinetic implications of ESLD are complex, patients with encephalopathy display an increased sensitivity to sedatives and analgesics.

Opioid metabolism is reduced in patients with liver disease, so dosing intervals should be increased to avoid drug accumulation. The clearance of the meperidine metabolite normeperidine is reduced in liver disease, which can lead to neurotoxicity [54]. The elimination of a single IV opioid bolus is less affected than a continuous infusion through redistribution to storage sites. Opioid dosages in patients with advanced disease should be reduced to avoid precipitating or worsening encephalopathy.

The intermediate duration neuromuscular blocking agents vecuronium and rocuronium are metabolized by the liver and exhibit a prolonged duration of action [55, 56]. Despite this, a resistance to the initial dose of neuromuscular blocker typically occurs due to elevated γ-globulin concentrations and an increase in the volume of distribution (due to edema and/or ascites). Atracurium and cisatracurium undergo organ-independent elimination and their durations of action are not affected by liver disease. Succinylcholine metabolism is altered due to reduced plasma cholinesterase activity in cirrhotic patients, but the clinical impact is rarely significant.

**Vasopressors and Volume Resuscitation**

In contrast to sedatives, patients with liver disease exhibit a reduced responsiveness to endogenous vasoconstrictors including angiotensin II, vasopressin, and norepinephrine [57]. Hyporesponsiveness to catecholamines may be modulated by the release of nitric oxide, prostacyclin, and other endothelial-derived factors in response to humoral and mechanical stimuli [58]. Many patients present with hyperdynamic circulation characterized by low systemic vascular resistance, borderline hypotension and elevated cardiac output. These patients frequently cannot tolerate induction or maintenance of anesthesia without vasopressor support. In patients undergoing abdominal surgery, fluids should be restricted (with or without CVP monitoring) in order to lower portal pressures.

When need for volume resuscitation arises, the fluid and blood products administered are similar in patients with and without liver disease, but with several notable exceptions. In ESLD, serum albumin function is quantitatively and qualitatively decreased [59]. Albumin has three major indications in the treatment of cirrhotic patients [60]:

1. After large volume (4–5 L) paracentesis [61]
2. The presence of spontaneous bacterial peritonitis to prevent renal impairment in patients with preexisting elevations of bilirubin or creatinine [62]
3. In conjunction with splanchnic vasoconstrictors for type I hepatorenal syndrome

In a randomized trial of terlipressin with and without albumin, a higher propor-tion (77%) of the group that received albumin showed a complete response com-pared to terlipressin alone (25%) [63]. In patients with hyponatremia, hypotonic sodium should be administered to avoid a rapid rise in serum sodium, which can be associated with central pontine demyelination and permanent neurologic injury.

**Transjugular Intrahepatic Portosystemic Shunt (TIPS) Procedure**

Sedation is commonly used to facilitate placement, although general anesthesia is preferred by some to limit patient movement, control diaphragmatic excursion, and reduce the risk of aspiration. Complications include pneumothorax or vascular injury during access to the jugular vein. Dysrhythmias can occur during catheter insertion and extrahepatic artery or portal vein puncture can result in significant hemorrhage [64].

**Hepatic Resection**

Hemorrhage remains a major complication in hepatic resections, although transfu-sion is necessary in less than 20% of cases [65, 66]. Newer transection techniques using ultrasonic dissectors, high-pressure water jets, and harmonic scalpels may be helpful, but they have not been proven to be superior to conventional clamp crush techniques [67–69]. Techniques to maintain CVP at normal or low (<5 cm $H_2O$) levels have been suggested to limit blood loss [70]. In a single-center, uncontrolled series of nearly 500 hepatic resections managed with low CVP, no cases of renal failure were attributed to the technique [71]. There is conflicting data regarding the correlation between low CVP technique and blood loss. Two series of living liver donor surgeries concluded that CVP is not a predictor of blood loss during hepatic resection [72, 73]. A recent meta-analysis found that low CVP does not decrease morbidity, but does reduce blood loss [74]. Another recent study found that fluid restriction, confirmed by high stroke volume variation, resulted in less blood loss [75]. Aside from CVP, vasopressors can reduce splanchnic pressure and decrease blood loss through their direct effects on splanchnic vessels [76].

Even in patients with normal preoperative coagulation profiles, the INR and platelet count can be abnormal after liver resection. The severity of the derangement correlates with the extent of the resection, peaks postoperative day one to two, and takes up to five or more days to resolve [77, 78]. This postoperative coagulopathy may be a contraindication to continuous epidural analgesia, increasing the risk of epidural hematoma during catheter removal. Some authors advise against preoperative epidural catheter placement, while others recommend correcting coag-ulation abnormalities prior to catheter discontinuation [79]. Using viscoelastic test-ing, brief hypercoagulability after liver resection despite prolonged prothrombin times have been reported [80]. Alternatives that avoid epidural catheter placement include intrathecal opioid and local anesthesia infusion systems [81].

# Conclusion

In general, contraindications to elective surgery in patients with ESLD include acute viral or alcoholic hepatitis, fulminant liver failure, Child's class C cirrhosis, severe coagulopathy due to splenic sequestration of platelets or prolongation of the INR despite vitamin K repletion, and severe extrahepatic complications secondary to hepatopulmonary syndrome, portopulmonary hypertension, hepatorenal syndrome, or cardiomyopathy [7]. Elective surgery is considered relatively safe with MELD scores below 11 and contraindicated until after liver transplantation when MELD exceeds 20 [15].

Preoperative optimization includes effective control of ascites through diuretics or paracentesis to improve oxygenation and increase functional residual capacity. Elevated INR is not an independent risk factor for increased perioperative bleeding. When available, viscoelastic testing may be a more accurate reflection of coagulopathy to guide repletion of clotting factors, fibrinogen, and platelets.

In the absence of particular contraindications (primarily significant coagulapthy), neuraxial, regional, as well as general anesthesia have all been successful in ESLD patients. Because of decreased hepatic metabolism and increased volume of distribution, initial dosing and dosing intervals will have to be adjusted, particularly for opioids and intermediate-acting neuromuscular blockers.

Advances in surgery, anesthesia, and intensive care have led to improved outcomes in patients with significant liver disease. These advances are related to comprehensive preoperative screening and preparation that avoids further hepatic injury. However, when deterioration occurs, liver transplantation should be considered early as it is the only definitive treatment for irreversible hepatic failure.

# References

1. Prevention CD and C. Hepatitis statistics: surveillance for viral hepatitis – United States. 2013. http://www.cdc.gov/hepatitis/statistics/2013surveillance/commentary.htm.
2. Prevention CD and C. Death rates by age and age-adjusted death rates for the 15 leading causes of death in 2013: United States. 1999–2013. http://www.cdc.gov/nchs/data/nvsr/nvsr64/nvsr64_02.pdf.
3. Csikesz NG, Nguyen LN, Tseng JF, Shah SA. Nationwide volume and mortality after elective surgery in cirrhotic patients. J Am Coll Surg. 2009;208(1):96–103. doi:10.1016/j.jamcollsurg.2008.09.006.
4. Ziser A, Plevak DJ, Wiesner RH, Rakela J, Offord KP, Brown DL. Morbidity and mortality in cirrhotic patients undergoing anesthesia and surgery. Anesthesiology. 1999;90(1):42–53. http://www.ncbi.nlm.nih.gov/entrez/query.fcgi?cmd=Retrieve&db=PubMed&dopt=Citation&list_uids=9915311
5. Powell-Jackson P, Greenway B, Williams R. Adverse effects of exploratory laparotomy in patients with unsuspected liver disease. Br J Surg. 1982;69(8):449–51. http://www.ncbi.nlm.nih.gov/pubmed/7104630
6. Rizvon MK, Chou CL. Surgery in the patient with liver disease. Med Clin North Am. 2003;87(1):211 - +. doi:10.1016/s0025-7125(02)00153-0.
7. Friedman LS, Xu J, Murphy SL, Kochanek KD, Bastian BA, Statistics V. Surgery in the patient with liver disease. Trans Am Clin Climatol Assoc. 2010;121(2):192–204. discussion 205.

http://www.ncbi.nlm.nih.gov/entrez/query.fcgi?cmd=Retrieve&db=PubMed&dopt=Citation &list_uids=20697561

8. Aranha GV, Sontag SJ, Greenlee HB. Cholecystectomy in cirrhotic patients: a formidable operation. Am J Surg. 1982;143(1):55–60. http://www.ncbi.nlm.nih.gov/pubmed/7053656

9. Doberneck RC, Sterling Jr WA, Allison DC. Morbidity and mortality after operation in non-bleeding cirrhotic patients. Am J Surg. 1983;146(3):306–9. http://www.ncbi.nlm.nih.gov/pubmed/6604465

10. Garrison RN, Cryer HM, Howard DA, Polk Jr HC. Clarification of risk factors for abdominal operations in patients with hepatic cirrhosis. Ann Surg. 1984;199(6):648–55. http://www.ncbi.nlm.nih.gov/pubmed/6732310

11. Mansour A, Watson W, Shayani V, Pickleman J. Abdominal operations in patients with cirrhosis: still a major surgical challenge. Surgery. 1997;122(4):730–6. http://www.ncbi.nlm.nih.gov/pubmed/9347849

12. Neeff H, Mariaskin D, Spangenberg H-C, Hopt UT, Makowiec F. Perioperative mortality after non-hepatic general surgery in patients with liver cirrhosis: an analysis of 138 operations in the 2000s using child and MELD scores. J Gastrointest Surg. 2011;15(1):1–11. doi:10.1007/s11605-010-1366-9.

13. Freeman RB, Wiesner RH, Harper A, et al. The new liver allocation system: moving toward evidence-based transplantation policy. Liver Transpl. 2002;8(9):851–8. doi:10.1053/jlts.2002.35927.

14. Northup PG, Wanamaker RC, Lee VD, Adams RB, Berg CL. Model for End-Stage Liver Disease (MELD) predicts nontransplant surgical mortality in patients with cirrhosis. Ann Surg. 2005;242(2):244–51. 00000658-200508000-00013 [pii]

15. Teh SH, Nagorney DM, Stevens SR, et al. Risk factors for mortality after surgery in patients with cirrhosis. Gastroenterology. 2007;132(4):1261–9. doi:10.1053/j.gastro.2007.01.040.

16. Raval Z, Harinstein ME, Skaro AI, et al. Cardiovascular risk assessment of the liver transplant candidate. J Am Coll Cardiol. 2011;58(3):223–31. doi:10.1016/j.jacc.2011.03.026.

17. Fede G, Privitera G, Tomaselli T, Spadaro L, Purrello F. Cardiovascular dysfunction in patients with liver cirrhosis. Ann Gastroenterol. 2015;28(1):31–40. http://www.ncbi.nlm.nih.gov/pubmed/25608575

18. Zimmon DS, Kessler RE. The portal pressure-blood volume relationship in cirrhosis. Gut. 1974;15(2):99–101. http://www.ncbi.nlm.nih.gov/pubmed/4820643

19. Nadim MK, Durand F, Kellum JA, et al. Management of the critically ill patient with cirrhosis: a multidisciplinary perspective. J Hepatol. 2016;64(3):717–35. doi:10.1016/j.jhep.2015.10.019.

20. Jia Q, Brown MJ, Clifford L, et al. Prophylactic plasma transfusion for surgical patients with abnormal preoperative coagulation tests: a single-institution propensity-adjusted cohort study. Lancet Haematol. 2016;3(3):e139–48. doi:10.1016/s2352-3026(15)00283-5.

21. Northup PG, McMahon MM, Ruhl AP, et al. Coagulopathy does not fully protect hospitalized cirrhosis patients from peripheral venous thromboembolism. Am J Gastroenterol. 2006;101(7):1524–28; quiz 1680. doi:AJG588 [pii]10.1111/j.1572-0241.2006.00588.x.

22. Tripodi A, Primignani M, Chantarangkul V, et al. An imbalance of pro- vs anti-coagulation factors in plasma from patients with cirrhosis. Gastroenterology. 2009;137(6):2105–11. doi:10.1053/j.gastro.2009.08.045.

23. Lisman T, Bakhtiari K, Pereboom IT, Hendriks HG, Meijers JC, Porte RJ. Normal to increased thrombin generation in patients undergoing liver transplantation despite prolonged conventional coagulation tests. J Hepatol. 2010;52(3):355–61. doi:10.1016/j.jhep.2009.12.001.

24. Viegas O, Stoelting RK. LDH5 changes after cholecystectomy or hysterectomy in patients receiving halothane, enflurane, or fentanyl. Anesthesiology. 1979;51(6):556–8. doi:10.1097/00000542-197912000-00017.

25. Shaikh AR, Muneer A. Laparoscopic cholecystectomy in cirrhotic patients. JSLS. 2009;13(4):592–6. doi:10.4293/108680809X12589999537959.

26. Curro G, Iapichino G, Melita G, Lorenzini C, Cucinotta E. Laparoscopic cholecystectomy in Child-Pugh class C cirrhotic patients. JSLS. 2005;9(3):311–5. http://www.ncbi.nlm.nih.gov/pubmed/16121878

27. Yeh CN, Chen MF, Jan YY. Laparoscopic cholecystectomy in 226 cirrhotic patients. Experience of a single center in Taiwan. Surg Endosc. 2002;16(11):1583–7. doi:10.1007/s00464-002-9026-0.

28. Azoulay D, Buabse F, Damiano I, et al. Neoadjuvant transjugular intrahepatic portosystemic shunt: a solution for extrahepatic abdominal operation in cirrhotic patients with severe portal hypertension. J Am Coll Surg. 2001;193(1):46–51. http://www.ncbi.nlm.nih.gov/pubmed/11442253

29. Marik PE, Baram M, Vahid B. Does central venous pressure predict fluid responsiveness? A systematic review of the literature and the tale of seven mares. Chest. 2008;134(1):172–8. doi:10.1378/chest.07-2331.

30. Mansour N, Lentschener C, Ozier Y. Do we really need a low central venous pressure in elective liver resection. Acta Anaesthesiol Scand. 2008;52(9):1306–07. doi:AAS1750 [pii]10.1111/j.1399-6576.2008.01750.x.

31. Schroeder RA, Kuo PC. Pro: low central venous pressure during liver transplantation – not too low. J Cardiothorac Vasc Anesth. 2008;22(2):311–4. doi:10.1053/j.jvca.2007.12.009.

32. Niemann CU, Feiner J, Behrends M, Eilers H, Ascher NL, Roberts JP. Central venous pressure monitoring during living right donor hepatectomy. Liver Transpl. 2007;13(2):266–71. doi:10.1002/lt.21051.

33. Spier BJ, Larue SJ, Teelin TC, et al. Review of complications in a series of patients with known gastro-esophageal varices undergoing transesophageal echocardiography. J Am Soc Echocardiogr. 2009;22(4):396–400. doi:10.1016/j.echo.2009.01.002.

34. Myo Bui CC, Worapot A, Xia W, et al. Gastroesophageal and hemorrhagic complications associated with intraoperative transesophageal echocardiography in patients with model for end-stage liver disease score 25 or higher. J Cardiothorac Vasc Anesth. 2015;29(3):594–7. doi:10.1053/j.jvca.2014.10.030.

35. Markin NW, Sharma A, Grant W, Shillcutt SK. The safety of transesophageal echocardiography in patients undergoing orthotopic liver transplantation. J Cardiothorac Vasc Anesth. 2015;29(3):588–93. doi:10.1053/j.jvca.2014.10.012.

36. Tripodi A. Tests of coagulation in liver disease. Clin Liver Dis. 2009;13(1):55 - +. doi:10.1016/j.cld.2008.09.002.

37. Tripodi A, Primignani M, Chantarangkul V, et al. Thrombin generation in patients with cirrhosis: the role of platelets. Hepatology. 2006;44(2):440–5. doi:10.1002/hep.21266.

38. Kennedy WF, Everett GB, Cobb LA, Allen GD. Simultaneous systemic and hepatic hemodynamic measurements during high spinal anesthesia in normal man. Anesth Analg Curr Res. 1970;49(6):1016 - &. <Go to ISI>://WOS:A1970H956200026

39. Kennedy WF, Everett GB, Cobb LA, Allen GD. Simultaneous systemic and hepatic hemodynamic measurements during high peridural anesthesia in normal man. Anesth Analg Curr Res. 1971;50(6):1069 - &. doi:10.1213/00000539-197150060-00029.

40. McDonnell JG, O'Donnell B, Curley G, Heffernan A, Power C, Laffey JG. The analgesic efficacy of transversus abdominis plane block after abdominal surgery: a prospective randomized controlled trial. Anesth Analg. 2007;104(1):193–7. doi:10.1213/01.ane.0000250223.49963.0f.

41. Niraj G, Kelkar A, Jeyapalan I, et al. Comparison of analgesic efficacy of subcostal transversus abdominis plane blocks with epidural analgesia following upper abdominal surgery. Anaesthesia. 2011;66(6):465–71. doi:10.1111/j.1365-2044.2011.06700.x.

42. Frink Jr EJ. The hepatic effects of sevoflurane. Anesth Analg. 1995;81(6 Suppl):S46–50. http://www.ncbi.nlm.nih.gov/entrez/query.fcgi?cmd=Retrieve&db=PubMed&dopt=Citation&list_uids=7486148

43. Schindler E, Muller M, Zickmann B, Kraus H, Reuner KH, Hempelmann G. Blood supply to the liver in the human after 1 MAC desflurane in comparison with isoflurane and halothane. Anasthesiol Intensivmed Notfallmed Schmerzther. 1996;31(6):344–8. doi:10.1055/s-2007-995933.

44. Matsumoto N, Koizumi M, Sugai M. Hepatolobectomy-induced depression of hepatic circulation and metabolism in the dog is counteracted by isoflurane, but not by halothane. Acta Anaesthesiol Scand. 1999;43(8):850–4. http://www.ncbi.nlm.nih.gov/pubmed/10492415

45. Crawford MW, Lerman J, Saldivia V, Carmichael FJ. Hemodynamic and organ blood flow responses to halothane and sevoflurane anesthesia during spontaneous ventilation. Anesth Analg. 1992;75(6):1000–6. http://www.ncbi.nlm.nih.gov/pubmed/1443679

46. Njoku D, Laster MJ, Gong DH, Eger 2nd EI, Reed GF, Martin JL. Biotransformation of halothane, enflurane, isoflurane, and desflurane to trifluoroacetylated liver proteins: association between protein acylation and hepatic injury. Anesth Analg. 1997;84(1):173–8. http://www.ncbi.nlm.nih.gov/pubmed/8989020

47. Sear JW, Prysroberts C, Dye A. Hepatic-function after anesthesia for major vascular reconstructive surgery – a comparison of 4 anesthetic techniques. Br J Anaesth. 1983;55(7):603–9. doi:10.1093/bja/55.7.603.

48. Nunn JF. Clinical aspects of the interaction between nitrous oxide and vitamin B12. Br J Anaesth. 1987;59(1):3–13. http://www.ncbi.nlm.nih.gov/pubmed/3548788

49. Parke TJ, Stevens JE, Rice AS, et al. Metabolic acidosis and fatal myocardial failure after propofol infusion in children: five case reports. BMJ. 1992;305(6854):613–6. http://www.ncbi.nlm.nih.gov/pubmed/1393073

50. Otterspoor LC, Kalkman CJ, Cremer OL. Update on the propofol infusion syndrome in ICU management of patients with head injury. Curr Opin Anaesthesiol. 2008;21(5):544–51. doi:10.1097/ACO.0b013e32830f44fb.

51. Thompson DR. Narcotic analgesic effects on the sphincter of oddi: a review of the data and therapeutic implications in treating pancreatitis. Am J Gastroenterol. 2001;96(4):1266–72. doi:10.1111/j.1572-0241.2001.03536.x.

52. Trouvin JH, Farinotti R, Haberer JP, Servin F, Chauvin M, Duvaldestin P. Pharmacokinetics of midazolam in anesthetized cirrhotic-patients. Br J Anaesth. 1988;60(7):762–7. doi:10.1093/bja/60.7.762.

53. Macgilchrist AJ, Birnie GG, Cook A, et al. Pharmacokinetics and pharmacodynamics of intravenous midazolam in patients with severe alcoholic cirrhosis. Gut. 1986;27(2):190–5. doi:10.1136/gut.27.2.190.

54. Tegeder I, Lotsch J, Geisslinger G. Pharmacokinetics of opioids in liver disease. Clin Pharmacokinet. 1999;37(1):17–40. http://www.ncbi.nlm.nih.gov/entrez/query.fcgi?cmd=Retrieve&db=PubMed&dopt=Citation&list_uids=10451781

55. Hunter JM, Parker CJ, Bell CF, Jones RS, Utting JE. The use of different doses of vecuronium in patients with liver dysfunction. Br J Anaesth. 1985;57(8):758–64. http://www.ncbi.nlm.nih.gov/pubmed/2861836

56. Magorian T, Wood P, Caldwell J, et al. The pharmacokinetics and neuromuscular effects of rocuronium bromide in patients with liver disease. Anesth Analg. 1995;80(4):754–9. http://www.ncbi.nlm.nih.gov/pubmed/7893030

57. Cahill PA. Vasoconstrictor responsiveness of portal hypertensive vessels. Clin Sci. 1999;96(1):3–4. doi:10.1042/cs19980297.

58. Cahill PA, Redmond EM, Sitzmann JV. Endothelial dysfunction in cirrhosis and portal hypertension. Pharmacol Ther. 2001;89(3):273–93. doi:10.1016/s0163-7258(01)00128-0.

59. Alves de Mattos A. Current indications for the use of albumin in the treatment of cirrhosis. Ann Hepatol. 2011;10(Suppl 1):S15–20. http://www.ncbi.nlm.nih.gov/pubmed/21566250

60. Bernardi M, Ricci CS, Zaccherini G. Role of human albumin in the management of complications of liver cirrhosis. J Clin Exp Hepatol. 2014;4(4):302–11. doi:10.1016/j.jceh.2014.08.007.

61. Runyon BA. Management of adult patients with ascites due to cirrhosis: an update. Hepatology. 2009;49(6):2087–107. doi:10.1002/hep.22853.

62. Terg R, Gadano A, Cartier M, et al. Serum creatinine and bilirubin predict renal failure and mortality in patients with spontaneous bacterial peritonitis: a retrospective study. Liver Int. 2009;29(3):415–9. doi:10.1111/j.1478-3231.2008.01877.x.

63. Ortega R, Gines P, Uriz J, et al. Terlipressin therapy with and without albumin for patients with hepatorenal syndrome: results of a prospective, nonrandomized study. Hepatology. 2002;36(4 Pt 1):941–8. doi:10.1053/jhep.2002.35819.

64. Quiroga J, Sangro B, Nunez M, et al. Transjugular intrahepatic portal-systemic shunt in the treatment of refractory ascites – effect on clinical, renal, humoral, and hemodynamic parameters. Hepatology. 1995;21(4):986–94. doi:10.1016/0270-9139(95)90245-7.

65. Lentschener C, Benhamou D, Mercier FJ, et al. Aprotinin reduces blood loss in patients under-going elective liver resection. Anesth Analg. 1997;84(4):875–81. http://www.ncbi.nlm.nih.gov/pubmed/9085974
66. Jones RM, Moulton CE, Hardy KJ. Central venous pressure and its effect on blood loss during liver resection. Br J Surg. 1998;85(8):1058–60. <Go to ISI>://WOS:000075280800006
67. Franco D. Liver surgery has become simpler. Eur J Anaesthesiol. 2002;19(11):777–9. doi:10.1017/s0265021502001254.
68. Lentschener C, Ozier Y. Anaesthesia for elective liver resection: some points should be revis-ited. Eur J Anaesthesiol. 2002;19(11):780–8. doi:10.1017/s0265021502001266.
69. Clavien PA, Petrowsky H, DeOliveira ML, Graf R. Strategies for safer liver surgery and partial liver transplantation. N Engl J Med. 2007;356(15):1545–59. doi:356/15/1545 [pii]10.1056/NEJMra065156.
70. Wang W-D, Liang L-J, Huang X-Q, Yin X-Y. Low central venous pressure reduces blood loss in hepatectomy. World J Gastroenterol. 2006;12(6):935–9. <Go to ISI>://WOS:000239994700015
71. Melendez JA, Arslan V, Fischer ME, et al. Perioperative outcomes of major hepatic resections under low central venous pressure anesthesia: blood loss, blood transfusion, and the risk of postoperative renal dysfunction. J Am Coll Surg. 1998;187(6):620–5. http://www.ncbi.nlm.nih.gov/entrez/query.fcgi?cmd=Retrieve&db=PubMed&dopt=Citation&list_uids=9849736
72. Kim YK, Chin JH, Kang SJ, et al. Association between central venous pressure and blood loss during hepatic resection in 984 living donors. Acta Anaesthesiol Scand. 2009;53(5):601–6. doi:10.1111/j.1399-6576.2009.01920.x.
73. Chhibber A, Dziak J, Kolano J, Norton JR, Lustik S. Anesthesia care for adult live donor hepatectomy: our experiences with 100 cases. Liver Transpl. 2007;13(4):537–42. doi:10.1002/lt.21074.
74. Hughes MJ, Ventham NT, Harrison EM, Wigmore SJ. Central venous pressure and liver resection: a systematic review and meta-analysis. HPB. 2015;17(10):863–71. doi:10.1111/hpb.12462.
75. Seo H, Jun IG, Ha TY, Hwang S, Lee SG, Kim YK. High stroke volume variation method by mannitol administration can decrease blood loss during donor hepatectomy. Medicine (Baltimore). 2016;95(2):e2328. doi:10.1097/MD.0000000000002328.
76. Massicotte L, Perrault MA, Denault AY, et al. Effects of phlebotomy and phenylephrine infu-sion on portal venous pressure and systemic hemodynamics during liver transplantation. Transplantation. 2010;89(8):920–7. doi:10.1097/TP.0b013e3181d7c40c.
77. Matot I, Scheinin O, Eid A, Jurim O. Epidural anesthesia and analgesia in liver resec-tion. Anesth Analg. 2002;95(5):1179–81. table of contents. http://www.ncbi.nlm.nih.gov/pubmed/12401587
78. Borromeo CJ, Stix MS, Lally A, Pomfret EA. Epidural catheter and increased prothrombin time after right lobe hepatectomy for living donor transplantation. Anesth Analg. 2000;91(5):1139–41. http://www.ncbi.nlm.nih.gov/pubmed/11049898
79. Elterman KG, Xiong Z. Coagulation profile changes and safety of epidural analgesia after hepa-tectomy: a retrospective study. J Anesth. 2015;29(3):367–72. doi:10.1007/s00540-014-1933-4.
80. Barton JS, Riha GM, Differding JA, et al. Coagulopathy after a liver resection: is it over diag-nosed and over treated? HPB. 2013;15(11):865–71. doi:10.1111/hpb.12051.
81. Lee SH, Gwak MS, Choi SJ, et al. Prospective, randomized study of ropivacaine wound infu-sion versus intrathecal morphine with intravenous fentanyl for analgesia in living donors for liver transplantation. Liver Transpl. 2013;19(9):1036–45. doi:10.1002/lt.23691.

# Chapter 6
# Nutrition Support of Patients with Cirrhosis

Jeanette Hasse and Manjushree Gautam

Metabolic aberrations and complications of liver failure directly affect the nutrition status of patients afflicted with cirrhosis. Nutrient metabolism is altered, nutrient requirements change, and the ability to for a patient to ingest adequate nutrients is often impaired. Therefore, it is vital to promptly assess the nutrition status of patients with cirrhosis and implement appropriate medical nutrition therapy. This chapter will provide insight into the nutrition management of patients with cirrhosis including assessing malnutrition, determining nutrient requirements, recognizing alterations in metabolism, identifying indications for nutrition support, and providing nutrition support to this medically complex patient population.

## Malnutrition and Cirrhosis

Malnutrition is common in patients with cirrhosis. In fact, malnutrition and severe muscle wasting has been identified as one of the most common complications of cirrhosis that adversely affects patient survival, quality of life, and recovery from infection or surgery [31]. The exact prevalence of malnutrition depends on the type and chronicity of liver disease, whether the patient has compensated or

J. Hasse, PhD, RD, LD, FADA, CNSC (✉)
Annette C. and Harold C. Simmons Transplant Institute, Baylor University Medical Center,
3410 Worth Street, Suite 950, Dallas, TX 75246, USA
e-mail: Jeanette.Hasse@BSWHealth.org

M. Gautam, MD, MAS
Department of Internal Medicine, Texas A&M College of Medicine, Bryan, TX 77807, USA

Simmons Transplant Institute, Baylor All Saints Medical Center,
1250 8th Avenue, Suite 515, Fort Worth, TX 76104, USA
e-mail: Manjushree.Gautam@BSWHealth.org

© Springer International Publishing AG 2017
B. Eghtesad, J. Fung (eds.), *Surgical Procedures on the Cirrhotic Patient*,
DOI 10.1007/978-3-319-52396-5_6

decompensated liver disease, and the markers used to identify malnutrition [46]. Assessing nutrition status in patients with cirrhosis is fraught with difficulties. Typical markers of malnutrition such as weight loss may be useful in patients with compensated liver disease. However, fluid retention (ascites and edema) can mask true weight in patients with decompensated liver disease. There are no laboratory markers of malnutrition; serum proteins are considered markers of inflammation rather than of nutrition [26, 27] and serum protein levels are depressed due to the inability of the liver to synthesize proteins. Conversely, serum albumin levels can be falsely elevated in patients who receive intravenous albumin infusions as a method to help control fluid overload.

Nutrition assessment of patients with cirrhosis is typically done using the Subjective Global Assessment (SGA) method. SGA includes three main parts: history, physical examination, and SGA rating [9]. The history section considers weight changes (including fluid shifts), dietary intake compared with normal, persistent gastrointestinal (GI) symptoms (e.g., nausea, vomiting, diarrhea, anorexia, early satiety), functional capacity (considering degree and duration of dysfunction), and medical diagnoses. The physical examination encompasses evaluation of fat and muscle stores as well as fluid retention and looking for signs of micronutrient deficiencies. The final section of SGA is the rating in which a patient is determined to be: (A) well nourished, (B) moderately (or suspected of being malnourished), or (C) severely malnourished. [9, 18]. SGA has been utilized successfully in patients with liver disease with acceptable interrater reliability [18]. Malnutrition, as assessed by SGA, has been found to been associated with worsening liver failure as measured by Child's score [44, 38] and has been identified as a marker of adverse outcomes and reduced survival in patients with liver disease [17, 38].

SGA is a simple, low-cost, bedside method to assess overall nutrition status but it is not accurate in quantifying body compartments, specifically fat vs. lean mass. Use of computed tomography (CT) and magnetic resonance imaging (MRI) scans can be used to assess body composition and has been utilized on a research basis for patients with cirrhosis. The scans, though ordered as part of a medical evaluation, can be used secondarily to determine body composition. Typically, abdominal scans are analyzed at the L3 level using specialized software to determine skeletal muscle vs. fat (subcutaneous, visceral, or intramuscular) mass. Multiple studies have utilized CT scans in patients with liver disease to assess body composition and show that reduced skeletal muscle mass is associated with increased mortality [8, 12, 21, 22, 29, 32, 43]. This technique has been particularly helpful in revealing that not all patients who are malnourished appear thin and cachectic. As the rate of obesity in the general population climbs, so has it increased in patients with cirrhosis. In fact, obesity and insulin resistance are strongly correlated with the incidence of nonalcoholic fatty liver disease (NAFLD), one of the most prominent causes of liver failure worldwide [49]. However, even in obese patients with a BMI >30–40 kg/m$^2$, the prevalence of sarcopenia as measured by CT scan has been shown to occur in >55% of patients with end-stage liver disease [8].

Novel body composition methods such as dual-energy X-ray absorptiometry, bioelectrical impedance analysis, bioimpedance spectroscopy, and air displacement plethysmography may have future applications but currently are not validated or used in a clinical setting for this specific population. At least one study has evaluated the use of ultrasound of the thigh muscle as a marker of sarcopenia in patients with liver disease [42]. Table 6.1 summarizes components of a comprehensive nutrition assessment for patients with cirrhosis.

**Table 6.1** Components of a comprehensive nutrition assessment for an adult patient with cirrhosis

| Component | Purpose | Specific elements |
|---|---|---|
| Physical assessment | Determine general nutrition condition including fat and muscle stores and fluid retention | Is the patient of appropriate weight for stature? Does the patient have noticeable ascites, edema, or other fluid retention? Is muscle wasting apparent? What are the patient's fat stores and where is the adipose tissue distributed? Is the patient jaundiced? Is the patient alert? Does the patient require oxygen, wheelchair, or other assistive device? |
| | Assess the degree and distribution of nutrient deficiencies | Evaluate degree and distribution of fat and/or muscle loss and fluid retention. Examine skin for color, texture, ecchymoses, etc. Examine nail beds and hair for symptoms of nutrient deficiencies. Assess the oral cavity for dental problems or signs of vitamin deficiencies. |
| History | Determine cause, degree, and duration of nutrient deficiencies | Obtain medical history of the type, degree, duration, and treatment of liver disease and associated complications. Inquire about patient's physical function. Obtain diet history to determine adequacy of intake. Note gastrointestinal symptoms (e.g., nausea, vomiting, diarrhea, early satiety) and other factors affecting appetite or intake. Question patient or caregiver about the use of nutrition supplements, vitamin or mineral supplements, and herbal or complementary products. Assess psychosocial and economic conditions to determine patient's ability to obtain food and comply with prescribed diet recommendation. |
| Anthropometric measurements | Provide objective measurements to evaluate and monitor progress | Fluid retention may have least effect on upper arm measurements. Anthropometric measurements are unlikely to be useful in the critical care setting. Anthropometric measurements have limitations in sensitivity and reliability but may be useful if monitored serially over time. Reliability is improved if all serial measruements are made by a single observer. |

(continued)

**Table 6.1** (continued)

| Component | Purpose | Specific elements |
|---|---|---|
| Functional status tests | Indirect measure of muscle function | Functional measurements such as hand-grip strength, sit-to-stand test, and 6-min walk are not useful in an acute setting. These tests may be useful in a chronic setting over a period of time to monitor muscle strength and function. |
| Laboratory tests | Provide detailed information; must be used selectively to avoid tests confounded by nonnutritional factors | Serum protein concentrations are not considered measures of nutrition status but of inflammation as they are acute phase reactants. Vitamin and mineral levels may be helpful to determine when micronutrients need to be supplemented or restricted. |
| Body composition measures | Give more accurate detail on lean vs. fat mass | CT and MRI scans of abdomen can be analyzed to determine fat and muscle content; typically measured at L3 level; tests are expensive and CT scan involves radiation. Full body dual energy X-ray absorptiometry (DXA) scans can provide accurate assessment of fat mass; not portable and can't be used at bedside. Bioelectrical impedance analysis (BIA) requires special equipment and can be used at bedside but standard BIA devices are not accurate when patients have fluid shifts; bioimpedance spectroscopy has not been validated in patients with cirrhosis. |

Adapted with permission from Hasse [52]

# Leading Causes of Malnutrition in Cirrhosis

As part of the evaluation of nutrition status, it is important to determine the cause of malnutrition so that interventions not only provide adequate nutrients but also address the root causes of malnutrition. The cause of malnutrition in this group of chronically ill patients is due to many factors that influence nutrient intake, metabolism, and expenditure (Table 6.2).

# Nutrient Metabolism

Because the liver is involved in numerous metabolic processes, cirrhosis can lead to metabolic alterations including increased protein catabolism, reduced hepatic and skeletal muscle glycogen synthesis, and a state of increased lipolysis [3].

**Table 6.2** Factors contributing to malnutrition in patients with chronic liver disease

| |
|---|
| *Inadequate nutrient intake* |
| ↑ levels of tumor necrosis factor-α & leptin → loss of appetite |
| Ascites → impaired gastric expansion → early satiety, delayed gastric emptying, bloating, abdominal distention |
| Hepatic encephalopathy → altered consciousness with decreased oral intake |
| Alcohol intake replaces nutrition |
| Nausea and vomiting |
| Restrictive diets (low-sodium, low-protein, fluid restriction) |
| Altered taste perception (zinc deficiency) |
| Socioeconomic constraints |
| *Metabolic Alterations* |
| Altered glucose, lipid, and protein metabolism |
| Altered pattern of energy consumption |
| Decreased glycogen levels and reduced ability to store nutrients |
| Insulin resistance |
| *Malabsorption* |
| Bile salt deficiency in cholestatic liver disease and cholestasis |
| Small bowel bacterial overgrowth |
| Portal hypertensive enteropathy |

Reprinted with permission from Hasse and DiCecco [19]

## Protein Alterations

Protein catabolism can be increased in patients with liver failure; therefore, protein should typically not be restricted even in the face of hepatic encephalopathy. Cordoba et al. randomized patients admitted to an intensive care unit to receive tube feeding with either protein at 1.2 g/kg body weight from the outset vs. 0 g protein initially gradually increasing up to 1.2 g/kg over a period of 2 weeks [4]. There was no difference in encephalopathy between the groups but there was increased protein breakdown in the low-protein group. Many factors such as infections, GI bleeds, electrolyte abnormalities, constipation, diuretic overdosing, medications, and hypoglycemia are most often associated with precipitation of hepatic encephalopathy rather than excessive dietary protein intake [24, 47].

Controversy exists with regards to benefit of branched-chain amino acid (BCAA) supplementation for hepatic encephalopathy. In a recent Cochrane Review, BCAAs were shown to have some beneficial effects on hepatic encephalopathy but results were not different between groups treated with BCAA or lactulose or rifaximin therapy [14]. In addition, BCAAs have not been found to improve nutrition or quality of life outcomes [14, 28, 50]. It has been suggested to utilize BCAA supplements when patients don't respond to other treatments for hepatic encephalopathy [24] and North American and Japanese consensus guidelines recommend use of BCAAs when other treatments fail [13, 47].

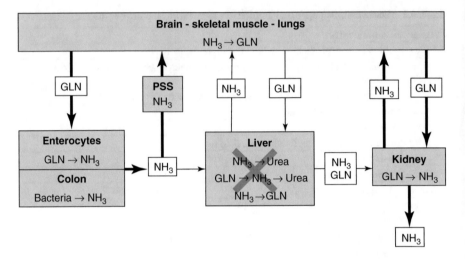

**Fig. 6.1** The role of glutamine (GLN) in ammonia detoxification in liver failure. In liver failure, ammonia escapes the urea cycle and is detoxified to GLN in the brain, skeletal muscle, and lungs. Enhanced GLN availability leads to enhanced GLN catabolism to ammonia in enterocytes and the kidneys. Thus GLN-ammonia cycling among tissues is activated. *PSS* Portal-systemic shunts (Used with permission from Holecek [20])

Glutamine is an amino acid involved in one of the proposed mechanisms of hepatic encephalopathy [20]. Ammonia can be converted to glutamine in muscle, brain, and lungs. However, glutamine released from muscle and brain is catabolized back to ammonia by enterocytes and kidneys leading to increased circulation of ammonia in the blood because the liver is unable to convert ammonia to urea (Fig. 6.1). Adverse effects of increased glutamine production include swelling of astrocytes and altered transmission in brain and catabolism of BCAAs in skeletal muscle [20].

Leucine has been singled out as a potential essential amino acid to aid in treating muscle wasting in patients with cirrhosis [30]. The mechanism is thought to be through activation of anabolic signaling via mammalian target of rapamycin (mTOR) [10, 11, 45]. The effect of specific amino acid supplementation other than BCAAs on nutrition status and patient outcomes has not been studied in the cirrhosis population.

## Glucose Alterations

Hyperglycemia is common in the early stages of cirrhosis. Glucose transport and peripheral glucose utilization are reduced in the early stages of cirrhosis. The rate of gluconeogenesis is increased leading to elevated blood glucose levels in the early stages of liver failure. Hyperglycemia may also occur due to impaired insulin sensitivity (especially common with NAFLD and hepatitis C) in spite of adequate or even elevated insulin levels. Insulin secretion worsens with increasing severity of liver disease, suggesting a detrimental effect of liver failure on pancreatic islets on its own [16]. In late stages of liver disease, hypoglycemia becomes more common due to depleting glycogen stores and decreasing gluconeogenic capacity.

## Lipid Alterations

The liver is central in the processing of lipoproteins. Steatosis occurs in nonalcoholic fatty liver disease (NAFLD) due to increased delivery of free fatty acids from adipose tissue to the liver, accelerated hepatic lipogenesis, reduced fatty acid oxidation in hepatocytes, and altered triglyceride export from the liver in the form of very-low-density lipoprotein (VLDL) cholesterol [5]. Insulin resistance is a contributing factor to these lipid alterations [5]. Alcoholic steatosis is caused by impaired ß-oxidation of fatty acids by mitochondria, increased de novo hepatic lipogenesis, and enhanced fatty acid uptake. VLDL secretion is also reduced [5]. On the other hand, hepatitis C is associated with hypolipidemia – reduced levels of total and low-density lipoprotein (LDL) cholesterol. Cholestatic liver disease leads to elevated total cholesterol levels but mainly in the form of lipoprotein-X. In patients with cirrhosis, lipoprotein metabolism usually reflects the degree of impairment in the liver [5].

With regards to digestion and absorption of dietary fat, steatorrhea can occur in patients with cholestatic liver disease due to a deficiency of bile salts in the intestine that aid in absorption. Steatorrhea can also contribute to fat-soluble vitamin deficiencies.

## Other Metabolic Derangements

Other metabolic derangements including electrolyte abnormalities may occur in liver failure. Hypervolemic hyponatremia is a common complication of advanced cirrhosis. It arises in part due to inappropriate secretion of antidiuretic hormone resulting in free water retention and is treated with a free water restriction (not supplementation of sodium). Severe hyponatremia can precipitate hepatic encephalopathy in patients with advanced liver disease. Functional renal dysfunction can occur in patients with cirrhosis of liver due to changes in renin-angiotensin system and sympathetic nervous system. This further exacerbates the electrolyte disturbances seen in patients with cirrhosis. Decreased pyruvate dehydrogenase activity is also noted with hepatic dysfunction [40]. This leads to impaired lactate utilization predisposing patients with cirrhosis to lactic acidosis.

Refeeding syndrome has been reported in malnourished patients who are treated with aggressive nutrition correction. Refeeding syndrome is characterized by onset usually within 5 days of feeding patients who are undernourished or have had impaired intake for at least 48 h [41]. Hypophosphatemia occurs in nearly all patients with about half of the patients also having low serum levels of magnesium or potassium [41]. Some patients can display low serum levels of all three electrolytes. Hypophosphatemia can contribute to hemolysis, rhabdomyolysis, paresthesias, tremors, and ATP depletion resulting in cardiac or respiratory failure [41]. This can further exacerbate the deficiency of potassium, phosphorus, magnesium, and vitamins often seen in patients with cirrhosis. Thiamine deficiency is already common in patients with cirrhosis (especially with chronic alcoholism, malabsorptive states, and malnutrition) and reintroduction of carbohydrate can exacerbate a further reduction in thiamine stores [34]. If a patient is at risk of refeeding syndrome, electrolyte levels should be checked and treated. Nutrition support should "start low and advance slow" while monitoring electrolyte levels and supplementing them as needed [7].

## Nutrient Needs

Nutrient requirements in a patient with end-stage liver disease are influenced by disease state, nutrition status, and other complicating factors. For example, patients with cholestatic liver diseases are more likely than patients with noncholestatic disease to have fat and fat-soluble vitamin malabsorption. Those who are malnourished have an increased caloric need compared with patients who are of normal or overweight status. Patients who have undergone surgery or those with fever and infection are likely to be hypermetabolic and have greater calorie and protein needs than those who are stable and without complicating factors. Patients with ascites can undergo large-volume paracentesis; protein needs can be increased as protein is lost with the ascitic fluid. Table 6.3 highlights general macronutrient recommendations.

**Table 6.3** General macronutrient considerations for individuals with cirrhosis

| Nutrient | Estimated Needs | Comments |
|---|---|---|
| Protein | 1–1.5 g/kg<br>Up to 2 g/kg for critical illness | Dependent upon nutrition status and comorbidities<br>Protein needs would be increased with surgery<br>Consider using dry weight or ideal body weight if patient is fluid-overloaded<br>Protein restriction is not recommended as it leads to muscle loss and does not improve outcomes<br>Protein can be lost with paracentesis |
| Calories | Usually 20–50% above basal | Dependent on nutrition status and losses<br>Indirect calorimetry is the most accurate way to determine actual calorie needs<br>Caloric restriction may be required for weight loss in face of obesity |
| Fat | As needed to provide adequate calories | Patients with cholestatic liver disease may experience fat malabsorption |
| Carbohydrate | Controlled carbohydrate intake if patient has diabetes mellitus or insulin resistance is present<br>Frequent meals and/or late evening snack to prevent hypoglycemia | Patients with liver disease or obesity may have insulin resistance and hyperglycemia<br>In severe or acute liver failure, hypoglycemia may ensue due to inability of the liver to store glycogen or undergo gluconeogenesis |
| Sodium | 2 g/day | If patient has fluid retention |
| Fluid | Restrict to 1000–1500 mL/day | If patient has hyponatremia |

Patients with chronic liver disease develop deficiencies of various micronutrients including magnesium, zinc, selenium, and vitamins. Possible mechanisms include poor appetite and dietary restrictions, altered metabolism, and poor absorption. Cholestatic liver diseases lead to malabsorption of fat-soluble vitamins (A, D, E, and K). Patients with alcoholic liver disease are at risk of poor absorption of potassium and magnesium and low levels of B vitamins. Zinc is mainly metabolized in the liver leading to its deficiency in chronic liver disease. Its deficiency can cause loss of appetite causing further malnutrition. Poor intake of potassium, zinc, calcium and vitamin C has been noted in patients with chronic hepatitis C in the absence of cirrhosis [15]. Iron stores could be depleted as a result of GI bleeds or anemia of chronic illness; on the other hand, iron supplementation should be avoided if the patient has hemosiderosis or hemochromatosis.

## Nutrition Support Indications

Because patients with cirrhosis are at high risk of malnutrition and heightened nutrient needs, inadequate oral intake should precipitate early consideration of nutrition support. Oral intake could be limited due to anorexia, nausea, vomiting, dysgeusia, or early satiety (commonly seen with tense ascites). When oral intake is inadequate, nutrition guidelines recommend prompt initiation of nutrition support for patients who are at high nutrition risk [26, 27]. In addition to cirrhotic patients having a poor appetite or early satiety, oral intake can be interrupted by complications such as hepatic encephalopathy and variceal bleeding. Patients with exacerbations of encephalopathy may not be alert enough to eat. In extreme cases, patients may require intubation to protect their airways in which case nutrition support would be required. Variceal bleeding can also cause an interruption in oral intake. Active bleeding is a contraindication for enteral feeding; if variceal banding is performed or a transjugular intrahepatic portosytemic shunt (TIPS) is placed, oral or enteral nutrition usually can be considered 48 h or longer after the procedure and if the bleeding has stopped. Other complications such as respiratory failure requiring mechanical ventilation warrant consideration of nutrition support. When nutrition support is indicted, EN is preferred over parenteral nutrition (PN). The benefits derived from early enteral nutrition (Table 6.4) outweigh the potential detrimental effects of parenteral nutrition on worsening liver function in patients with cirrhosis. Figure 6.2 from the American Society for Parenteral and Enteral Nutrition (ASPEN) outlines who is a candidate for EN vs. PN. The goal for nutrition support should be clearly defined before it is initiated – is it mainly to support a patient during an acute event or surgery or is it to improve a patient's condition to allow for repletion and eventual liver transplant [19].

**Table 6.4** Benefits of early enteral nutrition

| Nonnutrition benefits |
| --- |
| *Gastrointestinal responses* |
| Maintain gut integrity |
| Reduced gut/lung axis of inflammation |
| Enhance motility/contractility |
| Absorptive capacity |
| Maintain mass of GALT tissue |
| Support and maintain commensal bacteria |
| Production of secretory IgA |
| Trophic effect on epithelial cells |
| Reduced virulence of endogenous pathogenic organisms |
| *Immune responses* |
| Modulate key regulatory cells to enhance systemic immune function |
| Promote dominance of antiinflammatory Th2 over proinflammatory Th1 responses |
| Stimulate oral tolerance |
| Influence antiinflammatory nutrient receptors in the GI tract (duodenal vagal, colonic butyrate) |
| Maintain MALT tissue at all epithelial surfaces (lung, liver, lacrimal, genitourinary, and pulmonary) |
| Modulate adhesion molecules to attenuate transendothelial migration of macrophages and neutrophils |
| *Metabolic responses* |
| Promote insulin sensitivity through the stimulation of incretins |
| Reduce hyperglycemia (AGEs), muscle, and tissue glycosylation |
| Attenuating stress metabolism to enhance more physiologic fuel utilization |
| Nutrition benefits |
| Sufficient protein and calories |
| Provide micronutrient and antioxidants |
| Maintain lean body mass by providing substrate for optimal protein synthesis |
| Support cellular and subcellular (mitochondria) function |
| Stimulate protein synthesis to meet metabolic demand of the host |

Reprinted with permission from McClave [26])
*AGEs* advanced-glycolytic end products, *GALT* gut-associated lymphoid tissue, *GI* gastrointestinal, *MALT* mucosalassociated lymphoid tissue

# Nutrition Support Considerations for Patients with Cirrhosis

## *Enteral Nutrition*

If EN is indicated for a patient with cirrhosis, special consideration should be made for access route and formula choice. Short-term EN access is usually via a nasoenteric tube. Since patients with cirrhosis may be coagulopathic or have a history of epistaxis or esophageal varices, one should examine the risk vs. benefit of tube placement. A general practice is often to require an INR <2 and platelet count

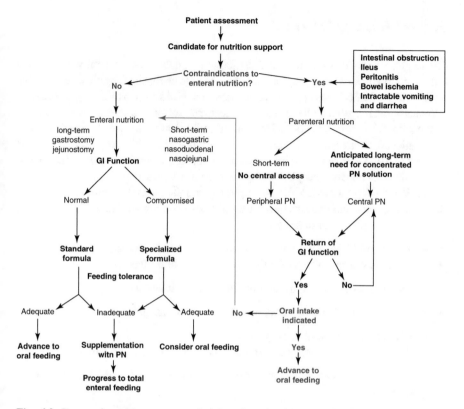

**Fig. 6.2** Route of nutrition support administration algorithm (Used with permission from Ukleja [51])

>50,000/uL before placement of a nasoenteric feeding tube. This is unrealistic for many patients with decompensated cirrhosis so infusion of platelets, fresh frozen plasma, or vitamin K may be required before tube placement [6]. Clearly if a patient is experiencing a GI bleed, EN should be withheld. A 24–48 h waiting period after GI bleed or endoscopic banding of esophageal varices is generally recommended before starting EN [1, 36].

Percutaneous endoscopic gastrostomy (PEG) tubes are contraindicated in patients with decompensated cirrhosis due to risks of ascites leakage, bleeding from the PEG site in the face of coagulopathy, peritonitis, impaired healing of the PEG tract, and gastric variceal bleed [2, 19, 21, 23, 25, 33, 35, 37, 48].

Controversy exists with regards to gastric vs. postpyloric delivery of EN in critically ill patients [26, 27, 39]. As per recent nutrition support guidelines, if patients are considered to be at high risk of aspiration, post-pyloric placement of a feeding tube is recommended [26, 27]. In patients with cirrhosis, those with severe hepatic encephalopathy would be considered at increased risk of aspiration as would those with a history of delayed gastric emptying.

## Enteral Formula Selection

There are a variety of EN formulas available commercially. Generally, a standard intact protein formula is appropriate for patients with cirrhosis; formulas are available in a variety of calorie and protein concentrations. Fluid overload and hypervolemic hyponatremia may dictate the use of a concentrated formula whereas development of acute kidney injury or hepatorenal syndrome could require the use of a renal formula with reduced electrolytes. As mentioned earlier, there are not strong data to support the use of BCAA formulas. Glutamine-supplemented formulas are not desirable in the presence of hepatic encephalopathy for reasons discussed earlier [20].

Table 6.5 summarizes EN formula options for patients with chronic liver disease. In addition, other publications have offered general recommendations for providing EN to patients with liver disease [19]:

- Maximize oral intake with nutrient-dense food, fluids, and supplements.
- Consider EN after 1 week of failure of adequate oral intake.

  – Consider earlier EN initiation in critical care situations.

- Place feeding tube (nasogastric, nasoduodenal, or nasojejunal).

  – Wait at least 24–48 h after GI bleed.
  – PEG tubes are generally contraindicated due to ascites and varices.

- Start EN at a low rate (especially if the patient is a refeeding risk), increasing to goal over several days.

  – Choose an intact protein formula considering a nutrient-dense product depending on nutrition needs and fluid status.
  – Specialty formulas may be used in cases of significant malabsorption (semi-elemental, elemental) or renal insufficiency (renal formula); data are lacking for use of immune-enhancing or BCAA formulas.

- Reassess frequently for tolerance, achievement of goal feedings, and improvement in nutrition and functional parameters.

## Parenteral Nutrition

PN is restricted for use with patients without a functional GI tract. Prolonged PN is known to cause PN-associated liver disease so utilizing PN in patients with preexisting liver disease increases the risk for worsening liver function. General guidelines for PN for patients with liver disease can be found in Table 6.6.

**Table 6.5** Enteral nutrition formula options for patients with chronic liver disease

| Enteral nutrition formula category | Indications and comments | Relative cost |
|---|---|---|
| Standard intact protein formulas | Requires normal digestion<br>Available in a variety of protein and calorie concentrations | $ |
| Nutrient-dense formulas | Requires normal digestion<br>Generally available as 1.5–2 kcal/mL concentrations<br>Useful in patients in whom fluid restriction is needed (e.g., hypervolemic hyponatremia, fluid retention, reduced urine output, early satiety issues, high nutrition requirements) | $ |
| Semielemental or partially hydrolyzed | Useful for patients who have impaired digestion<br>Available in a variety of protein and calorie concentrations<br>Often contain peptides and/or medium-chain triglycerides | $$ |
| Elemental | Useful when digestion is impaired or a very-low-fat formula is preferred<br>Contains amino acids and dextrose (vs. whole proteins and starches)<br>Usually high in carbohydrate which could contribute to hyperglycemia in patients with insulin impairment<br>Usually hypertonic which can reduce tolerance | $$$ |
| Renal | Requires normal digestion<br>Useful for patients with renal dysfunction and hyperkalemia or hyperphosphatemia<br>Usually fluid-restricted with reduced amounts of potassium and phosphorus | $$ |
| Immunoenhancing | Requires normal digestion<br>Have not been shown to be beneficial in patients with liver disease<br>Usually contain immunoenhancing nutrients such as fish oil, arginine, RNA<br>May affect insulin sensitivity and satiety<br>May temporarily increase serum ammonia levels but does not worsen symptoms of hepatic encephalopathy | $$$ |
| Branched-chain amino acid (BCAA) | Controversial as to benefit, but American and European guidelines suggest consideration of BCAA formulas in patients with encephalopathy refractory to other treatments or with a protein intolerance<br>Contains higher proportion of BCAAs and reduced amounts of aromatic amino acids and methionine<br>Usually with reduced electrolyte content | $$$ |

Used with permission from Hasse and DiCecco [19])
$ = low cost, $$ = moderate cost, $$$ = high cost

**Table 6.6** Considerations for providing parenteral nutrition (PN) to patients with cirrhosis

| Component | Comments |
| --- | --- |
| Volume | Volume restriction should be considered if the patient is hypervolemic. |
| Amino acid | Protein requirements should be determined by nutrition status and nutrient needs; do not restrict protein. |
| Glucose | Some patients will have insulin resistance and hyperglycemia; if needed, titrate insulin to maintain nonfasting serum glucose levels <180 mg/dL. Some patients with severe liver failure may have fasting hypoglycemia and require continuous glucose infusion which can be provided in PN. |
| Fat | Soy-based intravenous fat emulsions (IVFE) can contribute to liver dysfunction; usual dose is 1–2 g/kg. If PN is required long-term and liver function worsens with PN, alternative IVFE may be beneficial (e.g., olive-oil based IVFE, soy-MCT-olive oil-fish oil (SMOF) based IVFE). |
| Electrolytes | Sodium restriction and fluid restriction should be considered with fluid retention and hypervolemic hyponatremia. Adjust potassium, magnesium, and phosphorus based on laboratory values considering renal function, diuretic choices (potassium-sparing vs. potassium-wasting), and refeeding syndrome. |
| Vitamins | Provide daily multivitamin infusion. Patient may need additional thiamine and folate. |
| Trace elements | Provide daily trace elements. May need to withhold manganese and copper (excreted via bile) if levels are elevated. Additional zinc could be added if patient's level is low or if being used as an aid in treating encephalopathy. |

# Drug-Nutrient Interactions

When evaluating nutrition status and determining plans for nutrition therapy, it is paramount to also evaluate potential drug-nutrient interactions. Several commonly used medications to treat symptoms of liver disease have food or nutrient interactions. Lactulose is used as first line therapy for treatment of hepatic encephalopathy. It has several GI side effects including nausea, vomiting, and diarrhea. These side effects lead to poor appetite, and reduced oral intake contributing to worsening nutrition status. Diarrhea can cause loss of electrolytes including potassium. Furosemide and spironolactone are commonly used diuretics among patients with decompensated cirrhosis. Furosemide decreases the absorption of some of the important electrolytes including potassium, magnesium, and calcium. Conversely, spironolactone is renal sparing and hyperkalemia can occur especially in the face of renal dysfunction. Corticosteroids may be used for liver diseases such as autoimmune liver disease; chronic use of corticosteroids can lead to malabsorption of calcium and vitamin D. Use of cholestyramine and colestipol leads to fat malabsorption.

# Summary

Patients with cirrhosis present special challenges in providing nutrition support. The prevalence of malnutrition and alteration of metabolism associated with liver disease as well as how symptoms of end-stage liver disease and the treatment of those complications impact the nutrition needs and delivery of nutrition support. It is important to consider the risk or presence of malnutrition, metabolic aberrations, and altered nutrient needs when planning nutrition interventions for patients with cirrhosis. Finally, complications of cirrhosis can influence the route and type of nutrition support provided and drug-nutrient interactions should be accounted for in the medical nutrition therapy plan.

# References

1. Andus T. ESPEN guidelines on enteral nutrition: liver disease – tube feeding (TF) in patients with esophageal varices is not proven to be safe. Clin Nutr. 2007;26(2):272; author reply 273–4.
2. Baltz JG, Argo CK, Al-Osaimi AM, Northup PG. Mortality after percutaneous endoscopic gastrostomy in patients with cirrhosis: a case series. Gastrointest Endosc. 2010;72(5):1072–5. doi:10.1016/j.gie.2010.06.043.
3. Bémeur C, Butterworth RF. Nutrition in the management of cirrhosis and its neurological complications. J Clin Exp Hepatol. 2014;4(2):141–50. doi:10.1016/j.jceh.2013.05.008.
4. Córdoba J, López-Hellín J, Planas M, Sabín P, Sanpedro F, Castro F, Esteban R, Guardia J. Normal protein diet for episodic hepatic encephalopathy: results of a randomized study. J Hepatol. 2004;41(1):38–43.
5. Corey KE, Cohen DE. Lipid and lipoprotein metabolism in liver disease. In: De Groot LJ, Chrousos G, Dungan K, et al. Endotext [Internet]. South Dartmouth (MA): MDText.com, Inc.; 2000–2015 Jun 27. Available from: https://www.ncbi.nlm.nih.gov/books/NBK326742/. Accessed 28 Sept 2016.
6. Crippin JS. Is tube feeding an option in patients with liver disease? Nutr Clin Pract. 2006;21(3):296–8.
7. Crook MA. Refeeding syndrome: problems with definition and management. Nutrition. 2014;30(11–12):1448–55. doi:10.1016/j.nut.2014.03.026.
8. Cruz Jr RJ, Dew MA, Myaskovsky L, Goodpaster B, Fox K, Fontes P, DiMartini A. Objective radiologic assessment of body composition in patients with end-stage liver disease: going beyond the BMI. Transplantation. 2013;95(4):617–22. doi:10.1097/TP.0b013e31827a0f27.
9. Detsky AS, McLaughlin JR, Baker JP, Johnston N, Whittaker S, Mendelson RA, Jeejeebhoy KN. What is subjective global assessment of nutritional status? JPEN J Parenter Enteral Nutr. 1987;11(1):8–13.
10. Dreyer HC, Drummond MJ, Pennings B, Fujita S, Glynn EL, Chinkes DL, Dhanani S, Volpi E, Rasmussen BB. Leucine-enriched essential amino acid and carbohydrate ingestion following resistance exercise enhances mTOR signaling and protein synthesis in human muscle. Am J Physiol Endocrinol Metab. 2008;294(2):E392–400.
11. Drummond MJ, Rasmussen BB. Leucine-enriched nutrients and the regulation of mammalian target of rapamycin signalling and human skeletal muscle protein synthesis. Curr Opin Clin Nutr Metab Care. 2008;11(3):222–6. doi:10.1097/MCO.0b013e3282fa17fb.

12. Englesbe MJ, Patel SP, He K, Lynch RJ, Schaubel DE, Harbaugh C, Holcombe SA, Wang SC, Segev DL, Sonnenday CJ. Sarcopenia and mortality after liver transplantation. J Am Coll Surg. 2010;211(2):271–8. doi:10.1016/j.jamcollsurg.2010.03.039.

13. Fukui H, Saito H, Ueno Y, Uto H, Obara K, Sakaida I, Shibuya A, Seike M, Nagoshi S, Segawa M, Tsubouchi H, Moriwaki H, Kato A, Hashimoto E, Michitaka K, Murawaki T, Sugano K, Watanabe M, Shimosegawa T. Evidence-based clinical practice guidelines for liver cirrhosis 2015. J Gastroenterol. 2016;51(7):629–50.

14. Gluud LL, Dam G, Les I, Córdoba J, Marchesini G, Borre M, Aagaard NK, Vilstrup H. Branched-chain amino acids for people with hepatic encephalopathy. Cochrane Database Syst Rev. 2015;(2): CD001939. doi: 10.1002/14651858.CD001939.pub3.

15. Gottschall CB, Pereira TG, Rabito EI. Álvares-Da-Silva MR4. Nutritional status and dietary intake in non-cirrhotic adult chronic hepatitis C patients. Arq Gastroenterol. 2015;52(3):204–9.

16. Grancini V, Trombetta M, Lunati ME, Zimbalatti D, Boselli ML, Gatti S, Donato MF, Resi V, D'Ambrosio R, Aghemo A, Pugliese G, Bonadonna RC, Orsi E. Contribution of β-cell dysfunction and insulin resistance to cirrhosis-associated diabetes: role of severity of liver disease. J Hepatol. 2015;63(6):1484–90. doi:10.1016/j.jhep.2015.08.011.

17. Hasse J, Gautam M, Saracino G, Jennings L. Malnutrition reduces survival in patients awaiting liver transplantation. (Abstract) Presented at American Society for Parenteral and Enteral Nutrition Clinical Nutrition Week. 2015. http://pen.sagepub.com/content/suppl/2015/01/28/39.2.231.DC1/Clinical_Nutrition_Week_2015_Paper_Sessions_REV.pdf. Accessed 19 Sep 2016.

18. Hasse J, Strong S, Gorman MA, Liepa G. Subjective global assessment: alternative nutrition-assessment technique for liver-transplant candidates. Nutrition. 1993;9(4):339–43.

19. Hasse JM, DiCecco SR. Enteral nutrition in chronic liver disease: translating evidence into practice. Nutr Clin Pract. 2015;30(4):474–87. doi:10.1177/0884533615591058.

20. Holecek M. Evidence of a vicious cycle in glutamine synthesis and breakdown in pathogenesis of hepatic encephalopathy-therapeutic perspectives. Metab Brain Dis. 2014;29(1):9–17. doi:10.1007/s11011-013-9428-9.

21. Kaido T, Ogawa K, Fujimoto Y, et al. Impact of sarcopenia on survival in patients undergoing living donor liver transplantation. Am J Transplant. 2013;13(6):1549–56.

22. Krell RW, Kaul DR, Martin AR, Englesbe MJ, Sonnenday CJ, Cai S, Malani PN. Association between sarcopenia and the risk of serious infection among adults undergoing liver transplantation. Liver Transpl. 2013;19(12):1396–402. doi:10.1002/lt.23752.

23. Kynci JA, Chodash HB, Tsang T-K. PEG in a patient with ascites and varices. Gastrointest Endosc. 1995;42(1):100–1.

24. Leise MD, Poterucha JJ, Kamath PS, Kim WR. Management of hepatic encephalopathy in the hospital. Mayo Clin Proc. 2014;89(2):241–53. doi:10.1016/j.mayocp.2013.11.009.

25. Löser C, Aschl G, Hébuterne X, et al. ESPEN guidelines on artificial enteral nutrition-percutaneous endoscopic gastrostomy (PEG). Clin Nutr. 2005;24:848–61.

26. McClave SA, DiBaise JK, Mullin GE, Martindale RG. ACG clinical guideline: nutrition therapy in the adult hospitalized patient. Am J Gastroenterol. 2016;111(3):315–34. quiz 335 doi:10.1038/ajg.2016.28.

27. McClave SA, Taylor BE, Martindale RG, Warren MM, Johnson DR, Braunschweig C, Mc Carthy MS, Davanos E, Rice TW, Cresci GA, Gervasio JM, Sacks GS, Roberts PR, Compher C, Society of Critical Care Medicine; American Society for Parenteral and Enteral Nutrition. Guidelines for the Provision and Assessment of Nutrition Support Therapy in the Adult Critically Ill Patient: Society of Critical Care Medicine (SCCM) and American Society for Parenteral and Enteral Nutrition (A.S.P.E.N.). JPEN J Parenter Enteral Nutr. 2016;40(2):159–211. doi:10.1177/0148607115621863.

28. Metcalfe EL, Avenell A, Fraser A. Branched-chain amino acid supplementation in adults with cirrhosis and porto-systemic encephalopathy: systematic review. Clin Nutr. 2014;33(6):958–65. doi:10.1016/j.clnu.2014.02.011.

29. Meza-Junco J, Montano-Loza AJ, Baracos VE, Prado CM, Bain VG, Beaumont C, Esfandiari N, Lieffers JR, Sawyer MB. Sarcopenia as a prognostic index of nutritional status in concurrent cirrhosis and hepatocellular carcinoma. J Clin Gastroenterol. 2013;47(10):861–70. doi:10.1097/MCG.0b013e318293a825.

30. Montano-Loza AJ. Clinical relevance of sarcopenia in patients with cirrhosis. World J Gastroenterol. 2014a;20(25):8061–71.

31. Montano-Loza AJ. Muscle wasting: a nutritional criterion to prioritize patients for liver transplantation. Curr Opin Clin Nutr Metab Care. 2014b;17(3):219–25. doi:10.1097/MCO.0000000000000046.

32. Montano-Loza AJ, Meza-Junco J, Prado CM, Lieffers JR, Baracos VE, Bain VG, Sawyer MB. Muscle wasting is associated with mortality in patients with cirrhosis. Clin Gastroenterol Hepatol. 2012;10(2):166–73, 173.e1. doi:10.1016/j.cgh.2011.08.028.

33. O'Shea RS, Dasarathy S, McCullough AJ. Practice Guideline Committee of the American Association for the Study of Liver. Alcoholic liver disease. Hepatology. 2010;51(1):307–28.

34. Parli SE, Ruf KM, Magnuson B. Pathophysiology, treatment, and prevention of fluid and electrolyte abnormalities during refeeding syndrome. J Infus Nurs. 2014;37(3):197–202. doi:10.1097/NAN.0000000000000038.

35. Phillips MS, Ponsky JL. Overview of enteral and parenteral feeding access techniques: principles and practice. Surg Clin North Am. 2011;91(4):897–911.

36. Plauth M, Cabré E, Riggio O, Assis-Camilo M, Pirlich M, Kondrup J. ESPEN guidelines on enteral nutrition: liver disease. Clin Nutr. 2006;25(2):285–94.

37. Runyon BA. Practice guideline: management of adult patients with ascites due to cirrhosis. Update. 2012. AASLD website. http://www.aasld.org/sites/default/files/guideline_documents/adultascitesenhanced.pdf. Accessed 25 Sept 2016.

38. Sasidharan M, Nistala S, Narendhran RT, Murugesh M, Bhatia SJ, Rathi PM. Nutritional status and prognosis in cirrhotic patients. Trop Gastroenterol. 2012;33(4):257–64.

39. Schlein K. Gastric versus small bowel feeding in critically ill adults. Nutr Clin Pract. 2016;31(4):514–22.

40. Shangraw RE, Rabkin JM, Lopaschuk GD. Hepatic pyruvate dehydrogenase activity in humans: effect of cirrhosis, transplantation, and dichloroacetate. Am J Physiol. 1998;274(3 Pt 1):G569–77.

41. Skipper A. Refeeding syndrome or refeeding hypophosphatemia: a systematic review of cases. Nutr Clin Pract. 2012;27(1):34–40. doi:10.1177/0884533611427916.

42. Tandon P, Low G, Mourtzakis M, Zenith L, Myers RP, Abraldes JG, Shaheen AA, Qamar H, Mansoor N, Carbonneau M, Ismond K, Mann S, Alaboudy A, Ma M. A model to identify sarcopenia in patients with cirrhosis. Clin Gastroenterol Hepatol. 2016;14(10):1473–1480.e3. pii: S1542-3565(16)30198-7 doi:10.1016/j.cgh.2016.04.040.

43. Tandon P, Ney M, Irwin I, Ma MM, Gramlich L, Bain VG, Esfandiari N, Baracos V, Montano-Loza AJ, Myers RP. Severe muscle depletion in patients on the liver transplant wait list: its prevalence and independent prognostic value. Liver Transpl. 2012;18(10):1209–16. doi:10.1002/lt.23495.

44. Teiusanu A, Andrei M, Arbanas T, Nicolaie T, Diculescu M. Nutritional status in cirrhotic patients. Maedica (Buchar). 2012;7(4):284–9.

45. Tsien C, Davuluri G, Singh D, Allawy A, Ten Have GA, Thapaliya S, Schulze JM, Barnes D, McCullough AJ, Engelen MP, Deutz NE, Dasarathy S. Metabolic and molecular responses to leucine-enriched branched chain amino acid supplementation in the skeletal muscle of alcoholic cirrhosis. Hepatology. 2015;61(6):2018–29. doi:10.1002/hep.27717.

46. Vieira PM, De-Souza DA, Oliveira LC. Nutritional assessment in hepatic cirrhosis; clinical, anthropometric, biochemical and hematological parameters. Nutr Hosp. 2013;28(5):1615–21. doi:10.3305/nh.2013.28.5.6563.

47. Vilstrup H, Amodio P, Bajaj J, Cordoba J, Ferenci P, Mullen KD, Weissenborn K, Wong P. Hepatic encephalopathy in chronic liver disease: 2014 Practice Guideline by the American

Association for the Study of Liver Diseases and the European Association for the Study of the Liver. Hepatology. 2014;60(2):715–35. doi:10.1002/hep.27210.

48. Yarze JC. Peritonitis after PEG placement in patients with cirrhotic ascites. Gastrointest Endosc. 2011;73(5):1071.

49. Younossi ZM, Koenig AB, Abdelatif D, Fazel Y, Henry L, Wymer M. Global epidemiology of nonalcoholic fatty liver disease-Meta-analytic assessment of prevalence, incidence, and outcomes. Hepatology. 2016;64(1):73–84. doi:10.1002/hep.28431.

50. Zhu GQ, Shi KQ, Huang S, Wang LR, Lin YQ, Huang GQ, Chen YP, Braddock M, Zheng MH. Systematic review with network meta-analysis: the comparative effectiveness and safety of interventions in patients with overt hepatic encephalopathy. Aliment Pharmacol Ther. 2015;41(7):624–35. doi:10.1111/apt.13122.

51. Ukleja A, Freeman KL, Gilbert K, Kochevar M, Kraft MD, Russell MK, Shuster MH, Task force on standards for nutrition support: adult hospitalized patients, and the American Society for parenteral and enteral nutrition board of directors. Standards for nutrition support: adult hospitalized patients. Nutr Clin Pract. 2010;25(4):403–14. doi:10.1177/0884533610374200.

52. Hasse JM. Nutrition assessment and support of organ transplant recipients. JPEN J Parenter Enteral Nutr. 2001;25:120–31.

# Chapter 7
# Surgery in Patients with Hepatic Cirrhosis: Management of Portal Hypertension

Kareem Abu-Elmagd, Basem Soliman, Ajai Khanna, Masato Fujiki, Bijan Eghtesad, and Guilherme Costa

## Introduction

Portal hypertension (PH) is one of the most serious complications of hepatic cirrhosis and portomesenteric venous thrombosis [1]. The need for any major surgical procedure in these complex patients carries a relatively high morbidity and mortality. Of the major risk factors are marginal hepatic reserve, large gastrointestinal varices, and massive portomesenteric venous collaterals. Accordingly, thorough preoperative evaluation, personalized management strategy, and collaborative postoperative care are essential to achieve successful outcomes.

The primary focus of this chapter is to comprehensively address the pharmacologic, radiologic, and surgical management of PH in patients undergoing major abdominal, thoracic, and other complex surgical procedures. The proposed preemptive and active management strategies are discussed in the milieu of the pathophysiology of the portal hypertension and the coexisted pathology that is in need for surgical and other therapeutic interventions.

K. Abu-Elmagd, MD, PhD (✉)
Transplant Center, Cleveland Clinic, Cleveland, OH 44195, USA
e-mail: abuelmk@ccf.org

B. Soliman, MD, PhD • A. Khanna, MD, PhD • M. Fujiki, MD, PhD
B. Eghtesad, MD • G. Costa, MD, PhD
Transplant Center, Department of General Surgery, Cleveland Clinic, Cleveland, OH, USA

© Springer International Publishing AG 2017                                                    89
B. Eghtesad, J. Fung (eds.), *Surgical Procedures on the Cirrhotic Patient*,
DOI 10.1007/978-3-319-52396-5_7

# Pathophysiology

The term PH was first introduced in1902 describing large portosystemic abdominal collateral vessels in the setting of cirrhosis [2]. In 1937, the first time proposed concept of measuring the portal pressure was technically feasible through an intra-abdominal approach [3, 4]. In 1953, the percutaneous intrasplenic methodology was introduced as an alternative technique followed by direct and percutaneous intrahepatic portal pressure measurement [5]. With the recent evolution of the minimally invasive radiologic techniques, portal pressure measurements can be safely obtained to establish accurate diagnosis and guide appropriate therapy (Fig. 7.1).

In patients with hepatic cirrhosis, the diagnosis of PH is established when the hepatic venous pressure gradient (HVPG), calculated by the difference between the portal and the hepatic venous pressure, exceeds 5 mmHg. The clinical syndrome and its various complications commonly occur when the HVPG exceeds 10 mmHg [6]. In patients with presinusoidal PH particularly those with splenic and diffuse portomesenteric venous thrombosis, the HVPG is usually within a normal range. Computed Tomography (CT) and standard semi-quantitative selective visceral angiography are the gold standard for the accurate diagnosis and proper management of these complex patients (Fig. 7.2).

The clinical syndrome of PH includes gastroesophageal varices, ascites, spontaneous bacterial peritonitis, gastropathy, colopathy, hepatic hydrothorax, hepatorenal syndrome, hepatopulmonary syndrome, pulmonary hypertension, and cirrhotic cardiomyopathy [7–9]. The presence of one or more of these morbid events commonly influences the decision making process and overall results of any required major abdominal, thoracic and other surgical interventions. Of major consideration, is the interplay between the landscape of the PH complication and the required surgical procedure.

The development of gastrointestinal varices is one of the most serious consequences of PH. This life threatening complication occurs in 35–80% of cirrhotic patients [8, 10–12]. The risk of variceal bleeding ranges from 25% to 40% with a recurrence rate of 70% [8]. With the initial attack, mortality ranges from 30% to 50% with a high cumulative attrition rate. With major surgical interventions, the inevitable hemodynamic changes in the systemic and portal circulation with altered hepatic homeostasis could potentially provoke bleeding from silent or overt gut varies. As a result, a preemptive management strategy is desired to reduce risk of primary and recurrent variceal hemorrhage.

In addition to substantial gut varices, patients with splenic and diffuse portomesenteric venous thrombosis often develop respective segmental and extensive abdominal collaterals. These extra-anatomic vascular channels add great technical difficulties to any major abdominal surgery particularly in patients with complex pathology (Fig. 7.3). This ominous problem is commonly associated with increased risk of intraoperative bleeding due to innate thin vessel wall with turbulent flow pattern and high intravascular pressure. Other potential surgical complications include postoperative bleeding and anastomotic leaks due to mesenteric venous congestion with impaired tissue healing and altered gut homeostasis.

The development of complex life threatening abdominal and cardiothoracic disorders is not uncommon in patients with liver cirrhosis and PH. Defined hepatic lesions, pancreatic tumors, gastrointestinal neoplasms, colorectal malignancies, and other complex gut disorders are common coexisted diagnoses. In some of these patients, concomitant thrombosis of the portomesenteric venous system does occur due the proximity, aggressiveness, and thrombogenicity of the disease process. Cardiac revascularization, valve replacement, lung resection, and organ transplantation are the commonly required cardiothoracic procedures

**Fig. 7.1** The different routes to measure the portal pressure. Catheterization of one of the hepatic veins via the transjugular approach to measure the free and wedged hepatic venous pressure is the most commonly utilized methodology to calculate the portal pressure

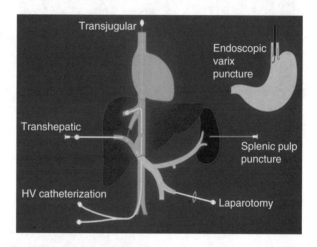

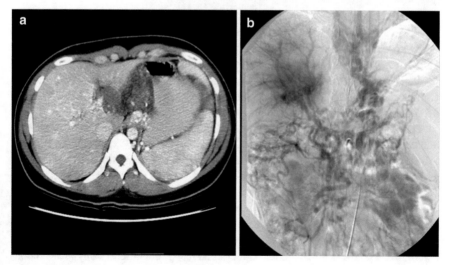

**Fig. 7.2** Radiologic imaging of the abdomen and portomesenteric venous system; (**a**) computed tomography (CT) with no radiologic features of hepatic cirrhosis and preserved liver volume. The observed portal vein thrombosis dictated the need for visceral angiography. (**b**) The venous phase of selective superior mesenteric arteriography demonstrating diffuse portomesenteric venous thrombosis with development of extensive abdominal collaterals. Note the presence of large gastroesophageal variceal collaterals with some hepatopedal flow

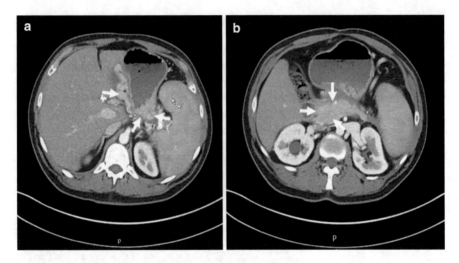

**Fig. 7.3** Abdominal computed tomography (CT) of a patient with recurrent life threatening Pancreatitis, splenic vein thrombosis, and brittle diabetes. (**a**) Massive gastric variceal and pancreatic collaterals (*arrows*). (**b**) Large pancreatic tumor with failed attempts of surgical resection at a local hospital. The patient underwent successful near total pancreatectomy combined with splenectomy and complete gastric devascularization

## Management Strategy

In patients with active gastroesophageal variceal hemorrhages and intra-abdominal bleeding, aggressive resuscitation along with simultaneous diagnostic and therapeutic measures must be promptly initiated. Emergent endoscopy and abdominal visceral angiography are the most reliable tools to identify and control variceal bleeding [8, 12, 13]. For those with intra-abdominal hemorrhage due to ruptured portosystemic collaterals or earlier surgical intervention, emergent surgical exploration is mandatory along with other treatment modalities.

The strategy of elective management is guided by the status of hepatic reserve and severity of portal hypertension. Adequate hepatic reserve is roughly measured by clinical and biochemical evidence of preserved hepatic functions with radiologically acceptable liver volume. The etiology and stage of liver damage is accurately defined by histopathologic examination of percutaneous or transjugular needle liver biopsy.

The level of PH is commonly assessed by the radiologic measurement of the HVPG. The coexistence of gut varices is better diagnosed by pan-endoscopic examination of the digestive tract. Upper endoscopy and colonoscopy are valuable in the respective detection of foregut and hindgut varices. For midgut and ectopic varices, push enteroscopy and capsule endoscopy have been the most useful investigative tools. Nonetheless, selective visceral angiographies better assess patency of the splanchnic arterial and portal venous circulation with detection of any associated vascular anomalies.

With suspected splenic and portomesenteric venous thrombosis, dedicated superior mesenteric, splenic, and inferior mesenteric angiographies are strongly recommended. The serial images of the venous phase characterize the collateral pattern, identify direction of flow, and semiquantitate the residual portal and preferential collateral flow (Fig. 7.2b). These valuable information are crucial for the proper management of patients who are in need for major abdominal surgical intervention.

Proper preoperative planning, fine surgical techniques, and collaborative postoperative care at highly specialized medical center are essential for successful outcome. Preemptive nonoperative PH treatment is recommended in high risk patients particularly those who are in need for extra-abdominal surgery. In contrast, simultaneous portal hypertensive and disease specific surgery is a good alternative for patients with abdominal pathology. With preoperative diagnosis of marginal hepatic reserve and postoperative development of liver failure, simultaneous or sequential organ transplantation should be promptly entertained.

# Therapeutic Modalities

The different modalities that are currently available for the treatment of gut varices and portomesenteric abdominal venous collaterals are categorized and described herein.

# *Pharmacologic Treatment*

The therapeutic efficacy of the currently available pharmacological agents is due to reduction of both portal blood flow and intrahepatic vascular resistance. They are more commonly used as an adjunct therapy. The indications, efficacy, and side effects of each agent are described herein.

### Vasopressin

Vasopressin is a potent splanchnic vasoconstrictor that is used for the management of acute life threatening variceal hemorrhage. It reduces HVPG and variceal pressure by 23% and 14%, respectively [14]. However, the potent systemic vasoconstrictive action of the drug is associated with numerous side effects that limit its use for very selected high risk patients and those who failed other therapeutic modalities. To improve the safety profile, the addition of nitroglycerin has been shown to mitigate many of its systemic side effects [15].

Terlipressin is a triglycyl lysine derivative of vasopressin. It produces less systemic vasoconstriction with reduced side effects. In addition, it has a longer half-life. Compared to placebo, Terlipressin has shown to better control active variceal bleeding and improved survival [16]. The drug has yet to be approved for clinical use in the United States but it is commonly utilized elsewhere worldwide [17]. Both Vasopressin and Terlipressin are valuable therapeutic options for patients with persistent active variceal bleeding particularly those with hemodynamic instability following any abdominal or thoracic surgery and not suitable candidates for any other portal hypertensive therapeutic interventions.

## Somatostatin

Somatostatin (SST) is a naturally occurring 14-amino acid peptide that causes splanchnic vasoconstriction and decreases portal blood flow. Despite its short half-life, SST is equally effective in controlling variceal hemorrhage compared to other pharmacologic agents and other treatment modalities such as balloon tamponade and endoscopic sclerotherapy [18, 19]. Despite its proven therapeutic efficacy, SST is not currently available in the United States.

Octreotide is a synthetic SST analogue that is routinely used in the United States as an adjunct therapy for the management of active variceal bleeding. The therapy is initiated from the outset and administered as continuous infusion because of its short half-life. The major therapeutic advantage of a short course of maintenance octreotide therapy is reduction in the risk of variceal rebleeding but without improvement in survival [20]. Despite the lack of current published data, it is our recommendation to use octreotide as a perioperative preemptive therapy for patients with endoscopic evidence of significant gut varices particularly in those with history of variceal bleeding.

## Beta Blocker

Nonselective beta blockers (NSBBs) are used extensively for primary and secondary prophylaxis of PH variceal bleeding. By producing unopposed alpha adrenergic vasoconstriction, it decreases portal pressure. It is most effective when the risk of bleeding is high by preventing the first attack and reducing the rate of recurrence. However, the role of NSBBs in preventing first time variceal bleeding among those at a low risk of variceal bleeding has yet to be determined. A meta-analysis of six randomized controlled trials showed that the incidences of large varices development, first upper-gastrointestinal bleeding, and death were similar between NSBB and placebo groups [21].

The most commonly used NSBBs in PHT patients are propranolol, carvedilol, and nadolol. Compared to propranolol, nadolol offers a longer half-life, once daily-use, and better tolerance by patients [10]. A recent meta-analysis showed that the carvedilol is more effective in decreasing HVPG than propranolol, and it may be as effective as endoscopic band ligation (EBL) in preventing variceal bleeding [22]. It is our recommendation to use NSBBs in all patients undergoing major abdominal surgery with coexisted gut varices.

## Nitrates

Nitrates have been used in combination with vasopressin in the setting of acute variceal hemorrhage (AVH). These drugs cause systemic hypotension, thereby decreasing vasopressin-associated vasoconstriction and portal pressure [10]. Nitrates can also be used with NSBB to prevent variceal rebleeding with greater HVPG reduction [23]. The most commonly used nitrate in PH patients is isosorbide mononitrate since it is long-acting with minimal first-pass metabolic clearance [10].

## Other Therapeutic Agents

### Statins

Simavastatin is used to decrease intrahepatic vascular resistance through nitrous oxide upregulation. In a double blinded placebo-controlled trial, simvastatin was associated with an 8% reduction of HVPG [24]. Another recent study proved the additive effect of simvastatin when used as adjunctive treatment in patients receiving standard therapy. It showed no effect on the rebleeding rate but improved survival [25].

### Antibiotics

Prophylactic antimicrobial therapy is commonly used in patients with acute variceal hemorrhage. The aim is to guard against bacterial translocation, bacterial infection, and aspiration pneumonia. Such a therapeutic strategy reduces the overall infectious morbidity and improves survival. Of the most commonly used drugs are quinolone and ceftriaxone [10].

## *Endoscopic Therapy*

The revisiting of endoscopic interventions with the introduction of advanced technology has revolutionized the management of gut varices in the majority of cirrhotics and selected patients with portomesenteric venous thrombosis [26, 27]. Over the last few decades, the efficacy of different endoscopic therapeutic modalities has been extensively studied and comprehensively published in the medical and surgical literature [13]. All of the currently published prospective and retrospective studies proved the superiority of endoscopic interventions particularly in patients with active variceal bleeding [13, 28]. The therapeutic efficacy of prophylactic and elective treatment in conjunction with other medical, radiologic, and surgical modalities has also been fully documented in the literature [29].

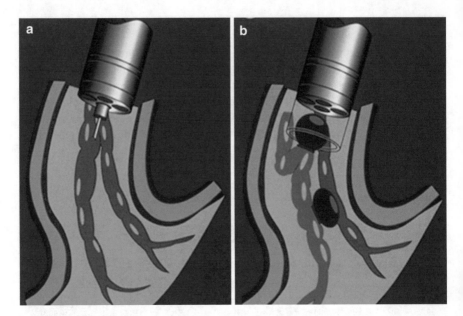

**Fig. 7.4** Endoscopic ablation of the esophageal varices with sclerotherapy (**a**) and band ligation (**b**)

Endoscopic band ligation (EBL) and sclerotherapy, when technically feasible, are lifesaving procedures for patients with active esophageal variceal bleeding along with comprehensive medical and pharmacologic therapy (Fig. 7.4). Both modalities are also effective as prophylactic and elective treatment with temporary and permanent obliteration of the esophageal varices. In selective cases, NSBBs is commonly used as an alternative or adjunct therapy.

When technically feasible, both sclerotherapy and EBL have a high therapeutic index with control of active bleeding in nearly 95% of patients with esophageal varices. However, both techniques are associated with a relatively high rebleeding rate of 50% [29]. Although commonly performed, the long-lasting prophylactic role of each procedure has yet to be fully documented.

Endoscopic therapy has certain technical limitations and significant side effects. With massive upper-gastrointestinal hemorrhage, poor visualization with the inability to identify and obliterate the bleeding varices is frequently witnessed [13, 29, 30]. One of the other major constraints is the inability to perform sclerotherapy or EBL in patients with gastric and enteric varices. The main side effects of endoscopic obliteration of the esophageal varices are induced hemorrhage, chest pain, dysphagia, odynophagia, ulceration of the mucosa, and esophageal perforation [29, 31]. However, recent data suggest that sclerotherapy guided with endoscopic ultrasound (EUS) increases the procedure's safety and efficacy [31].

Preemptive and elective EBL along with NSBBs are valuable therapeutic options for patients with large esophageal varices who are in need of major surgical intervention. For those with gastric, enteric, and ectopic varices, individualized radiologic and surgical treatments are alternative options as described later.

## Radiologic Interventions

Recent advances in the field of diagnostic and therapeutic intervention radiology added a new dimension to the effective management of patients with PH and gut varices. The procedures are mainly indicated for patients who failed or are not suitable candidates for endoscopic treatment. Of the commonly utilized procedures are intrahepatic portosystemic shunts, variceal obliteration, and collateral as well as splenic artery embolization.

The intrahepatic portosystemic shunt is the most commonly utilized radiologic procedure [32]. Along with the embolization techniques, these minimally invasive procedures are valuable therapeutic options for the emergent, elective, and prophylactic treatment of large gut varices and massive abdominal collaterals. The technical feasibility of the radiologic procedure is influenced by the altered vascular anatomy of the liver, site of gut varices, pattern of abdominal collaterals, and complexity of the associated abdominal pathology.

### Intrahepatic Shunts

The therapeutic goal of the radiologic shunts is to reduce the portosystemic gradient to 6–12 mm Hg. The transjugular intrahepatic portosystemic shunt (TIPS) is the most commonly performed procedure and is created within the liver between the portal and hepatic vein (Fig. 7.5). Direct intrahepatic portocaval shunt (DIPS) is another endovascular portocaval shunt that is technically more complex than TIPS. DIPS is specifically indicated for patients with thrombosed hepatic veins and other anatomical abnormalities that preclude the successful performance of the TIPS [33].

The major indications of radiologic shunts are active and recurrent variceal hemorrhage particularly in patients who failed pharmacological and endoscopic treatment. TIPS and DIPS are also indicated for patients with refractory ascites and hepatic hydrothorax as well as those with hepatorenal, Budd-Chiari, and hepatopul-

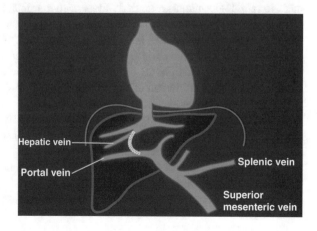

**Fig. 7.5** Transjugular intrahepatic portosystemic shunt (TIPS) between the portal and hepatic venous system. The radiologically created total shunt effectively decompresses the portal system by bypassing the high intrahepatic vascular resistance associated with cirrhosis

monary syndromes. Both procedures are most effective in patients with recurrent variceal hemorrhage and refractory ascites [6]. Nonetheless, these minimally invasive radiologic shunts are commonly used as a bridge to liver transplantation. The preemptive therapeutic role of radiologic shunts in patients with large gastrointestinal varices and significant abdominal collaterals has yet to be defined.

With a mortality rate mainly determined by calculated MELD (Model for End-Stage Liver Disease) score, intra-abdominal hemorrhage is the most serious procedural complication with an incidence ranging from 0.6% to 4.2% [34]. With diversion of portal flow, hepatic encephalopathy is common with an incidence ranging from 33% to 55% [35]. Stent dysfunction is another important complication with a primary patency rate of 50% at 1 year. However, some improvement has been achieved with the introduction of coated stents with a 1-year primary patency rate up to 88% [36]. Along with aggressive medical treatment of hepatic encephalopathy, diligent follow-up with serial Doppler ultrasound is strongly recommended for early detection and prompt treatment of shunt stenosis [6, 37].

### Variceal Obliteration and Collateral Embolization

The radiologic balloon-occluded retrograde transvenous obliteration (BRTO) procedure has been recently introduced for elective treatment of gastric varices. It is commonly utilized in Asia with a recurrent bleeding rate less than 5% [38, 39]. Moreover, BRTO can be performed in patients with poor hepatic reserve. Long-term complications include gastropathy and bleeding esophageal varices. A recent meta-analysis comparing TIPS and BRTO in patients with gastric varices showed no difference in incidences of technical failure and procedure-related complications. However, BRTO was associated with a lower rate of postoperative rebleeding and hepatic encephalopathy [40].

Percutaneous transhepatic embolization (PTE) has been shown to be effective in controlling acute portosystemic variceal bleeding [11]. However, the procedure is associated with a high risk of early rebleeding with an incidence of 37–65%. Accordingly, PTE is currently limited to patients who failed or are not suitable candidates to radiologic shunts particularly those with marginal hepatic reserve [41]. PTE is also indicated for patients with massive abdominal collaterals that are located in the vicinity of complex abdominal pathology with the intent of surgical resection.

Splenic artery embolization has been predominantly used in conjunction with other therapeutic modalities including radiologic shunts and endoscopic ablation. Complete or partial occlusion of the splenic arterial flow significantly reduces the portal and collateral venous flow. Infarction of 50–70% of the splenic cell mass is often required to achieve long term benefits particularly in patients with severe hypersplenism. Significant side effects include splenic abscess, bacterial peritonitis, and hepatic failure in patients with marginal reserve [42]. In addition, the gradual development of splenic arterial collaterals commonly erodes its long-term therapeutic benefits. Nonetheless, the procedure is highly recommended in patients with extensive gastric varices due to isolated splenic and diffuse portomesenteric venous thrombosis.

## Portal Hypertensive Surgery

Until the 1970s revisit of endoscopic sclerotherapy and the 1980s introduction of clinical liver transplantation, portal hypertensive surgery was the only available therapeutic modality for patients with cirrhosis and bleeding varices [43, 44]. Despite the 1960s and 1970s popularity of total shunts, the observed prohibitive risk of incapacitating hepatic encephalopathy triggered relentless efforts to introduce other surgical procedures with the aim to selectively decompress or ablate the gastroesophageal varices. Of these, are the selective shunt and the gastroesophageal devascularization procedures. By the mid-1980s, the results of liver transplantation had significantly improved and the organ replacement operation had become the standard of care for patients with end-stage liver disease including those with active and recurrent variceal hemorrhage. Meanwhile, the minimally invasive intrahepatic radiologic shunts were introduced with encouraging results [32]. As a result, portal hypertensive surgery has become less popular and only used after failure of the aforementioned therapeutic modalities. It is our current practice to use surgery as an elective treatment for patients with preserved hepatic functions and as a preemptive therapy for those receiving lifelong anticoagulation with significant gut varices.

Interesting data has recently emerged from a large meta-analysis comparing surgical and radiologic shunts [45]. The reviewers reported a higher rate of shunt stenosis (66%) and variceal rebleeding (28%) with TIPS compared to surgical shunts with a respective rate of 10% and 5%. The incidence of hepatic encephalopathy was also higher after TIPS (54%) compared to surgical shunts (32%). With similar overall mortality, the 5-year survival rate was better after shunt surgery [45]. Accordingly, more utilization of surgical shunts after failure of endoscopic therapy should be seriously considered particularly in low-operative-risk patients with adequate hepatic reserve [46].

### Total Shunts

The prototype of portosystemic shunts was first described by Eck in 1877 with the aim to totally decompress the splanchnic circulation and lower the portal pressure [47]. It involves dissection of the hepatic hilum with diversion of the portal blood flow to the systemic circulation. It is created by connecting the portal vein or one of its major branches to the inferior vena cava or one of its tributaries. The commonly utilized modalities were the end to side, side to side, and H-graft portocaval shunts. Despite its high therapeutic indices, a prohibitive risk of severe acute and chronic encephalopathy with the ultimate precipitation of hepatic failure is observed in most patients with patent shunt [48]. These sinister morbidities are due to the total diversion of the portal blood flow away from the hepatocytes.

In the 1980s, Sarfeh introduced the concept of partial portosystemic shunt by using an 8-mm polytetrafluoroethylene graft anastomosed between the portal vein and inferior vena cava (Fig. 7.6). The 8-mm H-graft portocaval shunt maintains

**Fig. 7.6** Partial portosystemic shunt with an 8-mm synthetic vascular graft anastomosed between the portal vein and inferior vena cava (Sarfeh shunt). The procedure reduces the portal pressure to a level that decompresses the gut varices with partial preservation of the portal flow (From Henderson [67] with permission)

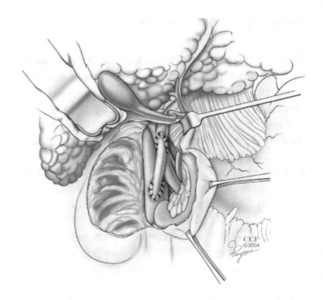

some portal flow to the liver and overcomes the high risk of hepatic encephalopathy commonly seen with the conventional total shunts. This new shunt modality provided excellent control of bleeding with a relatively low risk of encephalopathy and acceptable rate of long-term survival [49, 50]

## Selective Shunts

In the mid-1970s, the late Dean Warren introduced distal splenorenal shunt (DSRS) with the aim to selectively decompress the gastroesophageal varices with preservation of the portal flow (Fig. 7.7a). Despite its proven therapeutic efficacy, the procedure did not gain wide popularity due to the required high surgical skills [51, 52]. In addition, most of the published data demonstrated gradual loss of the proposed shunt selectively with the development of gastric, colosplenic, and pancreatic collaterals (Fig. 7.7b). Accordingly, a technical modification was introduced with the addition of complete splenopancreatic disconnection (Fig. 7.7c). With the increased utilization of the radiologic shunt among Child A/B patients, DSRS has been rarely utilized in recent years despite its relatively lower rates of encephalopathy and the minimal need for reintervention [53].

The seemingly superselective coronocaval shunt was introduced by Inokuchi to provide direct decompression of the gastroesophageal varices into the systemic circulation with better long-term shunt selectivity [54]. When technically feasible, the left gastric vein is dissected and anastomosed to the inferior vein cava. The operation did not gain much popularity because of the technical difficulties and the wide anatomic variations of the left gastric venous system among variceal bleeders [55].

Compared to total surgical shunts, selective shunts do not significantly influence the outcome of future liver transplantation [56]. Technical difficulties have been observed at

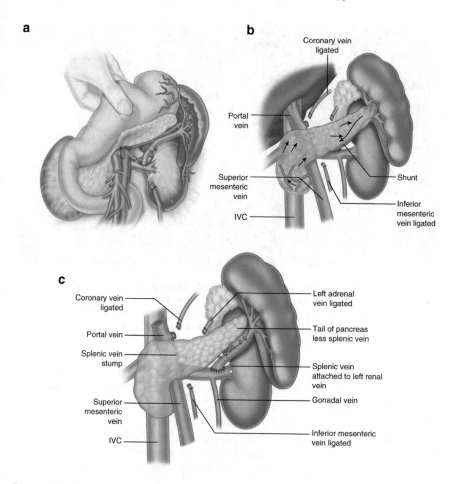

**Fig. 7.7** Distal splenorenal shunt (DSRS) with (**a**) selective decompression of the gastroesophageal varices, (**b**) development of postoperative portosystemic collaterals including pancreatic siphon, (**c**) the modified technique of splenopancreatic disconnection (**a**, From Henderson [67] with permission, **b** & **c**, from Warren [68] with permission)

a higher rate after total shunts particularly in patients with shunt and portal vein thrombosis. With selective shunts, the hepatic hilum remains intact with less risk of surgical bleeding and other technical complications [57, 58]. With patent DSRS, the shunt is commonly ligated soon before or immediately after reperfusion of the transplanted liver.

## Nonconventional Shunts

The management of diffuse portomesenteric venous thrombosis is a true challenge particularly in patients with hepatic cirrhosis and complex abdominal pathology. In most instances, both radiologic and endoscopic interventions are not technically feasible because of occlusion of the portal system with diffuse

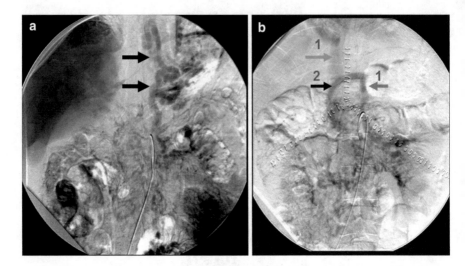

**Fig. 7.8** (**a**) Large gastroesophageal variceal collaterals (*black arrows*) in a patient with diffuse portomesenteric venous thrombosis and preserved hepatic functions. (**b**) Nonconventional porto-systemic shunt between a left gastric collateral and inferior vena cave using an 8-mm Gortex graft. Note the impressive decompression of the variceal collaterals (*1*) via the patent Gortex graft (*2*) with visualization of the inferior vena cava

gastric and enteric varices. With preserved hepatic functions, creation of a non-conventional portosystemic shunt should always be considered particularly in patients with sizeable variceal collaterals (Fig. 7.8). The procedure is also indicated as a preemptive therapy for patients requiring lifelong anticoagulation because of the forbidden risk of uncontrollable variceal gut hemorrhage. With the development of hepatic failure, modified liver or composite visceral transplantation is properly indicated without significant increase in morbidity and mortality.

## Gastroesophageal Devascularization

The gastroesophageal devascularization procedure along with splenectomy was first introduced by Hassab in Egypt [59, 60], and later by Sugiura in Japan [61]. The less extensive Hassab procedure includes gastric devascularization with ligation of the left gastric vascular pedicle, in the absence of an aberrant left replaced hepatic artery, along with splenectomy or splenic artery ligation (Fig. 7.9). The more extensive Sugiura operation involves esophageal transection with complete devascularization of the lower esophagus and stomach utilizing a thoracoabdominal approach. Because of its technical complexity, the procedure did not gain much popularity in the western hemisphere.

With preserved hepatic functions, gastric devascularization can be used for patients who are not shunt candidates and those with isolated splenic or diffuse

**Fig. 7.9** Gastroesophageal devascularization with splenectomy. Note ligation and transection of the gastroepiploic vascular arcades close to the gastric wall with complete disconnection of the short gastric vessels. Splenectomy should be avoided in the hypercoagulable patients particularly those with myeloproliferative disorders (From Henderson [67] with permission)

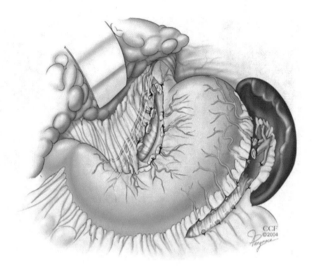

portomesenteric venous thrombosis. Compared to shunt surgery, the ablative procedure is associated with a lower incidence of encephalopathy but with higher rates of rebleeding and persistent ascites. Nonetheless, both surgical procedures have similar operative mortality and long-term survival [62]. With the need for major surgical intervention, gastric devascularization can be done as a first stage operation or simultaneously with the nonportal hypertensive abdominal surgery. The procedure does not preclude or significantly affect the outcome of future transplantation.

## *Hepatic and Composite Visceral Transplantation*

Allotransplantation has revolutionized the management of patients with organ failure. Simultaneous or sequential liver transplantation has been increasingly utilized for patients with poor hepatic reserve who are in need for major surgical interventions [63, 64]. With the coexistence of portomesenteric venous thrombosis, technical modification of the transplant procedure is required including portal vein thrombectomy or cavoportal hemitransposition (Fig. 7.10a).

In patients with concomitant gut failure and complex abdominal pathology, composite visceral transplantation with combined liver-intestine (Fig. 7.10b) or multivisceral transplantation (Fig. 7.10c) is often required. The organs are transplanted en bloc along with simultaneous replacement of the splanchnic arterial and portomesenteric venous system. Of the most common indications are chronic necrotizing pancreatitis, extensive desmoid tumors, and other locally aggressive abdominal neoplasms that are not amenable for resection without organ replacement [65, 66].

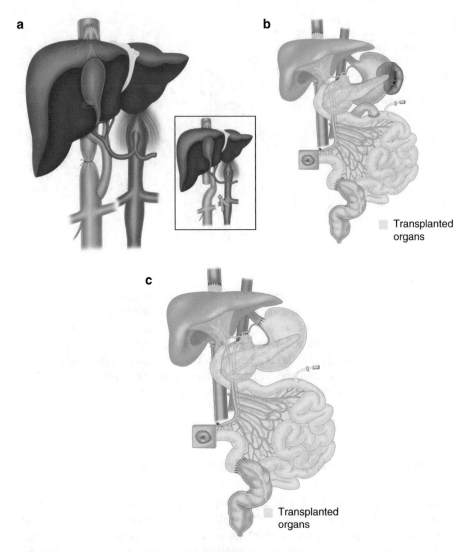

**Fig. 7.10** Organ transplantation for end stage liver disease in patients with portomesenteric venous thrombosis and complex abdominal pathology. (**a**) Isolated liver transplantation with cavoportal hemitransposition. (**b**) Combined liver and intestinal transplantation en bloc with the pancreas. (**c**) Full multivisceral transplantation including the stomach, duodenum, pancreas, intestine, and liver

## Summary

Thorough preoperative evaluation and comprehensive treatment strategy are crucial to the optimal management of patients with PH who are in need for major surgical intervention. The implementation of combined portal hypertensive therapy and planned surgical tactics with adoption of fine techniques is essential to achieve successful outcome. When indicated, simultaneous or sequential therapy should be considered. It is imperative to emphasize the need for collaborative postoperative care. Organ transplantation should be considered in patients with the preoperative diagnosis of marginal hepatic reserve and postoperative development of liver failure. Nonetheless, these complex patients should always be managed at tertiary medical centers with the ultimate goal to improve the overall outcome including value of health care.

**Disclosures** None

# References

1. Balducci G, Sterpetti AV, Ventura M. A short history of portal hypertension and of its management. J Gastroenterol Hepatol. 2016;31(3):541–5.
2. Gilbert DA-N. Les Fonctions hépatiques, par MM. A. Gilbert,... et P. Carnot. Paris: C. Naud; 1902.
3. Thompson WP, et al. Splenic vein pressure in congestive splenomegaly (Banti's syndrome). J Clin Invest. 1937;16(4):571.
4. Sandblom P. The history of portal hypertension. J R Soc Med. 1993;86(9):544–6.
5. Orrego-Matte H, et al. Measurement of intrahepatic pressure as index of portal pressure. Am J Med Sci. 1964;247:278–82.
6. Pillai AK, et al. Portal hypertension: a review of portosystemic collateral pathways and endovascular interventions. Clin Radiol. 2015;70(10):1047–59.
7. Gentilini P, Laffi G. Pathophysiology and treatment of ascites and the hepatorenal syndrome. Baillieres Clin Gastroenterol. 1992;6(3):581–607.
8. Vargas HE, Gerber D, Abu-Elmagd K. Management of portal hypertension-related bleeding. Surg Clin North Am. 1999;79(1):1–22.
9. Cadranel JF, et al. Hepatic hydrothorax. Presse Med. 2016;45(10):815–823.
10. Bhutta AQ, Garcia-Tsao G. The role of medical therapy for variceal bleeding. Gastrointest Endosc Clin N Am. 2015;25(3):479–90.
11. Garbuzenko DV. Current approaches to the management of patients with liver cirrhosis who have acute esophageal variceal bleeding. Curr Med Res Opin. 2016;32(3):467–75.
12. Cabrera L, Tandon P, Abraldes JG. An update on the management of acute esophageal variceal bleeding. Gastroenterol Hepatol. 2017;40(1):34–40.
13. Kapoor A, Dharel N, Sanyal AJ. Endoscopic diagnosis and therapy in gastroesophageal variceal bleeding. Gastrointest Endosc Clin N Am. 2015;25(3):491–507.
14. Bosch J, et al. Effects of vasopressin on the intravariceal pressure in patients with cirrhosis: comparison with the effects on portal pressure. Hepatology. 1988;8(4):861–5.
15. Groszmann RJ, et al. Nitroglycerin improves the hemodynamic response to vasopressin in portal hypertension. Hepatology. 1982;2(6):757–62.
16. Azam Z, et al. Short course adjuvant terlipressin in acute variceal bleeding: a randomized double blind dummy controlled trial. J Hepatol. 2012;56(4):819–24.
17. Rahimi RS, Guntipalli P, Rockey DC. Worldwide practices for pharmacologic therapy in esophageal variceal hemorrhage. Scand J Gastroenterol. 2014;49(2):131–7.
18. D'Amico G, Pagliaro L, Bosch J. The treatment of portal hypertension: a meta-analytic review. Hepatology. 1995;22(1):332–54.
19. Patch D, Burroughs AK. Advances in drug therapy for acute variceal haemorrhage. Baillieres Clin Gastroenterol. 1997;11(2):311–26.

20. Berreta J, et al. Endoscopic versus endoscopic plus octreotide treatment for acute variceal bleeding. Benefit according to severity at admission. Acta Gastroenterol Latinoam. 2013;43(2):89–97.
21. Qi XS, et al. Nonselective beta-blockers in cirrhotic patients with no or small varices: a meta-analysis. World J Gastroenterol. 2015;21(10):3100–8.
22. Li T, et al. Carvedilol for portal hypertension in cirrhosis: systematic review with meta-analysis. BMJ Open. 2016;6(5):e010902.
23. Albillos A, et al. Propranolol plus prazosin compared with propranolol plus isosorbide-5-mononitrate in the treatment of portal hypertension. Gastroenterology. 1998;115(1):116–23.
24. Abraldes JG, et al. Simvastatin lowers portal pressure in patients with cirrhosis and portal hypertension: a randomized controlled trial. Gastroenterology. 2009;136(5):1651–8.
25. Abraldes JG, et al. Addition of simvastatin to standard therapy for the prevention of variceal rebleeding does not reduce rebleeding but increases survival in patients with cirrhosis. Gastroenterology. 2016;150(5):1160–1170.e3.
26. Paquet KJ, Oberhammer E. Sclerotherapy of bleeding oesophageal varices by means of endoscopy. Endoscopy. 1978;10(1):7–12.
27. Palani CK, et al. Endoscopic sclerotherapy in acute variceal hemorrhage. Am J Surg. 1981;141(1):164–8.
28. Hui Ng NB, et al. Endoscopic evaluation in children with end-stage liver disease associated portal hypertension awaiting liver transplant. J Pediatr Gastroenterol Nutr. 2016;63(3):365–9.
29. Luigiano C, et al. Role of endoscopy in management of gastrointestinal complications of portal hypertension. World J Gastrointest Endosc. 2015;7(1):1–12.
30. Steevens C, et al. Massive duodenal variceal bleed; complication of extra hepatic portal hypertension: endoscopic management and literature review. World J Gastrointest Pharmacol Ther. 2015;6(4):248–52.
31. de Paulo GA, et al. Treatment of esophageal varices: a randomized controlled trial comparing endoscopic sclerotherapy and EUS-guided sclerotherapy of esophageal collateral veins. Gastrointest Endosc. 2006;63(3):396–402. quiz 463
32. Ring EJ, et al. Using transjugular intrahepatic portosystemic shunts to control variceal bleeding before liver transplantation. Ann Intern Med. 1992;116(4):304–9.
33. Petersen B. Intravascular ultrasound-guided direct intrahepatic portacaval shunt: description of technique and technical refinements. J Vasc Interv Radiol. 2003;14(1):21–32.
34. Tripathi D, et al. Ten years' follow-up of 472 patients following transjugular intrahepatic portosystemic stent-shunt insertion at a single centre. Eur J Gastroenterol Hepatol. 2004;16(1):9–18.
35. Riggio O, et al. Incidence, natural history, and risk factors of hepatic encephalopathy after transjugular intrahepatic portosystemic shunt with polytetrafluoroethylene-covered stent grafts. Am J Gastroenterol. 2008;103(11):2738–46.
36. Boyer TD, Haskal ZJ. American Association for the Study of Liver Diseases Practice Guidelines: the role of transjugular intrahepatic portosystemic shunt creation in the management of portal hypertension. J Vasc Interv Radiol. 2005;16(5):615–29.
37. Middleton WD, Teefey SA, Darcy MD. Doppler evaluation of transjugular intrahepatic portosystemic shunts. Ultrasound Q. 2003;19(2):56–70. quiz 108 – 10
38. Cho SK, et al. Balloon-occluded retrograde transvenous obliteration of gastric varices: outcomes and complications in 49 patients. AJR Am J Roentgenol. 2007;189(6):W365–72.
39. Patel A, Fischman AM, Saad WE. Balloon-occluded retrograde transvenous obliteration of gastric varices. AJR Am J Roentgenol. 2012;199(4):721–9.
40. Wang YB, et al. Balloon-occluded retrograde transvenous obliteration versus transjugular intrahepatic portosystemic shunt for treatment of gastric varices due to portal hypertension: a meta-analysis. J Gastroenterol Hepatol. 2016;31(4):727–33.
41. Smith-Laing G, et al. Role of percutaneous transhepatic obliteration of varices in the management of hemorrhage from gastroesophageal varices. Gastroenterology. 1981;80(5 pt 1):1031–6.
42. Zhu K, et al. Partial splenic embolization for hypersplenism in cirrhosis: a long-term outcome in 62 patients. Dig Liver Dis. 2009;41(6):411–6.

43. Marsh JW, et al. Liver transplantation today. Postgrad Med. 1987;81(5):13. -6, 19, 22-3
44. Adler M, et al. Prognosis of hepatic transplantation as a function of biological, immunological and functional preoperative findings. Acta Gastroenterol Belg. 1987;50(3):365–8.
45. Huang L, et al. Transjugular intrahepatic portosystemic shunt versus surgical shunting in the management of portal hypertension. Chin Med J (Engl). 2015;128(6):826–34.
46. Orloff MJ. Fifty-three years' experience with randomized clinical trials of emergency portacaval shunt for bleeding esophageal varices in Cirrhosis: 1958-2011. JAMA Surg. 2014;149(2):155–69.
47. Rocko JM, Swan KG. The Eck-Pavlov connection. Am Surg. 1985;51(11):641–4.
48. Stipa S, Balducci G, Ziparo V, Stipa F, Lucandri G. Total shunting and elective management of variceal bleeding. World J Surg. 1994;18:200–4.
49. Sarfeh IJ, Rypins EB, Mason GR. A systematic appraisal of portacaval H-graft diameters. Clinical and hemodynamic persepectives. Ann Surg. 1986;204:356–63.
50. Costa G, Cruz Jr RJ, Abu-Elmagd KM. Surgical shunt versus TIPS for treatment of variceal hemorrhage in the current era of liver and multivisceral transplantation. Surg Clin North Am. 2010;90(4):891–905.
51. Henderson JM, Warren WD. Selective variceal decompression: current status and recent advances. Adv Surg. 1984;18:81–115.
52. Henderson JM, Millikan WJ, Warren WD. The distal splenorenal shunt: an update. World J Surg. 1984;8(5):722–32.
53. Henderson JM, et al. Distal splenorenal shunt versus transjugular intrahepatic portal systematic shunt for variceal bleeding: a randomized trial. Gastroenterology. 2006;130(6):1643–51.
54. Inokuchi K, et al. New selective decompression of esophageal varices. By a left gastric venous-caval shunt. Arch Surg. 1970;100(2):157–62.
55. Inokuchi K, Sugimachi K. The selective shunt for variceal bleeding: a personal perspective. Am J Surg. 1990;160(1):48–53.
56. Harmantas A, et al. Selective vs total portosystemic shunts in the treatment of variceal hemorrhage in cirrhotic patients:: is there any advantage? Hepatol Res. 1999;14(2):144–53.
57. Shaked A, Busuttil RW. Liver transplantation in patients with portal vein thrombosis and central portacaval shunts. Ann Surg. 1991;214(6):696.
58. Aboujoud MS, et al. A comparison of treatment with transjugular intrahepatic portosystemic shunt or distal splenorenal shunt in the management of variceal bleeding prior to liver transplantation. Transplantation. 1995;59(2):226–9.
59. Hassab M. Gastroesophageal decongestion and splenectomy in the treatment of esophageal varices in bilharzial cirrhosis: further studies with a report on 355 operations. Surgery. 1967;61(2):169–76.
60. Hassab M. Nonshunt operations in portal hypertension without cirrhosis. Surg Gynecol Obstet. 1970;131(4):648.
61. Sugiura M, Futagawa S. Esophageal transection with paraesophagogastric devascularizations (the Sugiura procedure) in the treatment of esophageal varices. World J Surg. 1984;8(5):673–9.
62. Zong GQ, Fei Y, Liu RM. Comparison of effects of devascularization versus shunt on patients with portal hypertension: a meta-analysis. Chirurgia (Bucur). 2015;110(1):15–25.
63. Harrington PB, et al. Outcomes of patients who undergo cardiac surgical procedures after liver transplantation. Ann Thorac Surg. 2017;103(2):541–545.
64. Ceulemans LJ, et al. Combined liver-thoracic transplantation: single-center experience with introduction of the 'Liver-first' principle. Transpl Int. 2016;29(6):715–26.
65. Abu-Elmagd KM, et al. Five hundred intestinal and multivisceral transplantations at a single center: major advances with new challenges. Ann Surg. 2009;250(4):567–81.
66. Abu-Elmagd K. The concept of gut rehabilitation and the future of visceral transplantation. Nat Rev Gastroenterol Hepatol. 2015;12(2):108–20.
67. Henderson JM. Surgical therapies for management. Portal Hypertens. 2005:235–45.
68. Warren WD, Millikan WJ, Henderson JM, et al. Splenopancreatic disconnection: improved selectivity of distal splenorenal shunt. Ann Surg. 1986;204(4):347.

# Chapter 8
# Perioperative Critical Care of the Patient with Liver Disease Undergoing Nonhepatic Surgery

David J. Kramer

## Introduction

Patients with compensated liver disease are at increased risk of morbidity and mortality when undergoing anesthesia and surgery. Key concerns with hepatic decompensation include neurologic, cardiovascular, renal, respiratory dysfunction, coagulopathy, and infection.

## Risk Assessment

Risk assessment is based on a combination of the severity of liver dysfunction, intensity of surgical stress, comorbidities, and functional status. Liver dysfunction comprises synthetic dysfunction and portal hypertension. The Childs-Turcotte-Pugh score and the model for end-stage liver disease (MELD) gauge severity of liver dysfunction. Although controversy exists as to which score is better [1], they complement each other and present the clinician with a more robust understanding. The patient's functional status should also be considered. The Charlson comorbidity index [2] correlates with morbidity and mortality after surgery in cirrhotics [3], but the impact may be obscured by the status of MELD and American Society of Anesthesiologists (ASA) [4] in multivariate analysis. The ASA predicts short-term morbidity and mortality [4] but has limited discrimination as patients with chronic liver disease will be at least status III. MELD and CTP correlate with long-term

D.J. Kramer, MD, FACP
Aurora Critical Care Service, Aurora Health Care,
Suite 315, 2901 W. Kinnickinnic River Parkway, Milwaukee, WI 53215, USA

University of Wisconsin School of Medicine and Public Health, Madison, USA
e-mail: david.kramer@aurora.org

© Springer International Publishing AG 2017
B. Eghtesad, J. Fung (eds.), *Surgical Procedures on the Cirrhotic Patient*,
DOI 10.1007/978-3-319-52396-5_8

mortality, at 30, 90, and 365 days. Surgical stress is highest for intrathoracic, particularly cardiac and intra-abdominal procedures. However, procedures likely to result in significant blood loss and intraoperative hemodynamic instability should also be considered as high surgical stress. Surgery undertaken emergently increases this risk profile dramatically [5]. An online calculator is available to estimate the risk of major surgery in patients with cirrhosis. (http://www.mayoclinic.org/medical-professionals/model-end-stage-liver-disease/post-operative-mortality-risk-patients-cirrhosis )

## Risk Mitigation

### Hemodynamics and Renal Function

Liver injury which results from anesthesia and surgery is at least in part due to changes in hepatic hemodynamics. Increased hepatic venous resistance often coincides with decreased arterial perfusion pressure. Preoperative optimization requires assessment of the patient's cardiovascular status, renal function, and pulmonary function. Cirrhosis is associated with cardiomyopathy which is manifest by conduction abnormalities and diastolic dysfunction [6, 7]. Preoperative assessment with transthoracic echocardiography can be complemented by intraoperative transesophageal monitoring. In particular, right ventricular function can be assessed as intravascular volume and vasopressors are manipulated. Stress echocardiography is often used as a screen for hemodynamically significant coronary artery disease.

Patients with cirrhosis are often volume-overloaded with ascites and edema. Renal dysfunction is often masked as low creatinine and urea nitrogen may reflect sarcopenia and impaired ureagenesis rather than normal glomerular filtration rate (GFR). However, in early hepatorenal syndrome, the sodium avidity of the kidney indicates hypoperfusion, and echo demonstration of underfilling of the left ventricle will confirm intravascular volume contraction. This is often associated with significant arterial vasodilation which correlates with the severity of cirrhosis. Preoperative optimization includes restoration of perfusion pressure by increasing arterial tone and intravascular volume while controlling ascites and decreasing edema. Arterial vasodilation may reflect hypocalcemia and severe anemia as well as concomitant adrenal insufficiency [8, 9]. Hypoalbuminemia may be addressed with hyperoncotic albumin and judicious diuresis undertaken. Persistent arterial vasodilation may require vasopressor support. Terlipressin is not available in the United States but would be the first-choice agent in much of the world. Our preference is norepinephrine. Large-volume paracentesis may also be considered in an effort to optimize renal function once arterial tone and intravascular volume are optimized. The need for significant vasopressor support in advance of induction of anesthesia heralds an even higher risk of perioperative morbidity and mortality.

Electrolyte imbalance is common in cirrhosis. Hyponatremia, hypokalemia, hypomagnesemia, hypophosphatemia, and hypozincemia can be addressed preoperatively. Care should be taken to avoid exacerbating metabolic acidosis by administering hyperchloremic solutions. Balanced electrolyte solutions are commercially available. In addition, the relatively high chloride content of blood products including albumin can be counterbalanced by creating a solution of 0.45% sodium chloride with 50–75 mEq/L which is readily available and inexpensive. Over-rapid correction of hyponatremia which is associated with central pontine myelinolysis also can be avoided with this approach. Although colloid administration is controversial, patients with cirrhosis appear to benefit from albumin particularly in the settings of infection and renal failure. However, other colloids such as hydroxyethyl starch (Hetastarch) are associated with renal failure and relatively contraindicated in the setting.

## Neurologic Function

Hepatic encephalopathy develops with deteriorating liver function and worsening portosystemic shunting. It often heralds infectious complications or acute bleeding. Agitation, delirium, and altered nociception are typical. If the enteral route is available, we continue rifaximin and lactulose, and zinc if hypozincemia. We do not restrict protein but do occasionally use branched chain enriched formulae if encephalopathy is refractory to standard measures. We address environmental factors such as early mobilization of the patient out of bed, daylight during the daytime, and promote sleep hygiene with efforts to minimally disturb the patient at night. Local therapy such as repositioning, a heating pad, and/or lidocaine patch serve to minimize systemic narcotic requirements. Although we are hesitant to place epidural catheters in coagulopathic patients, regional anesthesia is often a very useful adjunct.

The metabolism of sedative hypnotics and narcotics is impaired in liver failure but unpredictably. We avoid benzodiazepines and minimize narcotics—treating as needed rather than with continuous infusions. Non-narcotic approaches are limited as nonsteroidal anti-inflammatory agents may increase the risk of GI bleeding. Acetaminophen is effective and can be administered parenterally if needed, but the total daily dose should be reduced in liver failure to 2 g. Ketamine is an excellent analgesic in small doses of 10–25 mg and does not cause respiratory depression or worsen hemodynamic instability. Gabapentin is an effective adjunct [10]. Even a single preoperative dose lowers narcotic requirements [11].

Hepatic encephalopathy seems to reduce the incidence of recall during anesthesia. Isoflurane and sevoflurane have minimal direct impact on hepatic function [12]. However, both may exacerbate arterial vasodilation and result in hypotension requiring vasopressors. Although the minimum alveolar concentration for volatile anesthetics is higher in chronic alcohol users, it is significantly lower in the setting of liver disease [13].

## Pulmonary Function

Respiratory function may be impaired in cirrhosis because of mechanical factors such as ascites and chest wall edema as well as altered respiratory drive related to hepatic encephalopathy. Gas exchange may also be affected by atelectasis, pulmonary edema, and pneumonia. In the absence of radiographic abnormalities, the diffusing capacity is often low and reflects intrapulmonary shunting due to hepatopulmonary syndrome, which can be demonstrated with echocardiography using microbubbles. In addition to optimizing the patient's volume status preoperatively, discontinuation of tobacco smoking and management of obstructive airways with appropriate bronchodilation are imperative. Once intubated and mechanically ventilated, such patients are particularly prone to lung injury. Consequently, a lung-protective ventilating strategy should be undertaken with low tidal volumes (6 mL/kg IBW) and PEEP [14]. We use the ARDS-Net high PEEP protocol [15] to titrate PEEP and $FiO_2$ and start with the PEEP set at BMI/4. The duration of intubation and mechanical ventilation should be minimized. This requires minimizing sedation in the ICU changing intraoperative anesthetic management. We attempt extubation within 6 h, in the OR if possible. We use noninvasive ventilation with CPAP or BiPAP until the patient can mobilize out of bed and cough effectively. These patients often have impaired gastric motility. Aspiration of gastric contents is often a life-ending event, prompting us to routinely decompress the stomach with a gastric tube until the patient can protect the airway.

## Nutrition

Malnutrition is common in liver failure [16], with muscle wasting and sarcopenia evident on exam and abdominal CT [17] even in obese patients with nonalcoholic fatty liver disease [18]. The MELD score fails to capture this comorbidity which correlates with weakness and risk of postoperative infection. Cirrhosis is a catabolic process which is difficult to reverse. However, if time permits, a trial of nutritional supplementation is indicated, with postpyloric placement of a small-bore feeding tube [19] if sufficient calories and protein cannot be reliably ingested per os. We aggressively treat hepatic encephalopathy rather than reduce protein. Vitamin deficiencies should be anticipated, particularly fat-soluble vitamins in cholestatic liver disease. Thiamine supplementation is indicated particularly in alcohol-induced liver disease.

## Liver Support

The potential for improvement in liver function should be assessed. Patients with acute viral hepatitis or untreated autoimmune hepatitis or alcoholic hepatitis are likely to improve with supportive care, specific treatments, and time. In such patients, elective surgery should be deferred. A combination of acute liver injury and the need for emergent surgery presents a high risk. There may be benefit for administration of N-acetylcysteine [20] .

Mechanical support for patients with liver failure is an area of intense interest. High-volume plasma exchange has recently been shown to be of benefit in acute liver failure [21]. Improvement in hemodynamics, encephalopathy, cholestasis, and ammonia levels results in acute or chronic liver failure in patients treated with MARS, although there is no improvement in survival [21, 22]. Data are insufficient to argue for routine prophylactic use or for attempted rescue with these approaches in the event hepatic decompensation occurs after surgery. The experience with other support devices such as ECMO and ventricular assist devices in liver failure has been dismal, and these interventions are unlikely to be of benefit.

## Portal Hypertension

Portal venous pressures and the transhepatic venous pressure gradient correlate with severity of cirrhosis and may be reflected in the degree of thrombocytopenia. Liver injury, perhaps due to ischemia or associated with acute inflammation, will increase resistance to portal flow. If portal flow is maintained despite higher resistance, portal pressures will rise. This will increase ascites production and will increase the risk of gastrointestinal and intra-abdominal hemorrhage. Preoperative placement of intrahepatic shunts (TIPS) has been advocated as a way of reducing the morbidity associated with portal hypertension [23]. However, small studies have failed to show benefit of preoperative placement of TIPS [24]. Furthermore, TIPS in advanced liver disease (MELD >14 or CTP "C") is associated with more rapid hepatic decompensation and is relatively contraindicated, particularly if liver transplantation is not an option. If a TIPS is placed, a period of 6–8 weeks should elapse before proceeding with surgery. This will allow decompression of the splanchnic vasculature. It also will allow hepatic decompensation to manifest, perhaps avoiding death after elective surgery.

## Hemostasis

The coagulopathy of liver disease includes depressed procoagulant and anticoagulant factors as well as thrombocytopenia. However, qualitative platelet dysfunction and unchecked fibrinolysis may also be factors. In addition, infection (even if low-grade) results in tissue inflammation and activation of coagulation pathways. Renal failure may exacerbate impaired platelet function. Conventional measures of coagulation often exaggerate the procoagulant factor deficiency with prolonged prothrombin time and INR. Fibrinogen levels can be assessed, but laboratory turnaround is often too slow to be of benefit. As a consequence, patients are transfused plasma, which may result in volume overload and increased hepatic congestion without effectively treating the coagulation deficit. Thromboelastography (TEG) offers real-time analysis of the patient's coagulation and guides more focused blood product transfusion [25]. Rotational thromboelastography is an emerging alternative. Hyperfibrinolysis can be recognized by TEG, but low-grade fibrinolysis likely often contributes to the bleeding diathesis in decompensated liver disease. ε-Aminocaproic acid (Amicar) is effective and safe in reversing hyperfibrinolysis [26]. Prophylactic use during surgery and in the ICU might be considered in the cirrhotic at high risk for bleeding.

## *Infection*

Liver failure is an immune-incompetent state. Postoperative infection is a feared complication, and the risks increase with the severity of liver disease and attendant comorbidities such as malnutrition, ascites, and renal failure. Perioperative antimicrobial prophylaxis for skin organisms may be augmented to cover bowel pathogens. Fungal pressure in these patients is high, and we have a low threshold for including antifungal agents such as fluconazole or micafungin. Accumulation of low protein (high serum—ascites albumin gradient, SAAG) with impaired opsonization of pathogens is a particular risk. Peritoneocentesis with supplemental albumin to maintain intravascular volume will decrease risk of infection and abdominal wound dehiscence. Ascitic neutrocytosis resolves rapidly (48 h) after surgery, and a rising ascites WBC thereafter may herald peritonitis [27]. We have a low threshold to include infection in the differential for any manifestation of hepatic decompensation. Cultures from all available sites, cell counts with differentials of ascites, and other drainage from surgical sites and stool leukocytes with *C. difficile* toxin assay are done if indicated. We minimize central venous and arterial access. We have a low threshold to initiate antimicrobial coverage—bacterial and fungal—with a commitment to discontinue in the absence of proven pathogen or site of infection. Procalcitonin may be misleading as a marker of infection as it is elevated in liver injury. However, elevated procalcitonin levels associated with infection diagnosed by other means will fall with effective therapy but may not normalize.

## End of Life

Improvements in surgical and anesthesia techniques mean that even high-risk patients are offered surgery, and they survive to reach the ICU. There, some will fare well. However, many suffer significant morbidity, and of these a high proportion die. This chapter has addressed risk mitigation strategies. It is vital that the patient and family understand that the options available to manage hepatic decompensation are limited. Realistic expectations must be established prior to surgery. An intensivist familiar with the perioperative management of such patients may be of particular value in this discussion. Prior to proceeding with surgery, the discussion should include when inappropriate medical care will be withheld. A practical example for discussion might be the patient who develops postoperative hepatic decompensation with intractable hemorrhage, for whom further surgical intervention is futile and will not benefit from continued blood product administration. Likewise, cardiac resuscitation in this setting is rarely medically appropriate. Even the candidate accepted for liver transplantation who acutely decompensated after nonhepatic surgery is unlikely to be transplanted successfully. This slim chance should not be used to provide medically inappropriate care.

# Conclusion

Surgery and anesthesia present significant risks of increased morbidity and mortality to the patient with liver disease. Risk assessment mandates an understanding of the cause and severity of liver disease, medical comorbidities, functional status of the patient, and the surgical stress of the planned procedure. Risk mitigation can be undertaken in elective case. Likewise, supportive strategies can be employed when emergent surgery precludes robust optimizations. Preoperative management includes counseling about the possible outcomes and the appropriate constraint of medical options to ensure best patient care.

# References

1. Farnsworth N, Fagan SP, Berger DH, Awad SS. Child-Turcotte-Pugh versus MELD score as a predictor of outcome after elective and emergent surgery in cirrhotic patients. Am J Surg. 2004;188(5):580–3.
2. Charlson ME, Pompei P, Ales KL, MacKenzie CR. A new method of classifying prognostic comorbidity in longitudinal studies: development and validation. J Chronic Dis. 1987;40:373–83.
3. Sato M, Tateishi R, Yasunaga H, Horiguchi H, Matsui H, Yoshida H, Fushimi K, Koike K. The ADOPT-LC score: a novel predictive index of in-hospital mortality of cirrhotic patients following surgical procedures based on a national survey. Hepatol Res. 2016: 1–9.
4. Teh SH, Nagorney DM, Stevens SR, Offord KP, Therneau TM, Plevak DJ, Talwalkar JA, Kim WR, Kamath PS. Risk factors for mortality after surgery in patients with cirrhosis. Gastroenterology. 2007;132(4):1261–9.
5. Havens JM, Columbus AB, Olufajo OA, Askari R, Salim A, Christopher KB. Association of model for end-stage liver disease score with mortality in emergency general surgery patients. JAMA Surg. 2016;151:e160789.
6. Fede G, Privitera G, Tomaselli T, Spadaro L, Purrello F. Cardiovascular dysfunction in patients with liver cirrhosis. Ann Gastroenterol. 2015;28(1):31–40.
7. Biancofiorea G, Mandell MS, Della RG. Perioperative considerations in patients with cirrhotic cardiomyopathy. Curr Opin Anaesthesiol. 2010;23:128–32.
8. Harry R, Auzinger G, Wendon J. The clinical importance of adrenal insufficiency in acute hepatic dysfunction. Hepatology. 2002;36:395–402.

9. Tsai MH, Peng YS, Chen YC, Liu NJ, Ho YP, Fang JT, Lien JM, Yang C, Chen PC, Wu CS. Adrenal insufficiency in patients with cirrhosis, severe sepsis and septic shock. Hepatology. 2006;43:673–81.

10. Doleman B, Heinink TP, Read DJ, Faleiro RJ, Lund JN, Williams JP. A systematic review and meta-regression analysis of prophylactic gabapentin for postoperative pain. Anaesthesia. 2015;70:1186–204.

11. Parsa AA, Sprouse-Blum AS, Jackowe DJ, Lee M, Oyama J, Parsa FD. Combined preoperative use of celecoxib and gabapentin in the management of postoperative pain. Aesthetic Plast Surg. 2009;33:98–103.

12. Nishiyama T, Fujimoto T, Hanaoka K. A comparison of liver function after hepatectomy in cirrhotic patients between sevoflurane and isoflurane in anesthesia with nitrous oxide and epidural block. Anesth Analg. 2004;98:990–3.

13. Yin Y, Yan M, Zhu T. Minimum alveolar concentration of sevoflurane in rabbits with liver fibrosis. Anesth Analg. 2012;114:561–5.

14. The Acute Respiratory Distress Syndrome Network. Ventilation with lower tidal volumes as compared with traditional tidal volumes for acute lung injury and the acute respiratory distress syndrome. N Engl J Med. 2000;342:1301–8.

15. Talmor D, Sarge T, Malhotra A, O'Donnell CR, Ritz R, Lisbon A, Novack V, Loring SH. Mechanical ventilation guided by esophageal pressure in acute lung injury. N Engl J Med. 2008;359:2095–104.

16. Peng S, Plank LD, McCall JL, Gillanders LK, McIlroy K, Gane EJ. Body composition, muscle function, and energy expenditure in patients with liver cirrhosis: a comprehensive study. Am J Clin Nutr. 2007;85:1257–66.

17. Giusto M, Lattanzi B, Albanese C, Galtieri A, Farcomeni A, Giannelli V, Lucidi C, Di Martino M, Catalano C, Merli M. Sarcopenia in liver cirrhosis: the role of computed tomography scan for the assessment of muscle mass compared with dual-energy X-ray absorptiometry and anthropometry. Eur J Gastroenterol Hepatol. 2015;27:328–34.

18. Carias S, Castellanos AL, Vilchez V, Nair R, Dela Cruz AC, Watkins J, Barrett T, Trushar P, Esser K, Gedaly R. Nonalcoholic steatohepatitis is strongly associated with sarcopenic obesity in patients with cirrhosis undergoing liver transplant evaluation. J Gastroenterol Hepatol. 2016;31:628–33.

19. Stephen A, SA MC, Taylor BE, Martindale RG, Warren MM, Johnson DR, Braunschweig C, MS MC, Davanos E, Rice TW, Cresci GA, Gervasio JM, Sacks GS, Roberts PR, Compher C, the Society of Critical Care Medicine and the American Society for Parenteral and Enteral Nutrition (A.S.P.E.N.). Guidelines for the provision and assessment of nutrition support therapy in the adult critically ill patient: Society of Critical Care Medicine (SCCM) and American Society for Parenteral and Enteral Nutrition (A.S.P.E.N.). J Parenter Enteral Nutr. 2016;40(2):159–211.

20. Lee WM, Hynan LS, Rossaro L, Fontana RJ, Stravitz RT, Larson AM, Davern TJ, Murray NG, McCashland T, Reisch JS, Robuck PR, the Acute Liver Failure Study Group. Intravenous N-Acetylcysteine improves transplant-free survival in early stage non-acetaminophen acute liver failure. Gastroenterology. 2009;137:856–64.

21. Larsen FS, Schmidt LE, Bernsmeier C, Rasmussen A, Isoniemi H, Patel VC, Triantafyllou E, Bernal W, Auzinger G, Shawcross D, Eefsen M, Bjerring PN, Clemmesen JO, Krister Hockerstedt K, Frederiksen HJ, Hansen BA, Antoniades CG, Wendon J. High-volume plasma exchange in patients with acute liver failure: an open randomised controlled trial. J Hepatol. 2016;64:69–78.

22. Sen S, Mookerjee RP, Cheshire LM, Davies NA, Williams R, Jalan R. Albumin dialysis reduces portal pressure acutely in patients with severe alcoholic hepatitis. J Hepatol. 2005;43:142–8.

23. Azoulay D, Buabse F, Damiano I, Smail A, Ichai P, Dannaoui M, et al. Neoadjuvant transjugular intrahepatic portosystemic shunt: a solution for extrahepatic abdominal operation in cirrhotic patients with severe portal hypertension. J Am Coll Surg. 2001;193:46–51.

24. Vinet E, Perreault P, Bouchard L, Bernard D, Wassef R, Richard C, et al. Transjugular intrahepatic portosystemic shunt before abdominal surgery in cirrhotic patients: a retrospective, comparative study. Can J Gastroenterol. 2006;20:401–4.
25. De Pietri L, Bianchini M, Montalti R, De Maria N, Di Maira T, Begliomini B, Gerunda GE, di Benedetto F, Garcia-Tsao G, Villa E. Thrombelastography-guided blood product use before invasive procedures in cirrhosis with severe coagulopathy: a randomized, controlled trial. Hepatology. 2016;63:566–73.
26. Gunawan B, Runyon B. The efficacy and safety of ε-aminocaproic acid treatment in patients with cirrhosis and hyperfibrinolysis. Aliment Pharmacol Ther. 2006;23:115–20.
27. Pungpapong S, Alvarez S, Hellinger WC, Kramer DJ, Willingham DL, Mendez JC, Nguyen JH, Hewitt WR, Aranda-Michel J, Harnois DM, Rosser BG, Hughes CB, Grewal HP, Satyanrayana R, Dickson RC, Steers JL, Keaveny AP. Peritonitis after liver transplantation: incidence, risk factors, microbiology profiles, and outcome. Liver Transpl. 2006;12(8):1244–52.

# Chapter 9
# Role of Minimally Invasive Surgery in Patients with Cirrhosis

**Naftali Presser and Jeffery L. Ponsky**

## Introduction

Cirrhosis, the end stage of progressive liver inflammation and fibrosis, poses a serious health risk to our society. A wide variety of disorders can contribute to the development of cirrhosis including viral hepatitis, alcohol-related liver disease, nonalcoholic fatty liver disease (NAFLD), nonalcoholic steatohepatitis (NASH), as well as a variety of metabolic derangements to name a few.

Cirrhosis in general and portal hypertension in particular have been associated with significant morbidity and mortality in patients undergoing a variety of surgical procedures. Csikesz et al. reviewed data from the national inpatient sample from 1998 to 2005. During this time, 22,659 patients with cirrhosis of whom 4214 patients had concomitant portal hypertension were reviewed. Four elective index operations were chosen including cholecystectomy, coronary artery bypass graft. These patients were compared to approximately 2.8 million others without said comorbidities during the same period. Mortality rates were significantly higher is those with cirrhosis and cirrhosis with additional portal hypertension compared to controls. Additionally, increased cost and length of hospital stay were identified emphasizing the increased difficulty of managing such patients [1]. Further studies demonstrated similar trends with increased in-hospital morbidity and mortality in

N. Presser, MD
Department of General Surgery, Digestive Disease Surgical Institute, Cleveland Clinic
Foundation, Cleveland, OH, USA
e-mail: Naftalipresser@yahoo.com

J.L. Ponsky, MD, FACS (✉)
Lerner College of Medicine, Department of General Surgery, Digestive Diseases Surgical
Institute, Cleveland Clinic Foundation, Cleveland, OH, USA

Cleveland Clinic Lerner College of Medicine, Digestive Disease and Surgery Institute,
9500 Euclid Avenue / A100, Cleveland, OH 44149, USA
e-mail: ponskyj@ccf.org

© Springer International Publishing AG 2017
B. Eghtesad, J. Fung (eds.), *Surgical Procedures on the Cirrhotic Patient*,
DOI 10.1007/978-3-319-52396-5_9

both elective and emergent cases [2]. As cirrhosis progresses and portal hypertension develops, morbidity and mortality rates increase further. Several scoring systems have been developed to stratify patients by the severity of their liver disease. The Childs–Pugh–Turcotte (CPT) system and the Model for End-Stage Liver Disease (MELD) scoring system represent the two most commonly utilized scales of the severity of liver disease. In one study of 92 patients undergoing elective and emergent surgery, mortality rates were 10, 30, and 82% respectively for Childs' class A, B, and C respectively [3]. In another compelling study, 772 patients undergoing major surgery were evaluated. Thirty-day mortality was found to increase with increasing MELD scores. In this study patients with a MELD score up to 7 had a 5.7% perioperative mortality, while patients with a MELD of $\geq 26$ had 90% mortality rates [4]. Both CPT and MELD can be used to stratify patients in order to assess feasibility and advisability of undertaking a surgical adventure in the nonemergent setting. While there is no specifically accepted maximum CPT or MELD score that necessarily precludes surgical intervention, these studies clearly demonstrate extremely high rates of mortality in patients who are CPT class C or with MELD scores in the 20s. As such, very careful consideration needs to be exercised as to which of these patients surgical interventions can be entertained, and which ones would any intervention be essentially futile. A variety of associated physiological derangements that area associated with cirrhosis predispose such patient to increased morbidity. Malnutrition, ascites, hyponatremia, coagulopathy in addition to associate renal and cardiac dysfunction that can often accompany cirrhosis all play a role in increasing the risk of complications and inhibiting the normal healing and recovery for such patients [5].

Laparoscopic surgery offers a variety of advantages over tradition open surgery. Numerous studies of various procedures have shown decrease post-operative pain, decreased -length of hospital stay, earlier return to work, often improvements in blood loss and infection rates [6–9]. Cirrhotics undergoing laparoscopic surgical are a unique surgical group. The possibility of small incisions, with less bleeding and less physiological stress is has the potential for improved tolerance of surgery in this high risk group. This improvement is balanced by the ability for patients with cirrhosis to tolerate the physiologic changes associated with laparoscopy. Laparoscopy requires the ability to insufflate the abdomen with gas. This pressurized gas causes a decrease in venous return to the right heart secondary to the increased intra-abdominal pressures. While a healthy person can tolerate this physiologic stress, cirrhotics, with there already vasodilated state could be more susceptible to this stress. Additionally, as the risk of bleeding is higher in cirrhotics compared to healthy controls, laparoscopy does not afford surgeons the same comfort in ability to control significant bleeding should it be encountered. Indeed in many series, one of the prime reasons for conversion to open surgery from laparoscopy is the onset of significant bleeding [10].

The remainder of this chapter will review some of the existing data for minimally invasive surgery performed in cirrhotics. We will address common procedures such as appendectomy and colon resection as well as procedures often linked to liver disease such as obesity related surgery and liver resections. We additionally will touch upon the data available for advanced endoscopic therapies in the cirrhotic patient. One of the most common procedures, the cholecystectomy, will be deferred. The next chapter is dedicated exclusively to this entity and as such we will only briefly touch upon this important procedure here.

## Laparoscopic Appendectomy and Colorectal Surgery

Laparoscopic appendectomy is one of the most common procedures performed by the general surgeon. Appendicitis, the primary etiology leading to appendectomy occurs in all groups including patients with liver cirrhosis. Despite this, there is limited data as to the safety and complications associated with appendectomy, open or laparoscopic, in the cirrhotic patient. One early population based study was performed in 2000 in Denmark. Analyzing data from the Danish National Patient Cohort, 22,840 patients between 1977 and 1993 were identified with cirrhosis of which 69 underwent appendectomy (both laparoscopic and open procedures). In comparison to healthy controls, the 30-day mortality was found to be 9% in patients with cirrhosis compared to 0.7% in controls [11]. Furthering this line of study, Tsugawa et al. compared patients undergoing open vs. laparoscopic appendectomy. 40 patients with cirrhosis underwent appendectomy. 25 underwent open surgery and 15 underwent laparoscopic appendectomy. Complications including bleeding and wound infections were decreased in the laparoscopic group. The investigators noted as well a decrease in hospital length of stay and decreased pain in the laparoscopic group. Despite these relatively small numbers, this represents the largest group of patients with cirrhosis undergoing appendectomy in the literature [12].

The literature for laparoscopic colectomy is similarly restricted, represented by a few small case series. In one of largest series to date Martinez et al. reviewed their 10 year experience of laparoscopic colorectal surgeries performed and identified 17 patients with cirrhosis. Twelve were Childs' A and 5 were Childs' B cirrhotics. Morbidity rates were 29%, [13] which was similar to the 30–48% rates seen in other groups [14, 15]. As with similar procedures, a correlation between MELD score and post-operative morbidity and mortality has been demonstrated highlighting once again the importance of careful patient selection in cirrhotics undergoing any surgical procedure [16].

## Obesity Surgery

Liver cirrhosis is a known complication of long term untreated obesity. Nonalcoholic fatty liver disease (NAFLD) and nonalcoholic steatohepatitis (NASH) are rapidly increasingly causes of liver disease in the obese population. The rates of NAFLD and NASH are estimated to be as high as 46% and 12% of the US population [17]. Increasingly, this has led to an increase in liver transplantation for NASH. Indeed,

NASH over the first decade of the century increased from 1.2% of liver transplants to 9.7%, ranking it third behind only hepatitis C and alcohol related liver disease [18]. Some have projected that these processes will become the leading cause of liver transplant in the United States by 2025 [19].

Laparoscopic bariatric surgery has become standard for surgical treatment of obesity. These surgeries include the Roux-en-Y gastric bypass, sleeve gastrectomy, gastric banding and bilio-pancreatic diversion/duodenal switch among others. The data of these procedures is scarce in the cirrhotic patient, typically, reports are the results of procedures performed where the patient is discovered intra-operatively to have cirrhosis. Increasingly, bariatric surgery is being considered in patients with known, early and well-compensated cirrhosis [20].

The largest early reports of bariatric surgery came out of the University of Pittsburgh in the early part of the last decade. Dallal et al. reported on a retrospective cohort of 2119 patients undergoing laparoscopic Roux-en-Y gastric bypass. Thirty of these patients were identified to have cirrhosis of which 27 were identified intra-operatively. The group was notable for increased rates of other metabolic derangements seen with obesity including increased rates of diabetes, hypertension and the patients tended to be heavier than their noncirrhotic counterparts. Overall complications were comparable between those patients with and without cirrhosis in the cohort with no significant bleeding complications or liver related complications [21]. Similarly, Shimizu et al. reported on a prospectively maintained cohort of patients undergoing bariatric surgery with cirrhosis. Twenty-three patients were part of the cohort, 12 with known preoperative cirrhosis and 11 with cirrhosis discovered intraoperatively. Surgeries undergone include 14 patients undergoing roux-en-Y gastric bypass, 8 undergoing sleeve gastrectomy and 1 undergoing adjustable gastric band placement. Once again cirrhotics had a disproportionately high prevalence of comorbidities including over 80% having diabetes and hypertension [22]. Outcomes in both the Dallal et al. study and Schimizi et al. highlight low complications rates achievable with laparoscopic bariatric surgery in the cirrhotic patient though it is important to note that all of these patients were well-compensated cirrhotics.

While laparoscopic bariatric surgery may be safe and have utility in select well-compensated patients, an interesting corollary to this is whether bariatric surgery may be helpful in improving the status of the ailing liver and thus stave off the progression to liver failure and cirrhosis before they take hold. In another report out of University of Pittsburgh, Mattar et al. reviewed 70 patients undergoing laparoscopic bariatric surgery with NAFLD in varying degrees from steatosis to more advanced fibrosis. Liver biopsy was performed at the time of surgery and repeat biopsy performed 15 ± 9 months after surgery. Steatosis dropped from 88% to 8%, inflammation from 23% to 2% and fibrosis from 37% to 13% all of which were significant changes. Overall grade of liver disease dropped in 82% of the cohort and stage improved in 39% of the patients [23].

Endoluminal bariatric procedures hold potential for patients who might otherwise be unable to undergo laparoscopic or open bariatric procedures but who are still in need of an effective weight loss procedure. Such techniques include endoluminal vertical gastroplasty, transoral gastroplasty, transoral endoscopic balloon placement. Currently the only technique with any reports in cirrhotic patients include the intragastric balloon in a small series of six patients. Choudhary et al. described six patients with decompensated cirrhosis awaiting liver transplant. The balloon was endoscopically inserted to allow for weight loss during the pretransplant period in hopes of maximizing the patients preliver transplant status [24]. While data for endoscopic balloon shows that it is not nearly as effective as other surgical modalities in promoting weight loss [25], it would be an interesting option for those unable or unwilling to undergo traditional weight loss surgeries.

## Endoscopy

Endoscopy is a mainstay in the treatment of the cirrhotic patient. Esophageal variceal bleeding, a prime cause of morbidity and mortality in the cirrhotic patient, are most often controlled endoscopically via banding, sclerotherapy or other endoscopically delivered interventions. Endoscopic variceal ligation has a role in the treatment of esophageal bleeding as well as prophylaxis to prevent bleeding in high-risk patient [26, 27]. Overall, outcomes from such interventions yield excellent outcomes with low complication rates. In one representative study of 300 patients with liver cirrhosis who underwent screening for esophageal varices, 101 patients underwent 259 bandings of which there were three episodes of post banding hemorrhage and one mild stricture of the esophagus [27].

While endoscopy itself is well established in the treatment of cirrhosis, especially with esophageal varices, there is less data for more complex treatments and interventions. Here we review of few such interventions.

Endoscopic retrograde cholangiopancreatography (ERCP) is used as a diagnostic and therapeutic modality in a variety of pancreatic and biliary pathologies. ERCP is used in a variety of pathologies found associated with cirrhosis. It has a diagnostic and therapeutic role in everything from the treatment of sclerosing cholangitis, to evaluation of pancreatic parenchyma if often co-existent chronic pancreatitis in alcoholic cirrhosis [28, 29]. In a recent review of the national inpatient sample for 2009, 1970 patients with a diagnosis of cirrhosis and undergoing ERCP were compared to a control group of 5790 randomly selected patients undergoing ERCP. Cirrhotics were more likely to have post ERCP bleeding (2.3% vs. 1.0%), pancreatitis (8.3% vs. 5.5%) compared to controls. Additionally, amongst cirrhotic patients undergoing ERCP, there were higher rates of bacterial peritonitis than those simply undergoing endoscopy (2.2 vs. 1.1%) [30].

Percutaneous endoscopic gastrostomy (PEG) is a technique that allows for a minimally invasive way of obtaining durable enteral access. Cirrhosis in general, and ascites in particular, has been viewed as a relative contraindication for PEG placement given the associated coagulopathy in such patients and propensity for ascitic leak around the tube tract. Cirrhotic patients are prone to significant malnutrition and as such would benefit greatly from the option of PEG placement in select cases. Blatz et al. reported a series of 26 patients with cirrhosis at a single institution who underwent PEG placement. There were 10 deaths at 30 days (38.5%) of which 2 were a direct cause of the PEG. Additionally, nine of the ten early deaths had significant ascites at the time of PEG [31]. This series highlights the concern with PEG placement in cirrhotics and the high associate complications with this procedure. Several methods have been utilized to overcome these challenges including pre-PEG paracentesis and associated perito-venous shunting [32, 33]. There remains a severe paucity of data in these areas and despite improvements in surgical technique and instrumentation, the poor early experiences with some of these techniques will make it that much more difficult to develop good quality studies which will advance the field but not put patients at undue risk.

# Hepatobiliary Surgery

Laparoscopic cholecystectomy is one of the most common procedures performed by the general surgeon today. Cirrhotics fall prey to this disease process like other noncirrhotics and indeed some cirrhosis associated conditions can predispose patients to cholelithiasis and cirrhosis development like significant long-standing obesity. Numerous studies have highlighted the utility and safety of laparoscopic cholecystectomy in cirrhotic patients and the technique has been increasingly applied to sicker and more advanced cirrhotics. Defining the boundaries of this technique and proper patient selection is the current challenge for the field. The next chapter deals extensively with biliary disease and laparoscopic cholecystectomy so we will defer detailed discussion on this topic until then.

A disproportionate number of liver resection surgeries are performed in patients with underlying cirrhosis. Cirrhosis predisposed the patient from development of hepatocellular carcinoma, a leading cause of liver resection. Traditionally, this already difficult procedure was performed in an open fashion. Recently groups have begun to challenge the notion that laparoscopy was not a viable option in such patients.

Worhunsky et al. reported on a single surgeon series of 167 patients undergoing laparoscopic liver resection between 2008 and 2015. The patients were subdivided into those with cirrhosis ($n = 48$) and those with normal hepatic function/parenchyma ($n = 119$). Of the patients with cirrhosis, 85% were Childs' class A. While they found higher rates of complications in cirrhotics (38 vs. 13%), the rates of major complications (Clavien-Dindo III and IV), liver related morbidity, and mortality were similar between the groups. A few important caveats to this study must be noted. First, only 4 of the 29 patients with cirrhosis underwent what they defined as major hepatic resections (two left lobectomies, one posterior sectionectomy, one anterior sectionectomy). Additionally, more patients required hand assist technique to prevent conversion to open. Finally, the surgeon tended to do precoagulation of the parenchyma using a bipolar device in most of the cirrhotic patients compared with healthy parenchyma (65 vs. 15%) [34]. Takahara et al. reported a group of patients undergoing laparoscopic liver resection, both those with cirrhosis ($n = 60$) and those without ($n = 58$). Their findings also supported the possible use of laparoscopy in this population. There were similar findings of operative success and operative blood loss. Again this study has to be qualified in that the majority of patients in the cirrhotic laparoscopic group were undergoing wedge resection and not more significant liver resections [7]. In an attempt to extend the utility of laparoscopy to every more advanced stages of cirrhosis, Brystka et al. did a retrospective study of 232 liver resections in patients with hepatitis B and C–related hepatocellular carcinoma. They identified 16 patients with Childs' B and C cirrhosis. When analyzing this group they reported similar complication rates and 5-year survival between this small group with more advanced cirrhosis compared to those with less advanced or no cirrhosis [35]. A meta-analysis performed by Chen et al. compared laparoscopic and open hepatectomy in patients with HCC in the setting of cirrhosis. They included seven studies in their review including 828 patients. They found decreased blood loss, postoperative complications, length of hospital stay, and wider tumor margins in the laparoscopic group. There was no difference in disease-free survival or in overall survival. They concluded that laparoscopy was safe and had improved outcomes compared with open surgery [36]. While certainly interesting, no distinction is made to separate the degree of resection needed (major hepatectomy vs. wedge resections) or the degree of cirrhosis (e.g. Childs' class). As such, numerous questions still remain as to which patients we can safely apply this trend toward an increasingly laparoscopic approach to liver resection.

## Conclusions

As we have tried to show from the studies presented here, minimally invasive surgery, particularly laparoscopy, has data, albeit mostly from smaller case series, supporting the carefully applied use in the cirrhotic. The benefits associated with minimally invasive surgery can allow for a safe operative intervention when such results may or may not be achievable with an open technique. They may allow for less physiologic stress, decreased bleeding, and less complications in the postoperative period. As these techniques continue to evolve, we can anticipate their roles in the ever-increasing population of patients with liver disease to evolve as well.

## References

1. Csikesz NG, Nguyen LN, Tseng JF, Shah SA. Nationwide volume and mortality after elective surgery in cirrhotic patients. J Am Coll Surg. 2009;208(1):96–103.
2. Neeff H, Mariaskin D, Spangenberg HC, Hopt UT, Makowiec F. Perioperative mortality after non-hepatic general surgery in patients with liver cirrhosis: an analysis of 138 operations in the 2000s using Child and MELD scores. J Gastrointest Surg. 2011;15(1):1–11.
3. Mansour A, Watson W, Shayani V, Pickleman J. Abdominal operations in patients with cirrhosis: still a major surgical challenge. Surgery. 1997 Oct;122(4):730–5.

4. Teh SH, Nagorney DM, Stevens SR, Offord KP, Therneau TM, Plevak DJ, Talwalkar JA, Kim WR, Kamath PS. Risk factors for mortality after surgery in patients with cirrhosis. Gastroenterology. 2007;132(4):1261–9.
5. Lopez-Delgado JC, Ballus J, Esteve F, Betancur-Zambrano NL, Corral-Velez V, Mañez R, Betbese AJ, Roncal JA, Javierre C. Outcomes of abdominal surgery in patients with liver cirrhosis. World J Gastroenterol. 2016;22(9):2657–67.
6. Sauerland S, Jaschinski T, Neugebauer EA. Laparoscopic versus open surgery for suspected appendicitis. Cochrane Database Syst Rev. 2010;10:CD001546.
7. Takahara T, Wakabayashi G, Nitta H, Hasegawa Y, Katagiri H, Takeda D, Makabe K, Sasaki A. Laparoscopic liver resection for hepatocellular carcinoma with cirrhosis in a single institution. Hepatobiliary Surg Nutr. 2015;4(6):398–405.
8. Braga M, Vignali A, Gianotti L, Zuliani W, Radaelli G, Gruarin P, Dellabona P, et al. Laparoscopic versus open colorectal surgery: a randomized trial on short-term outcome. Ann Surg. 236:759–67.
9. Dwivedi A, Chahin F, Agrawal S, Chau WY, Tootla A, Tootla F, Silva YJ. Laparoscopic colectomy vs. open colectomy for sigmoid diverticular disease. Dis Colon Rectum. 45:1309–15.
10. Delis S, Bakoyiannis A, Madariaga J, Bramis J, Tassopoulos N, Dervenis C. Laparoscopic cholecystectomy in cirrhotic patients: the value of MELD score and Child-Pugh classification in predicting outcome. Surg Endosc. 2010;24(2):407–12.
11. Poulsen TL, Thulstrup AM, Sørensen HT, Vilstrup H. Appendicectomy and perioperative mortality in patients with liver cirrhosis. Br J Surg. 2000;87(12):1664–5.
12. Tsugawa K, Koyanagi N, Hashizume M, Tomikawa M, Ayukawa K, Akahoshi K, Sugimachi K. A comparison of an open and laparoscopic appendectomy for patients with liver cirrhosis. Surg Laparosc Endosc Percutan Tech. 2001;11(3):189–94.
13. Martínez JL, Rivas H, Delgado S, Castells A, Pique JM, Lacy AM. Laparoscopic-assisted colectomy in patients with liver cirrhosis. Surg Endosc. 2004;18(7):1071–4.
14. Garrison RN, Cryer HM, Howard DA, Polk Jr HC. Clarification of risk factors for abdominal operations in patients with hepatic cirrhosis. Ann Surg. 199:648–55.
15. Metcalf AM, Dozois RR, Wolff BG, Beart Jr RW. The surgical risk of colectomy in patients with cirrhosis. Dis Colon Rectum. 1987;30:529–31.
16. Hedrick TL, Swenson BR, Friel CM. Model for End-stage Liver Disease (MELD) in predicting postoperative mortality of patients undergoing colorectal surgery. Am Surg. 2013;79(4):347–52.
17. Petros Z, Eberhard LR. Liver transplantation and non-alcoholic fatty liver disease. World J Gastroenterol. 2014;20(42):15532–8.
18. Charlton MR, Burns JM, Pedersen RA, Watt KD, Heimbach JK, Dierkhising RA. Frequency and outcomes of liver transplantation for nonalcoholic steatohepatitis in the United States. Gastroenterology. 2011;141:1249–53.
19. Reino DC, Weigle KE, Dutson EP, Bodzin AS, Lunsford KE, Busuttil RW. Liver transplantation and sleeve gastrectomy in the medically complicated obese: new challenges on the horizon. World J Hepatol. 2015;7(21):2315–8.
20. Pestana L, Swain J, Dierkhising R, Kendrick ML, Kamath PS, Watt KD. Bariatric surgery in patients with cirrhosis with and without portal hypertension: a single-center experience. Mayo Clin Proc. 2015;90(2):209–15.
21. Dallal RM, Mattar SG, Lord JL, Watson AR, Cottam DR, Eid GM, Hamad G, Rabinovitz M, Schauer PR. Results of laparoscopic gastric bypass in patients with cirrhosis. Obes Surg. 2004;14(1):47–53.
22. Shimizu H, Phuong V, Maia M, Kroh M, Chand B, Schauer PR, Brethauer SA. Bariatric surgery in patients with liver cirrhosis. Surg Obes Relat Dis. 2013;9(1):1–6.
23. Mattar SG, Velcu LM, Rabinovitz M, Demetris AJ, Krasinskas AM, Barinas-Mitchell E, Eid GM, Ramanathan R, Taylor DS, Schauer PR. Surgically-induced weight loss significantly improves nonalcoholic fatty liver disease and the metabolic syndrome. Ann Surg. 2005;242(4):610–7.

24. Choudhary NS, Puri R, Saraf N, Saigal S, Kumar N, Rai R, Rastogi A, Goja S, Bhangui P, Ramchandra SK, Raut V, Sud R, Soin A. Intragastric balloon as a novel modality for weight loss in patients with cirrhosis and morbid obesity awaiting liver transplantation. Indian J Gastroenterol. 2016;35:113–6.
25. Imaz I, Martínez-Cervell C, García-Alvarez EE, Sendra-Gutiérrez JM, González-Enríquez J. Safety and effectiveness of the intragastric balloon for obesity. A meta-analysis Obes Surg. 2008;18:841–6.
26. Imperiale TF, Chalasani N. A meta-analysis of endoscopic variceal ligation for primary prophylaxis of esophageal variceal bleeding. Hepatology. 2001;33:802–7.
27. Lim EJ, Gow PJ, Angus PW. Endoscopic variceal ligation for primary prophylaxis of esophageal variceal hemorrhage in pre-liver transplant patients. Liver Transpl. 2009;15(11):1508–13.
28. De Vries B, Weersma RK. Endoscopic assessment of primary sclerosing cholangitis. Endoscopic assessment of primary sclerosing cholangitis. Minerva Gastroenterol Dietol. 2016;62(1):49–62.
29. Hastier P, Buckley MJ, Francois E, Peten EP, Dumas R, Caroli-Bosc FX, Delmont JP. A prospective study of pancreatic disease in patients with alcoholic cirrhosis: comparative diagnostic value of ERCP and EUS and long-term significance of isolated parenchymal abnormalities. Gastrointest Endosc. 1999 Jun;49(6):705–9.
30. Inamdar S, Berzin TM, Berkowitz J, Sejapl DV, Sawhney MS, Chutanni R, Pleskow DK, Trindade AJ. Decompensated cirrhosis may be a risk factor for adverse events in endoscopic retrograde cholangiopancreatography. Liver Int. 2016;36:1457–63.
31. Baltz JG, Argo CK, Al-Osaimi AM, Northup PG. Mortality after percutaneous endoscopic gastrostomy in patients with cirrhosis: a case series. Gastrointest Endosc. 2010;72(5):1072–5.
32. Moriwaki Y, Otani J, Okuda J, Niwano T, Sawada Y, Nitta T, Ohshima C. Successful nutritional support for a dysphagic patient with massive cirrhotic ascites and intrathoracic stomach using percutaneous endoscopic gastrostomy (PEG). Nutrition. 2014;30(11–12):1456–9.
33. Lee MJ, Saini S, Brink JA, Morrison MC, Hahn PF, Mueller PR. Malignant small bowel obstruction and ascites: not a contraindication to percutaneous gastrostomy. Clin Radiol. 1991;44:332–4.
34. Worhunsky DJ, Dua MM, Tran TB, Siu B, Poultsides GA, Norton JA, Visser BC. Laparoscopic hepatectomy in cirrhotics: safe if you adjust technique. Surg Endosc. 2016;19; 4307–14.
35. Brytska N, Han HS, Shehta A, Yoon YS, Cho JY, Choi Y. Laparoscopic liver resection for hepatitis B and C virus-related hepatocellular carcinoma in patients with Child B or C cirrhosis. Hepatobiliary Surg Nutr. 2015;4(6):373–8.
36. Chen J, Bai T, Zhang Y, Xie ZB, Wang XB, Wu FX, Li LQ. The safety and efficacy of laparoscopic and open hepatectomy in hepatocellular carcinoma patients with liver cirrhosis: a systematic review. Int J Clin Exp Med. 2015;8(11):20679–89.

Chapter 10
# Cholecystitis, Cholelithiasis, and Cholecystectomy in Cirrhotic Patients

**Kenneth D. Chavin, Gabriel R. Chedister, Vinayak S. Rohan, and Arun P. Palanisamy**

## Introduction

Like many other ailments that can be attributed to or worsened by liver cirrhosis, disease of the gallbladder has been shown to be more common in patients with cirrhosis. While gallstones are found in approximately 10–15% of the general population in developed countries, prevalence of gallstones in cirrhotic patients can be as high as 25–30%, twice the rate [1–4]. The reason for increased prevalence of gallstones in cirrhotic patients is multifactorial, with some factors associated with the causes of the cirrhotic liver disease and some the sequelae. These gallstones can cause further complications in patients with an already morbid illness. Due to many patient factors and associated comorbidities, management of gallbladder disease in cirrhotic patients requires careful consideration in determining the best course for each individual patient. The care of these patients may include both nonoperative as well as operative interventions, where an evolution of surgical technique has proven that laparoscopic cholecystectomy, previously thought to be contraindicated in cirrhotic patients, can be of benefit.

K.D. Chavin, MD, PhD (✉) • A.P. Palanisamy, PhD
Department of Surgery, Case Western Reserve University, Cleveland, OH, USA
e-mail: Kenneth.chavin@uhhospitals.org; arun.palanisamy@case.edu

G.R. Chedister, MD • V.S. Rohan, MD
Medical University of South Carolina, Charleston, SC CSB409, USA
e-mail: chediste@musc.edu; rohanv@musc.edu

© Springer International Publishing AG 2017                                    129
B. Eghtesad, J. Fung (eds.), *Surgical Procedures on the Cirrhotic Patient*,
DOI 10.1007/978-3-319-52396-5_10

# Pathogenesis of Gallstones in the Cirrhotic Patient

There are many factors that lead to the increased prevalence of gallstones in cirrhotic patients. The same conditions that can lead to cirrhosis have been linked to gallstone development. Chronic Hepatitis C viral infections (HCV), alcohol abuse, as well as nonalcoholic fatty liver disease (NAFLD), each of which can lead to cirrhosis, are risk factors for gallstones with increased risk associated with advanced stages of each disease. Like the general population, the prevalence of gallstones increases with age in cirrhotic patients, but cirrhotic patients have a more even distribution between the sexes. The rate of symptomatic versus asymptomatic gallstones is similar for cirrhotic patients and noncirrhotic patients, with the majority of gallstones being asymptomatic [5]. Cirrhotic patients who are female, of advanced age, have a family history of gallstones, or have cirrhosis due to viral infection, however, have been shown to have greater rates of symptomatic gallbladder disease [1].

While cholesterol stones are predominant in the general population, they represent only about 15% of stones in cirrhotic patients, with black pigmented stones making up the majority [1]. The black pigmented stones develop due to a number of factors associated with the cirrhotic pathophysiology. Portal hypertension, commonly associated with cirrhosis, often results in hypersplenism, which in turn leads to increased hemolysis [5]. This, coupled with impaired bile acid synthesis by the liver, leads to the supersaturation of calcium bilirubinate in the bile. This supersaturation is further compounded by induced enterohepatic cycling of unconjugated bilirubin due to the reduced bile salt concentrations as well as alcoholic abuse and low-protein diets, leading to precipitation of the black pigmented stones.

Reductions of gallbladder motility and decreased emptying in the setting of supersaturation also play a significant role in lithogenesis. Patients with cirrhosis have larger fasting gallbladder volumes and hypomotility as a result of liver disease [1]. Edema in the wall of the gallbladder from venous congestion, secondary to portal hypertension, and decreased serum albumin are thought to play a role in decreased gallbladder contractability. Impaired hepatic metabolic functions resulting in increased plasma levels of estrogen, progesterone, and other intestinal peptide hormones (vasoactive intestinal peptide, somatostatin, glucagon, pancreatic polypeptide) also result in hypomotility through inhibition of gallbladder smooth muscle [1, 6]. This decreased motility results in longer retention of contents in the gallbladder and greater opportunity for precipitation of stones.

## Cholelithiasis in the Cirrhotic

### *Patient Presentation*

While the prevalence of gallstones is increased in cirrhotics, many do not report any symptoms from the stones. Symptomatic gallbladder disease can present in the cirrhotic patient much as it does in patients without liver disease. Signs and symptoms of symptomatic gallbladder disease need to be approached with care in cirrhotic patients, as liver disease adds additional considerations to the differential diagnosis. Postprandial right upper quadrant pain, nausea, and emesis are common symptoms associated with both gallbladder and chronic liver diseases. Spontaneous bacterial peritonitis in patients with ascites can also present with symptoms similar to gallbladder disease [7]. This necessitates the need to carefully consider the diagnosis in cirrhotic patients.

## Assessment and Work–Up

Work-up for a patient presenting with symptomatic gallbladder disease should include a thorough history and physical focusing on both gallbladder and liver disease. Vitals should be examined with added concern for patients with fever and other signs of systemic inflammatory response syndrome. A right upper quadrant ultrasound to evaluate for the presence of stones, signs of acute cholecystitis, obstruction of the common bile duct, and other related pathologies is warranted. Laboratory values including complete blood count, basic metabolic panel, liver function tests, and prothrombin time are also needed [6]. It is not only important to make the diagnosis of gallbladder disease but also to determine the extent of liver disease in the cirrhotic patient, as this plays a key role in the treatment decisions for the patient and also the overall prognosis.

Determination of Child-Turcotte-Pugh (CTP) score as well as Model for End-stage Liver Disease (MELD) is important to help determine the appropriate course of care. While there is some debate as to which is a better predictor of outcome for surgery in chronic liver patients, the CTP score (total bilirubin, serum albumin, prothrombin time, ascites, hepatic encephalopathy) and MELD (total bilirubin, serum creatinine, INR) are both good adjuncts to help decide if a patient is appropriate for surgical intervention. Surgical intervention should be considered for patients with CTP class A and B or with MELD scores of <8 [5]. Mortality rates for patients undergoing surgery have been shown to be 0.5% for patients in CTP class A and 3% for patients in CTP class B. MELD similarly shows increasing risk with increasing scores—mortality rates of 0% for patients with a score <8% and 6% for scores >8. A MELD score of 14 or greater was found to be a better predictor of poor outcome than CTP class C, for which surgical intervention for gallbladder disease is unwise with reported mortality of 23–50% and morbidity as high as 75% after cholecystectomy [8, 9].

The patient's cardiovascular, hepatic, and nutritional status need to be optimized prior to cholecystectomy. Fluid and electrolyte balances need to be corrected. Thrombocytopenia should be corrected with the administration of platelets to ensure a platelet count of >50,000. Coagulopathies should be managed with vitamin K, fresh frozen plasma, and cryoprecipitate as appropriate to reduce the risk of bleeding. Branched chain amino acids may help to bolster nutritional status and prevent encephalopathy. If a patient has continued to consume alcohol, they should be counseled to abstain preoperatively, as continued consumption has been proven to contribute to poorer postoperative outcomes [8].

In addition to the right upper quadrant ultrasound, additional preoperative imaging is of great benefit for surgical planning. Computed tomography or magnetic resonance imaging can determine the presence of a recanalized umbilical vein, abdominal wall varices, and other additional pathologies that might affect surgical approach. Abdominal wall ultrasonography can also be used to identify and mark any large abdominal wall or periumbilical varices that should be avoided. Upper endoscopy to evaluate for varices can also be considered for patients with portal hypertension. Wedged hepatic vein pressure and hepatic vein pressure gradient can be used to assess the portal hypertension. Patients with advanced CTP score or MELD of 14 or greater should be evaluated for liver transplantation.

## Treatment

Patients with symptomatic gallstones or biliary colic and CTP class A and B should be strongly considered for elective surgical intervention sooner rather than later. Emergency surgery for progression of gallbladder disease is associated with higher mortality and morbidity in cirrhotic patients, so it is potentially of great benefit to operate early prior to additional complications [8]. Early surgical intervention, prior to progression of hepatic disease, might also lessen the risk of having to consider operative intervention in CTP class C patients who are extremely poor candidates. Elective surgery also allows for better presurgical optimization of patients, which provides the best chance for a positive outcome. Acute cholecystitis in chronic liver disease patients in CTP class A and B, as in noncirrhotic patients, is an indication for urgent surgical intervention. There is however a number of considerations that chronic liver disease requires prior to operative intervention.

Patients who either fall in CTP class C or with higher MELD scores should be considered for surgical intervention for gallbladder disease in only rare circumstances. Patients with symptomatic gallstones should be medically optimized with the goal of getting them to CTP class B, where intervention does not carry as high of a risk or temporizing them until a possible transplantation surgery. Acute cholecystitis in the setting of advanced liver disease warrants admission to the ICU with aggressive medical management and intravenous antibiotics [7]. Biliary decompression via percutaneous transhepatic cholangiography (PTC) drain or percutaneous cholecystostomy should be considered for patients who do not improve, especially if the patient is waiting for liver transplantation [2, 8]. Percutaneous decompression allows for control of local infection and inflammation and may allow for a delayed surgical intervention under better circumstances [10].

## Cholecystectomy

Cholecystectomy is currently the most common surgical procedure performed on cirrhotic patients [11]. Laparoscopic cholecystectomy, with its many advantages over open intervention, is the most commonly utilized procedure today, but this was not always the case. Through the early laparoscopic era, cirrhotic liver disease was thought to be a contraindication to laparoscopic cholecystectomy [2, 7]; however, since the reports in the early 1990s, various studies have shown the laparoscopic approach to be a critically important tool in the treatment of symptomatic gallbladder disease with many significant advantages to open cholecystectomy in appropriate patients. The laparoscopic cholecystectomy has shorter surgical times, less intraoperative complications, reduced chance of contamination of ascites, and less bleeding requiring fewer transfusions [9, 12]. Additionally, cirrhotic patients who undergo laparoscopic cholecystectomy have less postoperative wound infections, wound dehiscence, incisional hernias, and a lower rate of postoperative adhesions, which aids in future potential liver transplantations [2, 12].

## *Procedure*

After preoperative imaging to determine the presence of enlarged collateral vessels, access to the abdomen is gained using the open Hassan technique with the initial port placed in an infraumbilical location. The open Hassan technique is preferred over the Veress needle technique, due to higher risks of bleeding from interrupted collaterals associated with the latter [3]. A transmural ligation technique can be utilized in the event of sectioning and bleeding of abdominal wall varices or a recanalized umbilical vein. The infraumbilical access location is preferred as this is not normally a site of variceal formation.

$CO_2$ pneumoperitoneum can then be introduced via the infraumbilical port, but care should be taken to maintain lower intra-abdominal pressures. Higher intraabdominal working pressures, in the setting of portal hypertension and poor physiological reserve of the cirrhotic liver, can lead to decreased blood flow to the liver, perturbations in the patient's vitals, and ischemia/reperfusion injury (IRI) to the liver. This fact also makes it important to gradually decrease the pneumoperitoneum pressure at the completion of the laparoscopic procedure to ensure added protection from IRI injury [9]. One of the potential benefits of the laparoscopic cholecystectomy is the fact that the pressure from $CO_2$ pneumoperitoneum helps to tamponade venous bleeding during the procedure, allowing better visualization. The surgical team must balance this fact and the need for lower working pressures to ensure continued hepatic blood flow.

Additional laparoscopic access ports can then be inserted as appropriate under direct visualization aided by transillumination, where light from the laparoscope and visualization of the external abdominal wall can help to avoid enlarged vessels. This technique is not always possible when the body habitus and the depth of the abdominal wall prevent transillumination. The subxiphoid access port should be placed to the right of the midline to avoid any recanalized collaterals present in the falciform ligament. The surgical team should also consider placing additional port sites to aid in the retraction of an often enlarged and fibrotic liver. A left lumbar port at the level of the umbilicus may allow additional blunt retraction of an enlarged right or quadrate lobe. An additional port to the right of the epigastric/subxiphoid port may also be useful in the better retraction of a difficult right lobe. The surgical team might also find retraction of the duodenum useful in better visualization.

Once adequate access to the abdomen is gained, it is important to carefully assess the intra-abdominal theater. One of the benefits of utilizing the laparoscope is that it allows for magnification of the surgical field [3]. This helps facilitate evaluation for enlarged collaterals in the gallbladder bed, omental adhesions to the gallbladder, and in the porta hepatis, as well as aberrant anatomy that can make dissection treacherous. The conversion to open rate for laparoscopic cholecystectomy is documented as anywhere from 0% to 15.7% [9], and is largely contributed to the above-listed difficulties. Indications for conversion to an open procedure include bleeding that cannot be controlled laparoscopically, inability to define anatomy, and uncertainty of safety. If, for any reason, the surgical team has doubts about completing via the laparoscopic approach, conversion should be considered.

It is not uncommon for portal hypertension and chronic liver disease to result in neovascularity, pericholecystic fibrosis, and/or inflammation in the hilar region, which can make careful dissection and identification of structures in the critical view difficult. In this event, a dome-down or fundus-first dissection technique can be utilized. This technique allows for dissection, while ensuring the safety of any large collaterals in the porta hepatis. On occasions when dome-down approach fails to provide for safe dissection, subtotal cholecystectomy should be considered. Laparoscopic subtotal cholecystectomy (LSC) has been described with three variations, each designed to address different variables in presentation encountered during cholecystectomy in cirrhotic patients. LSC I, accomplished by gallbladder removal while leaving the posterior wall of the gallbladder in place, is employed for increased vascularity in the gallbladder bed. LSC II, division of the infundibulum, is used when identification of critical anatomy in the hilar region is difficult or uncertain, making dissection impossible. Finally, LSC III is the combination of LSC I and II. Care should be taken to perform mucosectomy or electrofulguration of mucosa and to retrieve any spilled stones and suction-irrigate spilled bile as to prevent infectious seeding of ascitic fluid.

The need for meticulous hemostasis during cholecystectomy in cirrhotic patients is paramount. There are a number of adjuncts that allow the surgical team to accomplish this as best as possible. Utilization of harmonic ACE shears (Ethicon Endo-Surgery, Cincinnati, OH) to accomplish dissection during laparoscopic cholecystectomy in cirrhotic patients has been shown to result in less blood loss, shorter operative times, and prevention of postoperative bile leakage [4]. Harmonic shears are also very useful during LSC to help seal the transected stump and reduce bile and stone spillage into the abdomen. Utilizing surgical clips, in addition to the harmonic shears, was also shown to decrease morbidity rates from 15–35% to 8.3–25% when clips were utilized [11]. The use of Argon beam coagulation, thrombin spray, and Gelfoam (Pfizer, New York, NY) can also assist in ensuring hemostasis.

Use of surgical drain following cholecystectomy remains a controversial issue. While many prefer to not leave drains in cirrhotic patients due to concern for increased ascites and secondary spontaneous bacterial peritonitis, there are some that advocate placement of a drain. If there is concern for bleeding and/or bile leakage at the end of the cholecystectomy, placement of a drain may be warranted. In this event, it is advised to remove the drain within 24–48 h to attempt to prevent further associated complications.

At the conclusion of the laparoscopic cholecystectomy, care should be taken to achieve hemostasis, remove all spilled stones, and irrigate and suction out as much spilled bile as possible. Port sites should be removed under direct visualization utilizing the laparoscope to ensure lack of bleeding, and should be closed using nonabsorbable suture to prevent leakage of ascites [6]. Pneumoperitoneum should be gradually relieved to prevent any further exacerbation of ischemia and reperfusion injury to the liver. Any ascitic fluid that was evacuated in order to perform the surgical procedure can be replaced with albumin.

While laparoscopic cholecystectomy is appropriate and can be successful in treating gallbladder disease in many cirrhotic patients, there are indications for either primary open cholecystectomy or conversion to open cholecystectomy after an attempted laparoscopic approach. Patients with suspected or known gallbladder cancer, or inability to tolerate pnuemoperitoneum due to hemodynamic instability or cardiopulmonary comorbidities, are candidates for primary open cholecystectomy. Conversion from laparoscopic to open cholecystectomy should be considered when scar tissue from previous upper abdominal surgery precludes safe dissection, Mirrizi syndrome obscures anatomy, anatomy is unidentifiable via a laparoscopic approach, or bleeding is uncontrollable laparoscopically. Open cholecystectomy can be performed by either the top–down, fundus-first method, or the bottom–up technique. The top–down method is particularly useful when there are enlarged vessels in the porta hepatis.

The most common postoperative complication following laparoscopic cholecystectomy in cirrhotic patients is reported to be infections, and accounted for 36% of the morbidity from the procedure [6]. Decompensation secondary to chronic liver disease and the stress from the surgical procedure are also of concern; however, patients undergoing laparoscopic cholecystectomy have been shown to have either no change or mild elevations of CTP scores, which speaks to the safety of the procedure in cirrhotic patients [5]. Other complications similar in nature to ones suffered by noncirrhotics, such as postoperative bile leaks, can be managed by endoscopic retrograde cholangiopancreatography and stenting or other appropriate interventions.

# References

1. Acalovschi M. Gallstones in patients with liver cirrhosis: incidence, etiology, clinical and therapeutical aspects. World J Gastroenterol. 2014;20(23):7277–85.
2. Lledo JB, et al. Laparoscopic cholecystectomy and liver cirrhosis. Surg Laparosc Endosc Percutan Tech. 2011;21(6):391–5.
3. McGillicuddy JW, et al. Is cirrhosis a contraindication to laparoscopic cholecystectomy? Am Surg. 2015;81(1):52–5.

4. Bessa SS, et al. Laparoscopic cholecystectomy in cirrhotics: a prospective randomized study comparing the conventional diathermy and the harmonic scalpel for gallbladder dissection. J Laparoendosc Adv Surg Tech A. 2011;21(1):1–5.
5. Hamad MA, et al. Laparoscopic versus open cholecystectomy in patients with liver cirrhosis: a prospective, randomized study. J Laparoendosc Adv Surg Tech A. 2010;20(5):405–9.
6. Quillin 3rd RC, et al. Laparoscopic cholecystectomy in the cirrhotic patient: predictors of outcome. Surgery. 2013;153(5):634–40.
7. Nguyen KT, et al. Cirrhosis is not a contraindication to laparoscopic cholecystectomy: results and practical recommendations. HPB (Oxford). 2011;13(3):192–7.
8. Bhangui P, et al. Assessment of risk for non-hepatic surgery in cirrhotic patients. J Hepatol. 2012;57(4):874–84.
9. Machado NO. Laparoscopic cholecystectomy in cirrhotics. JSLS. 2012;16(3):392–400.
10. Yao Z, et al. Delayed laparoscopic cholecystectomy is safe and effective for acute severe calculous cholecystitis in patients with advanced cirrhosis: a single center experience. Gastroenterol Res Pract. 2014;2014:178908.
11. de Goede B, et al. Morbidity and mortality related to non-hepatic surgery in patients with liver cirrhosis: a systematic review. Best Pract Res Clin Gastroenterol. 2012;26(1):47–59.
12. Poggio JL, et al. A comparison of laparoscopic and open cholecystectomy in patients with compensated cirrhosis and symptomatic gallstone disease. Surgery. 2000;127(4):405–11.

# Chapter 11
# Pancreatic Surgery in Patients with Cirrhosis

Nelson A. Royall and R. Matthew Walsh

**Objectives**
1. To develop an understanding of the considerations for management of pancreatic malignancies in the setting of cirrhosis or prior liver transplantation
2. To develop an understanding of the role of surgery and methods for selectively applying surgery to maximize overall and disease-specific survival for patients with cirrhosis or prior liver transplantation in the setting of pancreatic malignancies
3. To describe the relative frequency of incidental pancreatic cystic lesions and how to apply existing management algorithms to the population of patients with cirrhosis and prior liver transplantation
4. To describe the management principles for chronic pancreatitis in the setting of cirrhosis or prior liver transplantation and the selective indications for surgical interventions

## Introduction

Surgical management of pancreatic disease is a challenging aspect of surgical practice. Even among experienced high-volume surgeons, complications and mortalities occur with a greater frequency than for most other operations in

N.A. Royall, MD
Cleveland Clinic Foundation, Cleveland, OH 44195, USA

R.M. Walsh, MD (✉)
Department of General Surgery, Academic Department of Surgery, Cleveland Clinic Foundation, 9500 Euclid Ave, A10-0422, Cleveland, OH 44195, USA
e-mail: walshm@ccf.org

© Springer International Publishing AG 2017
B. Eghtesad, J. Fung (eds.), *Surgical Procedures on the Cirrhotic Patient*,
DOI 10.1007/978-3-319-52396-5_11

general surgery. With the exception of genetic or hereditary disorders and some pediatric malignancies, pancreatic disease is most commonly seen in advanced age groups throughout the world. The combination of medical comorbidities, technically challenging procedures, and high relative operative morbidities makes surgery for pancreatic disease in the general population a formidable proposition.

Within the spectrum of patients with pancreatic disease lies those with liver dysfunction, not an uncommon occurrence. Underlying liver dysfunction in the general population, recognized as an incidental finding during evaluation for other diseases, is common. Unfortunately, for those patients undergoing evaluation or planned surgical therapy for pancreatic disease who are found to have liver cirrhosis, the relative risk of any surgical procedure increases and their potential treatment options may also decrease. As will be noted later in this chapter, the incidental finding of cirrhosis in a patient with a pancreatic adenocarcinoma can drastically limit the presumed safety of some promising chemotherapeutic agents. Furthermore, given the already limited practice of appropriate referral to pancreatic surgeons for resectable pancreatic tumors, the concomitant diagnosis of cirrhosis may further worsen the referral of these patients for a potentially curative treatment.

Another common situation is the identification of pancreatic disease during the evaluation or treatment for liver cirrhosis. In the most frequent scenario, those patients who are being evaluated for liver transplantation or followed for liver transplant may be identified to have changes within their pancreas covering the spectrum from benign cystic disease and chronic pancreatitis to malignant masses. The challenge in these scenarios spans decisions to abort consideration of some treatment options, for example, liver transplantation versus consideration of treatment options for the pancreatic disease at some point during treatment of their liver cirrhosis. In the rare event, some patients may necessitate concurrent pancreatic and hepatic surgical therapies. The surgical decision-making for these patients must be deliberate and thoughtful due to the relative paucity of existing evidence. Evidence for management of these patients has only developed in a limited number of centers.

The purpose of this chapter is to discuss common surgical pancreatic diseases encountered in patients with either cirrhosis or a history of liver transplantation. The specific aims of the chapter will be to describe standard therapies for these common pancreatic diseases and methods from the authors' experience in applying these standards to this unique patient population. As mentioned earlier, the overall lack of reported experiences in this patient population has led surgeons to develop a wide variety of level III evidence-based practices. The approach described in this chapter attempts to identify those patients who can be managed with traditional standards of care and those who must have a more tailored treatment algorithm.

# Main Ideas

## *Pancreatic Malignancies*

### Pancreatic Ductal Adenocarcinoma

The most common malignancy of the pancreas is ductal adenocarcinoma. This is the 12th most common malignancy is the United States with an estimated 53,000 new cases diagnosed per year. However, the mortality is disproportionately high compared to other malignancies and represents the third most common cause of cancer-related death in the United States. Unlike many cancer diagnoses, the overall incidence is also increasing over the past decade with a growth from 11.0 to 12.7 cases per 100,000 between 1993 and 2013.

The development of novel chemotherapeutic regimens in addition to significantly increased experience with surgical techniques has led to an overall improvement in the generally poor long-term survival of many pancreatic cancer patients. Historically 5-year overall survival for pancreatic adenocarcinoma was 3.6%; however, with newer therapies, this has improved to 7.6%. The most significant improvement in long-term survival has come in those with resectable localized disease which represents approximately 9–10% of all new pancreatic adenocarcinoma diagnoses. In these patients, the expected 5-year overall survival is estimated to be 29.3%, with significantly higher reported outcomes in those patients who are medically suitable for surgery. The addition of neoadjuvant or adjuvant therapies has also been reported to significantly improve overall survival for this subpopulation. In contrast, those patients with locoregional or locally advanced disease, lymph node invasion, or vascular invasion have a more limited 5-year overall survival estimated at 11.1%. The development of neoadjuvant therapies has played a particular role in prolonging survival in this subpopulation, as modern chemotherapy regimens have demonstrated newfound response rates not previously seen with historical regimens. Finally, those patients with metastatic disease represent the majority of patients presenting with pancreatic adenocarcinoma with approximately 52% presenting at this stage. Despite advances in the treatment for pancreatic adenocarcinoma in the past several decades, this subpopulation remains a significant challenge and is reflected by a 5-year overall survival of only 2.6%. More specifically, the median survival for a patient diagnosed with stage IV pancreatic adenocarcinoma is estimated to be only 4.5 months, as shown in Fig. 11.1.

In patients with underlying cirrhosis, pancreatic adenocarcinoma is more likely to occur than in the general population. As seen with cancers of hepatic origin, pancreatic adenocarcinoma occurs at a significantly higher likelihood in cirrhotic patients with alcoholic etiology as compared to other causes. In the United Kingdom, patients with cirrhosis were found to have an approximately ninefold increased risk for the development of pancreatic adenocarcinoma, except in

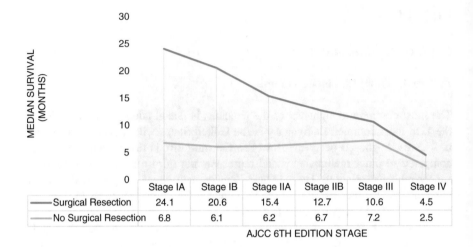

| | Stage IA | Stage IB | Stage IIA | Stage IIB | Stage III | Stage IV |
|---|---|---|---|---|---|---|
| Surgical Resection | 24.1 | 20.6 | 15.4 | 12.7 | 10.6 | 4.5 |
| No Surgical Resection | 6.8 | 6.1 | 6.2 | 6.7 | 7.2 | 2.5 |

AJCC 6TH EDITION STAGE

Surgical Resection ——— No Surgical Resection

**Fig. 11.1** Estimated median survival in months for patients diagnosed with pancreatic adenocarcinoma. The impact of surgical resection is demonstrated to be greatest in those patients who are diagnosed with local or resectable disease. The impact of neoadjuvant therapies in prolonging overall survival in those patients with borderline resectable or locally advanced disease has been demonstrated in multiple retrospective studies. Those patients with metastatic disease are most likely to have limited benefit from current therapies (Data derived from Bilimoria Karl Y, et al. Validation of the 6th edition AJCC pancreatic cancer staging system. *Cancer.* 2007;110(4):738–44)

patients with primary biliary cirrhosis who were not found to have an elevated risk. The relative risk for development of pancreatic adenocarcinoma in cirrhotics may be only partially attributable to a history of acute or chronic pancreatitis, of which the presence of chronic pancreatitis is associated with a markedly elevated risk for eventual pancreatic adenocarcinoma of 27% compared to 5%, respectively.

Three of the largest case series to date have reported on surgical outcomes for patients with Child's A and B cirrhosis with resectable pancreatic adenocarcinoma. These studies provide current evidence to support individual experiences for appropriate selection and anticipated outcomes in this population. In each series (El Nakeeb et al., Regimbeau et al., and Busquet et al.), the survival for patients who underwent resection demonstrated improved survival compared to historical outcomes; however, there were discordant findings regarding the comparison of outcomes to noncirrhotic patients. Specifically, Regimbeau et al. found that in their series the patients with cirrhosis had similar 3-year overall survival and disease-free survival (50% and 18%, respectively) compared to noncirrhotic patients (44% and 34%, respectively). In contrast, the series by El Nakeeb reported a decreased 3-year survival in the cirrhotic patients of 3% versus 19% with similar median survival of 19 months and 24 months, respectively. The likely rationale for this difference is the high rate of adjuvant therapy adherence by the cirrhotic patients in the Regimbeau study of 76%, compared to 74% in noncirrhotic patients. This exemplifies the importance of adjuvant or neoadjuvant therapy in conjunction with surgery for the management of cirrhotic patients, similar to noncirrhotic patients.

## Initial Evaluation and Staging Assessment

Critical to the determination of the management of pancreatic adenocarcinoma involves an accurate assessment of the resectability of the primary tumor and identification of metastatic disease. The classification of resectability of a pancreatic adenocarcinoma is currently divided into three groups: (1) resectable, (2) borderline resectable, and (3) locally advanced unresectable. Definitions for what tumor characteristics qualify in each group have variability based upon the criteria produced from each of the three main publications on the management of pancreatic adenocarcinoma. Table 11.1 details the criteria for determining the resectability of each primary tumor from each of the major published guidelines.

The key component of assessing the resectability comes through proper selection of diagnostic imaging. Based upon current guidelines, the recommended

**Table 11.1** Published criteria for determination of the resectability of a pancreatic adenocarcinoma from the International Hepato-Pancreato-Biliary Association (IHPBA)/Society of Surgical Oncology (SSO)/Surgery of the Alimentary Tract (SSAT), National Comprehensive Cancer Network (NCCN), and MD Anderson Cancer Center (MDACC)

|  | AHPBA/SSO/SSAT | NCCN 2016 | MDACC |
|---|---|---|---|
| Resectable | No venous or arterial abutment of SMV/PV or SMA or CHA/CA | No arterial abutment Abutment of SMV/PV | No arterial abutment Abutment of SMV/PV |
| Borderline resectable | Abutment/encasement/ occlusion of SMV/PV Abutment of SMA/ CHA Short-segment encasement of CHA No abutment of CA | Abutment/encasement/ occlusion of SMV/PV Abutment of SMA/CHA or CA Encasement of CA (body/tail tumors only) | Encasement/occlusion of SMV/PV Abutment of SMA or CHA/CA or IVC Short-segment encasement of CHA |
| Unresectable | Unreconstructable SMV/PV Encasement of SMA Long-segment encasement of CHA Abutment of CA | Unreconstructable SMV/PV Encasement of SMA or first jejunal SMA branch Abutment of aorta | Unreconstructable SMV/PV Encasement of SMA or CA Long-segment encasement of CHA |

Abutment is defined as less than or equal to 180° contact with the target vessel (variable definition including contour irregularity of the vessel). Encasement is defined as > 180° contact with the target vessel. *SMV* superior mesenteric vein, *PV* portal vein, *SMA* superior mesenteric artery, *CHA* common hepatic artery, *CA* celiac artery, *IVC* inferior vena cava study should be either a multidimensional computed tomography (MDCT) using a pancreas-specific protocol of intravenous and oral contrast, or magnetic resonance imaging (MRI) using a pancreas-specific protocol of intravenous contrast. CT pancreas protocols based upon the American Pancreatic Association guidelines should be obtained using slice thickness no larger than 3 mm (goal of 0.5–1 mm), a pancreas parenchymal arterial phase and a portal venous phase, and neutral oral contrast in order to maximize the sensitivity for pancreatic masses. Similar guidelines for MRI pancreas protocols include maximal slice thickness of 6 mm on T1-weighted in-phase and opposed-phase gradient echo (GRE), T2-weighted fat-suppressed fast-spin echo (FSE), and diffusion-weighted imaging (DWI), as well as 2–3 mm thickness for pre- and post-gadolinium contrast T1-weighted fat-suppressed echo (phases: pancreas parenchyma, portal venous, equilibrium) and T2-weighted MRCP. A benefit of MRI imaging for staging is the improved resolution for subcentimeter hepatic metastases which can be most readily seen on DWI series with proper processing software. Recent retrospective studies have demonstrated the potential improved recognition of patients with these subcentimeter metastases not appreciated on traditional pancreatic CT imaging through MRI.

In the setting of combined chronic kidney disease with hepatic insufficiency, a decision to omit intravenous contrast can have a significant impact on the reliability of staging imaging. As mentioned previously, understaging due to failed identification of metastases or locally advanced disease may lead to an unfortunate decision to proceed with surgical resection in a patient population unlikely to benefit from the effort. An effort to ameliorate renal risks using precontrast volume expansion, N-acetylcysteine, or even temporary hemodialysis in selected patients should be made to allow proper imaging with intravenous contrast in the staging phase for all patients.

Other variables which have been assessed to attempt to improve accurate preoperative stratification of patients most likely to benefit from upfront surgical resection include serum CA 19-9 and CT/PET. Serum CA 19-9 is of particular interest in many pancreatobiliary tumors due to its common production by tumors of this cell lineage. CA 19-9 is a glycopeptide which is produced in a majority of pancreatic ductal adenocarcinoma patients, with the exception of approximately 10% of patients who lack the Lewis antigen and therefore are unable to produce CA 19-9 regardless of tumor burden. Unfortunately, CA 19-9 can be elevated with a range of hepatopancreatobiliary diseases including cirrhosis and biliary obstruction. Studies which have attempted to identify a role of elevated CA 19-9 have intentionally excluded patients with cirrhosis or underlying hepatopancreatobiliary diseases to avoid the risk for false positives. The role of CA 19-9 as a decision tool in the setting of cirrhosis is therefore not currently recommended. Additionally, CT/PET has been suggested in some small retrospective series to have a potential role of identification of metastatic pancreatic disease. These studies however have been limited to a significant false-positive rate with specific false positives identified in the liver and regional lymph nodes. Furthermore, in the setting of dysplastic nodules commonly seen in cirrhosis, additional false positives in the liver would be expected due to their typically FDG-avid state on CT/PET. The decision-making ability of these adjunctive tests is therefore even more limited in the setting of cirrhosis patients and should not be used as a tool to differentiate treatment options for these patients with pancreatic adenocarcinoma.

A final consideration for pretreatment evaluation of pancreatic adenocarcinoma is the medical status of the patient. Significant experience has been gained in the surgical management of patients of greater ages and higher medical comorbidity risk within the past two decades. Current high-volume centers have demonstrated the feasibility of pancreatectomy procedures for pancreatic adenocarcinoma in these traditionally high-risk patient populations with near-equivalent morbidity and mortality. The main determinant that has been shown to be of importance in patient selection is the associated frailty assessment. Multiple methods have been described to report aspects of medical frailty across cardiovascular, pulmonary, and metabolic assessments. The ideal method to define frailty in the setting of ductal adenocarcinoma has yet to be determined. Further, in the setting of underlying cirrhosis or chronic immunosuppression for liver transplantation, the frailty of a patient may be the primary determinant for determining whether upfront surgery is appropriate. In these higher risk patients with surgically resectable tumors, a medical frailty assessment should be made to determine if neoadjuvant therapy is necessary to allow for an interval intervention to optimize frailty prior to any surgical intervention.

## Neoadjuvant Therapy

The use of neoadjuvant therapy implies the intention to proceed with surgical resection following completion of the intervention. Development of neoadjuvant therapies occurred in response to the lack of patients with surgically resectable disease and overall lack of increased survival despite effective surgical resection. The intent of initial neoadjuvant therapies was to make locally advanced and unresectable tumors surgical candidates, given some survival benefit seen with resection. Subsequent advances in neoadjuvant therapy for borderline resectable and locally advanced tumors have been demonstrated mostly through retrospective or prospective observational studies. A limitation of a majority of these neoadjuvant therapy studies has been the lack of an intention-to-treat analysis demonstrating survival benefit from neoadjuvant therapy versus traditional upfront surgery with adjuvant therapy. More importantly, the role of neoadjuvant in the setting of resectable disease has yet to yield a demonstrable improvement in survival and therefore remains limited to clinical trials.

Within neoadjuvant therapies, the main applied interventions are chemotherapy alone, radiation with a chemotherapy agent as a radiosensitizing agent (chemoradiation), or a combination of the two modalities. Historical evaluation of radiation alone was demonstrated to have a limited role in the subset of locally advanced and borderline resectable patients. The historical benefit seen in initial studies evaluating chemoradiation has more recently been questioned compared to the survival benefit seen with chemotherapy alone. In combined regimens of chemotherapy followed by chemoradiation, there has yet to be a demonstrated clear survival benefit by the addition of chemoradiation. Specifically, as applied to those patients with cirrhosis, the consideration for radiation field reduction and potential hepatotoxicity must be accounted for. Without a clear survival benefit and potential significant risk beyond those patients with well-compensated Child's A cirrhosis, the use of chemoradiation should likely be avoided unless a clear benefit can be demonstrated.

A major development for neoadjuvant therapies has been seen in recent years with modified FOLFIRINOX regimens to borderline resectable and locally advanced populations. The modified FOLFIRINOX regimen relies on a 25% dose reduction of irinotecan and 5-FU to reduce the high toxicity of the initial FOLFIRINOX regimens utilized in the study of metastatic pancreatic adenocarcinoma patients. Despite this dose reduction, the associated hepatotoxicity of irinotecan and oxaliplatin generally prevents the use of this regimen to cirrhotic patients beyond those with well-compensated Child's A class. Use of the modified FOLFIRINOX regimen in previously transplanted patients has not been evaluated to date, although the potential application would seem safe from a toxicity standpoint. Given the absence of alternative highly active chemotherapy regimens, the use of FOLFIRINOX may be warranted despite these hypothetical risks of liver injury. Another current regimen which has recently been demonstrated to yield significant survival advantages is the gemcitabine and nab-paclitaxel regimen. This regimen was demonstrated in the metastatic setting to improve overall survival from 6.6 months to 8.7 months in the MPACT trial and has also been extrapolated to the neoadjuvant setting more recently. Current evidence for this regimen in neoadjuvant setting is currently in development with ongoing studies to evaluate its efficacy. However, given the lack of underlying hepatotoxicity associated with gemcitabine and nab-paclitaxel, the use of this regimen may be preferred in the cirrhotic and liver transplantation population for neoadjuvant therapy.

Overall patients with borderline resectable or locally advanced pancreatic adenocarcinoma clearly have a survival benefit to neoadjuvant chemotherapy and possibly the addition of chemoradiation in well-selected patients. As has been shown, the implementation of neoadjuvant therapy is associated with an elevated likelihood to complete systemic and surgical therapies compared to upfront surgery. This benefit in particular is useful for those with cirrhosis who are prone to additional hepatic decompensation following a pancreatoduodenectomy, given the underlying perioperative risk for decompensation as well as progressive hepatic insufficiency from protein malabsorption associated with the reconstruction. As newer studies attempt to evaluate the benefit of patients with resectable pancreatic adenocarcinoma treated with modern neoadjuvant regimens, this pathway and its associated benefits may aid in the treatment of those cirrhosis patients who otherwise would be capable of undergoing surgical resection, but unfit to complete adjuvant therapy to yield the greatest survival benefit.

## *Pancreatectomy Procedures*

Surgical management for pancreatic adenocarcinoma should be attempted in patients with resectable tumors and those with borderline resectable or locally advanced, who are anticipated to be capable of achieving an R0 resection. Given the inability to assess for venous or arterial invasion following neoadjuvant therapies using imaging studies and the unreliability of CA19-9 in predicting resectability, beyond the presence of metastases, those who have completed neoadjuvant therapy and are medically fit for surgery should be offered resection. General considerations for surgical resection of pancreatic adenocarcinoma should be the decision to use a diagnostic laparoscopy prior to proceeding with attempted resection. Historical rates of positive liver/peritoneal findings from diagnostic laparoscopy for pancreatic adenocarcinoma were up to 21% across all patients without radiographic peritoneal metastases. More modern imaging techniques however likely have led to this rate being lower, although many consider a diagnostic laparoscopy prior to resection as an important method to prevent unnecessary open exploration and potential resection. The use of diagnostic laparoscopy therefore remains an important component of surgical exploration for cirrhotic patients, given their inherent increased perioperative morbidity and mortality.

Standard resection principles for pancreatectomy should be applied regardless of the underlying liver function, as shown in Table 11.2. The technical procedure of performing a pancreatoduodenectomy or distal pancreatectomy and splenectomy is beyond the focus of this chapter. Standard resection techniques are appropriate to apply, and attention to oncological standards should be emphasized with avoidance of atypical resections or inadequate procedures simply due to underlying liver dysfunction or prior transplantation. One challenge in reported series of cirrhotic patients undergoing pancreatectomy is the risk for a lower lymph node yield. Reasons for this traditionally lower number of nodal tissue are likely due to concern for the risk of intraoperative hemorrhage with extensive dissection. With respect to the safety of venous resection in the setting of cirrhotic patients, small series have demonstrated the safety of venous resection in the setting of cirrhosis both with and without portal hypertension. Outcomes of these patients have led to increased intraoperative blood loss and operative duration, although this is not significantly different than is seen in noncirrhotic patients.

General factors likely to be encountered in the setting of cirrhosis include both anatomical and physiological changes. Anatomical changes which may alter the operative conduct and safety of the procedure relate to portal hypertension. In the setting of cirrhosis with portal hypertension, the development of engorged portal and mesenteric veins can obscure surgical planes with an increased propensity for hemorrhage. Dissection of the portal structures and superior mesenteric vein borders, which normally have small caliber vessels, is more likely to be of significant caliber and inadequately controlled with electrodissection techniques. The underlying pressurization of these vessels may cause the caliber to be inadequate for

**Table 11.2** Standard recommendations for performance of a pancreaticoduodenectomy or distal pancreatectomy and splenectomy for pancreatic ductal adenocarcinoma

| Surgical factor | Pancreaticoduodenectomy | Distal pancreatectomy and splenectomy |
|---|---|---|
| Target margin | R0 | R0 |
| En Bloc organ resection | Rare; acceptable if R0 obtained | Possible (up to 40%); Acceptable if R0 obtained |
| Vein resection | Common; should not be combined with arterial resection | Rare; can be combined with arterial resection |
| Arterial resection | Rare; should be avoided if gross invasion | Common; should be performed if no aorta involvement |
| Lymphadenectomy | Regional only | Regional only |
| Margin assessment | SMA (retroperitoneal/uncinate) Posterior PV groove Proximal PV Distal PV Pancreatic neck (transection) Common bile duct Anterior pancreas Proximal enteric Distal enteric | Proximal pancreatic (transection) Anterior peripancreatic (cephalad) Posterior peripancreatic (Caudad) |
| Minimally invasive approach | Possible noninferior oncological outcomes Highly selected patients only Technically challenging | Noninferior oncological outcomes Decreased length of stay |

vessel-sealing bipolar technologies, which some surgeons prefer to employ along these margins. Furthermore, in the setting of portal vein or mesenteric obstruction leading to collateralization of portal venous branches, the lesser sac can be dangerously replaced with thin-walled venous structures. Entrance into the lesser sac and attempted mobilization of the pancreatic neck can produce significant hemorrhage if these overlying vessels remain pressurized. Current recommendations for patients with portal vein obstruction or thrombosis are against surgical resection, although a report on complex venous reconstruction and decompression of collateral veins has been reported in a highly selected group of 11 patients from the Medical College of Wisconsin group following neoadjuvant therapies. The implications for portal occlusion in this setting however were related to the underlying pancreatic cancer, and therefore how these outcomes apply to those patients with chronic cavernous changes is uncertain.

Other factors which are unique to patients who have underlying cirrhosis in pancreatic surgery are those relating to physiological alterations. As mentioned in other chapters, an underlying bleeding diathesis predisposes to significant increases in intraoperative hemorrhage. In a series of patients with both Child's A and B cirrhosis undergoing pancreaticoduodenectomy, El Nakeeb et al. reported a significant increase in operative blood loss as well as need for blood transfusion in the cirrhosis subpopulation. Additionally, they identified the presence of portal hypertension as a significant factor associated with bleeding and need for transfusion. When controlled for portal hypertension (median 1000 mL), the operative blood loss and need for transfusion were similar between cirrhotic patients without portal hypertension (median 300 mL) and noncirrhotic patients (median 200 mL). This suggests that the bleeding diathesis may not be the major risk factor for hemorrhage in these patients compared to the anatomical changes associated with portal hypertension alone. Additionally, the development of ascites either preoperatively or postoperatively has the potential to impact surgical outcomes. Although not specifically evaluated in the existing series on cirrhotic patients, the presence of ascites has the potential to increase infectious complications which are clearly demonstrated to increase pancreatojejunostomy anastomotic leakage rates. Given the absence of level I or II evidence establishing a difference in the leak rate between pancreatogastrostomy and pancreatojejunostomy, no recommendation can be made for a preference of either anastomotic method.

In the setting of prior liver transplantation, the presence of prior surgical changes in the biliary and arterial supply to the liver requires unique attention to operative technique. One significant consideration is the method for biliary reconstitution in the setting of a prior hepatoenterostomy for liver transplantation. In these patients, the absence of regional nodal continuity makes meaningful nodal staging in the region of the hepatoduodenal ligament of lower impact on overall survival. The inherent risk for inadvertent devascularization of the transplanted extrahepatic biliary tree makes this dissection of potential risk beyond the potential benefit. Additionally, if a prior hepatoenterostomy has been performed in the Roux-en-Y fashion, the need to take down this anastomosis is of questionable benefit. Unfortunately, the presence of a short Roux limb or inability to gain adequate limb laxity to perform a pancreatic anastomosis proximal to the hepatoenterostomy makes it likely to require a takedown of the limb with re-formation of the hepatoenterostomy in traditional order with the pancreatojejunostomy. In the absence of a prior hepatoenterostomy, the standard reconstruction of the biliary continuity can be performed. Adequate resection of the extrahepatic common hepatic duct with limited dissection of the preserved duct to prevent regional biliary ischemia is important in this setting. Clearly thoughtful preoperative planning in consort with the transplantation team is essential in this setting.

Surgical outcomes following pancreatectomy for pancreatic adenocarcinoma are associated with a relatively high rate of overall morbidity but low mortality. Recent advances in perioperative management, preoperative optimization, and improved centralization have likely led to the reduction in severity of complications following pancreatoduodenectomy with a majority of complications consisting of Clavien I or II, whereas more serious complications such as those requiring reoperation are less frequent. Reported mortality across all patients undergoing pancreatoduodenectomy has been reported to be generally <5%. When evaluating the series by El Nakeeb, Regimbeau, and Busquets on cirrhotic patients undergoing pancreaticoduodenectomy, there is clearly an elevated risk for serious complications (Clavien III or higher). Factors which have been shown to be associated with

**Table 11.3** List of medical and surgical factors which can be used to select appropriate surgical candidates for definitive pancreatectomy procedures for pancreatic adenocarcinoma

| Acceptable for surgery | Not acceptable for surgery |
|---|---|
| Child's A cirrhosis | Child's B or C cirrhosis |
| Normal portal venous pressure (exception in those with prior TIPS or surgical shunt may be acceptable risk) | Portal hypertension |
| Patent or reconstructable portal/mesenteric vein | Unreconstructable portal/mesenteric vein or cavernous transformation |
| Low-volume medically controlled ascites | Uncontrolled or moderate or high-volume ascites |
| | Hepatopulmonary or portopulmonary syndrome |
| | Recent bleeding from esophageal varices |
| | Uncontrolled hepatic encephalopathy |
| | Medical noncompliance |

an elevated risk among those with cirrhosis are portal hypertension and Child's B cirrhosis. For these reasons, surgical resection in these patients should be considered high risk for both pancreatectomy-related and cirrhosis-related complications. More specifically, the reported postoperative risk for hepatic decompensation following pancreaticoduodenectomy in patients with Child's B cirrhosis is approximately 36% compared to only 8% in Child's A cirrhosis patients. Mortality in those patients with Child's B was 50–55% compared to 4–9.5% in Child's A patients. The risk for hepatic decompensation in patients with portal hypertension is approximately 12.5% compared to 3.9% in those without. Mortality in patients with portal hypertension is similarly elevated at 9–25% compared to 4–7.8% in those without. Table 11.3 summarizes our recommendations for selection of patients with cirrhosis who are most likely to have an acceptable operative and perioperative risk profile for pancreatectomy for ductal adenocarcinoma.

## Pancreatic Neuroendocrine Tumor (pNET)

Gastroenteropancreatic neuroendocrine tumors (GEP-NET) are a group of specialized tumors which are believed to originate from neural crest and endodermal cells in the gastrointestinal tract. Within this group of tumors exist pancreatic neuroendocrine tumors (pNET) which originate specifically from cells which differentiate into islets of Langerhans cells. Overall, GEP-NET are a rare group of tumors with an estimated incidence of about 0.02–0.08%. Within this group, pNET represents an even smaller incidence of about 0.005–0.01%. Of all pancreatic tumors, pNET represents approximately 1–10%, although the overall incidence of pNET is increasing, as with other GEP-NET.

pNET tumors are classified into whether they produce hormones capable of leading to clinically significant syndromes. Within pNET tumors, those which are nonfunctional represent the significant majority of about 60–90%. With the increasing incidence of pNET over the past several decades, the prevalence of functional and nonfunctional pNET has remained approximately the same. There has however been an increasing incidence of diagnosed nonfunctional pNET lesions likely associated with increased imaging sensitivity and utilization. While there is a known increased risk for the development of pNET lesions with inherited genetic syndromes, the majority of pNET occur sporadically. Furthermore, even though there is a far greater percentage of functional pNET occurring in genetic syndromes, both the majority of functional pNET occur sporadically, and the majority of pNET in hereditary syndromes are nonfunctional. The known hereditary syndromes with associated elevated risk for pNET lesions are: Multiple Endocrine Neoplasia Type 1 (MEN1), von Hippel Lindau disease (VHL), von Recklinghausen's syndrome or Neurofibromatosis type 1, and tuberous sclerosis. The inherited syndrome with the greatest likelihood for the development of a pNET is MEN1, with approximately 50% developing a functional pNET and nearly 100% developing nonfunctional pNET during their lifetime.

Common to pNET lesions is the production of cellular products which aid in the surveillance and diagnosis of these tumors. Unlike neuroendocrine tumors of the midgut, a majority of pNET do not express serotonin or its similar metabolites. Rather, these tumors can be followed by measuring serum chromogranin A, pancreatic polypeptide, neuron-specific enolase, neurotensin, or protein S. Most often, the serial measurement of chromogranin A is sufficient as a marker for progressive or recurrent disease. In the setting of new pancreatic lesion of uncertain etiology, the elevation of chromogranin A and pancreatic polypeptide suggests the presence of a neuroendocrine tumor rather than adenocarcinoma, although it is not entirely specific for pancreatic origin.

There remains significant variability in the reporting and staging for pNET lesions. The best known predictors for survival in pNET involve the tumor size, grade, lymph node invasion, and presence of metastases which are reflected in most classification systems used. In the seventh edition of the AJCC staging system, however, the TNM classification for pNET is the same as that of adenocarcinoma. More importantly however are the recognition of the grading systems published by both the North American NeuroEndocrine Tumor Society (NANETS) and European NeuroEndocrine Tumor Society (ENETS) which classify tumors by grade: based upon the Ki-67 index, mitotic count, and level of differentiation. It is important to understand that with pNET lesions the survival is markedly prolonged compared to adenocarcinoma with median survival ranging from 14 to 112 months between stage IV and stage I, respectively. Therefore, the management of pNET in patients with cirrhosis must consider that the anticipated disease-specific survival related to the pNET is greater than that of the patient's underlying cirrhosis and other comorbidities without transplantation. In the setting of prior liver transplantation, the principles guiding therapy must be to intervene only on those lesions which have the greatest likelihood for eventual metastases, in order to prevent metastases to the liver which may impact the liver transplant function.

## Management of Functional pNET

Functional pancreatic neuroendocrine tumors are often identified based upon their clinical symptoms which are either a constellation of a recognized syndrome or more commonly refractory symptoms. Of the clinical syndromes, the most common are shown in Table 11.4. As can be seen from Table 11.4, the most common functional pNET is an insulinoma. These tumors typically are singular with the exception of MEN1 patients who have approximately 10% likelihood of multifocal insulinoma lesions. Unlike almost all other pNET lesions, localization of insulinomas using somatostatin receptor scintigraphy is not reliable, given that only 30% of these lesions express the somatostatin receptors required for this modality. Historically, the use of arterial stimulation tests using calcium has been suggested to be the most sensitive method for identifying insulinomas, although a majority of these lesions can be readily identified on CT or MRI imaging using pancreatic protocols described earlier. The management of these lesions is generally enucleation, given the often benign clinical course. In the setting of cirrhosis or prior transplantation, this should only be attempted if a reasonable survival is anticipated related to the underlying medical conditions and well-compensated Child's A cirrhosis without portal hypertension. In those patients not suitable for local resection, insulin antisecretory agents can be used to minimize hypoglycemia events such as diazoxide.

Gastrinomas represent the second most common type of functional pNET. Unlike insulinomas, there is a higher rate of metastases in gastrinomas approaching 60% in some series. Further, a greater percentage (up to one-third) of patients with

**Table 11.4** Summary of common clinical syndromes and their suspected hormonal mediators for functional pancreatic neuroendocrine tumors (pNET)

| Syndrome | Incidence (per 100,000/year) | Hormonal mediator | Clinical symptoms |
|---|---|---|---|
| Insulinoma | 1–32 | Insulin | Recurrent hypoglycemia |
| Gastrinoma (Zollinger-Ellison syndrome) | 0.5–21.5 | Gastrin | Pain Diarrhea Gastritis/ulcers/esophagitis |
| VIPoma (Verner-Morrison syndrome) | 0.05–0.2 | Vasoactive intestinal peptide | Diarrhea Dehydration |
| Glucagonoma | 0.01–0.1 | Glucagon | Rash Refractory hyperglycemia Weight loss |
| Somatostatinoma | <0.01 | Somatostatin | Hyperglycemia Cholestasis Diarrhea |

Overall, these functional tumors are estimated to represent about 10–40% of pNET lesions. Their incidence in patients with cirrhosis or prior transplantation is unreported, although likely follows similar to the general population gastrinoma are likely to have the MEN1 syndrome. Despite the higher likelihood of progression to metastatic disease in gastrinoma, there remains a prolonged clinical course which can reach up to 90% of patients at 10 years. Localization is more challenging for these lesions due to the small diameter of many gastrinoma tumors. However, with the development of improved CT and MRI imaging in addition to EUS, up to 75% of lesions may be identified. More recently, a somatostatin-based CT/SPECT study has been developed which has shown higher sensitivity for identifying gastrinoma lesions and should be utilized to localize the tumor as the technology disseminates. As with insulinoma lesions, the ideal management for gastrinomas is enucleation and possibly tumor debulking in the setting of liver metastases. The likelihood for metastases, as well as the ability to control symptoms using proton pump inhibitors, makes the need for surgical resection less. Therefore, in patients with high surgical risk such as those beyond Child's A or with portal hypertension, the use of medical therapy alone would be adequate. In patients with a prior liver transplantation, if there is no demonstrated metastatic disease, these lesions can likely be followed until their risk for metastasis begins to increase. This would follow the existing guidelines for those patients with MEN1 who are not recommended for resection until the primary lesion reaches 2 cm in diameter, at which time the risk for metastases begins to increase. The challenge in the setting of resection for gastrinoma lesions is the need to perform a duodenotomy which has a greater likelihood for postoperative leak or fistula in the setting of immunosuppression. Therefore, if the lesion is clearly localized to the pancreas, this traditionally critical step should be excluded.

## *Management of Nonfunctional pNET*

The presence of nonfunctional pNET lesions is of uncertain significance to those patients with cirrhosis or prior liver transplantation. The approach to management of pNET lesions is based primarily upon the size of the tumors, which predicts the likelihood for locoregional metastases. For those tumors which arise sporadically, they are often single with a variable risk for metastases depending on several factors. The ability to predict the presence of metastases in these sporadic tumors is mostly predicated on the size of the lesion, with those <1.0 cm diameter having a risk of metastases of about 4%. In this setting, the existing evidence is clear that resection for nonfunctional pNET is not warranted regardless of the clinical status of the patient. The risk for metastases increases with increasing size of the lesion and is generally warranted for patients with tumors >2.0 cm diameter, given the risk increases to >20% for locoregional metastases. The management of lesions between 1.0 and 2.0 cm is more uncertain with current guidelines from the European Neuroendocrine Tumor Society (ENETS) recommending observation for nonfunctional pNET unless the diameter is >2.0 cm. The management for a patient with underlying cirrhosis should utilize a more cautious approach than that proposed for the general population based upon the long survival associated with these neuroendocrine tumors. Even in those patients with nonfunctional pNET lesions >2.0 cm diameter, the anticipated benefit with respect to survival is expected to be low. The survival of these patients would be limited to that of the underlying cirrhosis and other medical comorbidities. Although debulking techniques for metastatic disease can be used to improve overall survival for these nonfunctional pNET lesions as with functional tumors, the clinical benefit is even less clear in the setting of cirrhosis. Rather than a surgical approach, medical therapies should be utilized in the cirrhotic population, given the inability to tolerate the significant hepatic parenchymal loss that is often required with metastatic lesions to the liver.

**Other Pancreatic Malignancies**

Less common pancreatic malignancies may occur regardless of the status of a patient's hepatic status or prior liver transplantation. Less common primary tumors of the pancreas which are not clearly related to cirrhosis or prior liver transplantation are undifferentiated carcinoma, squamous-type carcinoma, colloid carcinoma, medullary carcinoma, pancreatoblastoma, solid pseudopapillary neoplasm, and acinar cell carcinoma. The management of each of these tumors should be similar to that of ductal adenocarcinoma with respect to determining suitability for resection. Unfortunately, many of these rare tumors are often diagnosed at a late stage as well, and therefore not surgical candidates, regardless of liver status. An exception is solid pseudopapillary neoplasms which are most often seen in young females and grow to large size without malignant features oftentimes. If a solid pseudopapillary neoplasm was suspected, the role of surgery could be significant as these tumors tend to compress adjacent structures including the superior mesenteric vein and portal vein which could produce a degree of portal insufficiency independently.

Additionally, pancreatic metastases which occur rarely can occur and represent approximately 5% of all pancreatic malignancies. The most common tumors which develop pancreatic metastases are renal cell carcinoma, sarcoma, and colorectal carcinoma. Experience with surgical resection for pancreatic metastases is limited, and the demonstrated survival benefit has only been through retrospective series. Therefore, in the presence of cirrhosis or prior liver transplantation, the role of pancreatectomy is unlikely to be justified. General recommendations for patients in this setting would be for systemic therapies for primary management of their disease rather than attempt a pancreatectomy with uncertain survival benefit.

## Cystic Lesions of the Pancreas

Pancreatic cystic lesions are common findings which have become more prevalent with increasing quality of imaging and utilization in medical care. Among patients with underlying cirrhosis, the presumed incidence is believed to be similar to the baseline population, given the lack of any effect of liver disease on pancreatic cystic lesions. A greater likelihood of identification of pancreatic cystic lesions occurs in cirrhotic patients due to the use of routine abdominal imaging with similar small slice thickness through the region of the liver which includes the pancreas. Among transplant evaluation patients, the reported incidence of pancreatic cystic lesions is approximately 3%, of which mucinous cystic lesions are thought to represent approximately half. Those patients who then undergo liver transplantation are similarly likely to have an incidental pancreatic cyst identified with an additional 3% identified following transplant for a cumulative incidence of 6% among cirrhotic patients who eventually undergo transplantation.

Of the numerous described types of cystic lesions of the pancreas, most can be broadly classified into either those which are neoplastic or those which are not. Of the nonneoplastic types of pancreatic cysts, the most common are associated with postinflammatory pancreatic pseudocysts following acute pancreatitis and pancreatic trauma. Pancreatic cysts in this setting are not true cysts, rather representing either pancreatic pseudocysts or walled-off necrosis as defined by the Revised Atlanta Classification. Management of these lesions will be discussed later under the Pancreatitis section. Neoplastic cysts can be then further subclassified into those with benign, variable, or malignant characteristic. Of the cysts which have near-uniform benign characteristics are serous cystadenoma, acinar cell cystadenoma, dermoid cyst, cystic hamartoma, and Von Hippel-Lindau associated cystic neoplasms. The management of these cysts does not typically involve resection or serial follow-up imaging. In the setting of identification of these cystic lesions in a cirrhotic or prior liver transplantation patient, there would be no further follow-up or intervention warranted.

Neoplastic mucinous cysts have either variable or malignant characteristics that are more concerning. Cysts with variable natural history include mucinous cystic neoplasms (MCN), intraductal papillary mucinous neoplasms (IPMN), cystic pancreatic neuroendocrine tumors, and solid pseudopapillary tumors. Similarly, cysts with defined malignant behavior are cystic ductal adenocarcinoma and cystic pancreatoblastoma. The management of these lesions will be discussed in the following subsections. In general, the risk for a malignant process must be evaluated in the context of these patients with cirrhosis or prior liver transplantation, as the risk of surgery and potential improved survival benefit compared to that of their baseline underlying medical conditions. More specifically, the therapy must not attempt to cure a disease, which is unlikely to be the cause of death of a patient.

## Mucinous Pancreatic Cysts

Of the cystic lesions of the pancreas, approximately 30% are mucinous neoplasms. Within mucinous pancreatic cystic neoplasms are subclassifications, of which intraductal papillary mucinous neoplasms (IPMN) and mucinous cystic neoplasms (MCN) are the most common. IPMN is far more common compared to MCN among cystic lesions, representing 20% of all cystic lesions and 67% of all mucinous cystic lesions. The clinical significance of the mucinous cystic lesions of the pancreas is their high relative risk for either the development of an invasive carcinoma within the cyst or development of a primary ductal adenocarcinoma in other regions of the gland. Variable reports have suggested the possibility that the carcinoma arising from either IPMN or MCN may behave in a more indolent fashion compared to pancreatic ductal adenocarcinoma. To date, there is molecular evidence which suggests the progression to IPMN or MCN with an associated invasive carcinoma that involves different cellular targets than those of pancreatic ductal adenocarcinoma. The relative rarity of these lesions with invasive carcinoma has made definitive evidence to support a clinical difference compared to ductal adenocarcinoma hard to definitively demonstrate. Furthermore, the lack of clear definitions until the Baltimore definitions reported in 2015 for cystic neoplasms has made characterization difficult, given the prior definitions used which led to confusion of malignancy and invasive terminology in reported series. One additional concerning feature for these neoplasms is the elevated relative risk for development of a concomitant or distinct pancreatic ductal adenocarcinoma. The risk for these concomitant ductal adenocarcinoma lesions is believed to be approximately 4% for a synchronous, and up to 11% when followed serially. Typical findings for these concomitant ductal adenocarcinomas are those of primary ductal adenocarcinomas such as progressive diabetes mellitus, jaundice, or elevated serum CA19-9.

Intraductal papillary mucinous neoplasms arise from ductal endothelial cells which can be located within either the: (1) main pancreatic duct (main duct type), (2) branches of the main pancreatic duct (branch duct type), or a combination of the two (mixed type). Papillary projections within the duct are seen, as these tumors grow within the duct unless there is an associated invasive component. The pattern of ductal involvement is one of the most predictive factors for determining risk for development of an invasive carcinoma, with the main duct type having a 40–50% likelihood at the time of resection. In comparison, the rate of invasive carcinoma in branch duct is 17%. Mixed-type tumors appear to have a similar risk for the development of an invasive carcinoma as the main duct type (about 45%), suggesting a possible biological mechanism of progression of a branch duct neoplasm to involvement of the main duct as the etiology of this mixed type. Histological subtypes of IPMN are also of clinical interest and consist of either gastric, intestinal, pancreatobiliary, or oncocytic. Of these subtypes, gastric is most commonly associated with the lowest risk for development of an invasive carcinoma and also to be of the branch duct type. In contrast, the intestinal and pancreatobiliary types are more often seen with progression to development of an invasive carcinoma and of the main duct type. The type of carcinoma (tubular vs. colloid) has also been shown to correlate with both the ductal involvement pattern and the histological subtype, which may account for the previously discussed potential difference in survival for these cancers.

Classification criteria for IPMN lesions as either main duct, branch duct, or mixed is based upon imaging characteristics. Imaging findings supportive of a main duct type are segmental or diffuse dilation of the main pancreatic duct (>9 mm diameter), whereas side branch appears as a cyst with communication to a nondilated main pancreatic duct. Findings of both ductal dilation and a side-branch cystic lesion communicating with the main duct suggest a mixed type. Well-accepted criteria for standard patients have been adopted from two consensus conferences (Sendai and Fukouka). The most recent updated guidelines recommend resection of all main duct and mixed-type IPMN lesions due to the >50% risk for an invasive or malignant component.

In contrast, side-branch lesions are generally observed serially due to a limited yearly risk for development of malignancy (2–3% per year). Goals of monitoring are to identify features predictive of an underlying malignancy categorized as either high-risk stigmata (symptoms associated to the cyst, enhancing solid component, main duct >10 mm) or development of worrisome features (acute pancreatitis related to the cyst, size >3 cm, thickened/enhancing walls, main duct >5 mm, mural nodule, or change in the main duct with distal atrophy). If the high-risk stigmata develop, recommendations for resection are appropriate given the likely associated underlying malignancy. However, if only worrisome features develop while under surveillance, recommendations are for endoscopic ultrasound to better delineate noninvasive imaging findings from false-positive findings that are characteristic of IPMN lesions. Endoscopic ultrasound findings of a mural nodule, main duct involvement, or fine needle aspiration cytology with suspicious (high-grade dysplasia) or malignant cells warrant resection, given a similarly high relative risk for underlying malignancy. In the absence of these endoscopic findings or worrisome features, continued surveillance at intervals dependent on the size of the lesion with CT or MRI and endoscopic ultrasound can be continued, given a low relative risk of a malignancy.

The role of liver cirrhosis in the decision to proceed with pancreatic resection is currently uncertain. The guidelines which have been developed only recently and have not been demonstrated to lead to improved outcomes for patients with pancreatic mucinous cysts cannot be directly applied to the high-risk cirrhosis population. Predictive tools to determine the likelihood of an underlying malignancy in the setting of a mucinous cyst should be similarly applied to cirrhosis patients to allow for the most accurate assessment of risk for the patient. In the absence of clear markers for malignancy, the role of prophylactic pancreatic surgery must be balanced with the risk for decreased overall survival from the risks for major pancreatic surgery. The development of improved predictive methods may aid in this population. For example, the recent developments of combined molecular and pathological fluid analysis may eventually show an improved predictive ability for the risk of malignancy than prior evaluations limited by radiographic and cytology results alone.

Limited pancreatic resections have been proposed for high-risk medical patients to limit their overall surgical risk; however, these series have failed to definitively demonstrate a clear benefit. Of particular interest is that use of enucleation is associated with a higher risk for pancreatic fistula compared to traditional resection techniques. As mentioned earlier in the chapter, selection criteria for well-compensated Child's A cirrhosis patients without portal hypertension or other high-risk associated diagnoses from cirrhosis are likely at a relatively similar risk profile to the baseline population and can be considered for a traditional resection in the setting of a high-risk mucinous cystic lesion, such as a main duct IPMN or MCN. However, in those patients with Child's B cirrhosis, portal hypertension, or other high-risk diagnoses, these patients are more likely to succumb to complications of surgery than benefit from the prophylactic surgery. Even in the setting of an associated pancreatic malignancy, the overall survival for these high-risk patients is unlikely to be increased by pancreatectomy. Thus, the role of pancreatic resection in cirrhosis patients must be clearly defined for the patient and more cautiously applied to this subpopulation than those with traditional ductal adenocarcinoma.

In evaluating the impact of chronic immunosuppression from liver transplantation, there has not been evidence suggesting that mucinous cystic lesions have a higher risk for progression or development of an invasive or malignant component. In a retrospective study of liver transplantation patients, Lennon et al. demonstrated no difference in the development of high risk or worrisome features compared to a control population (17.4% and 16.4%, respectively). Further, in this series, the only factor associated with development of progression of the lesion was early age of diagnosis which is similar to that seen in studies on normal patient populations. Of the patients in this series who developed high-risk or worrisome features, none of them underwent resection and were alive at a median follow-up of 32.9 months. In a similar series by Ngamruengphong et al. four patients were found either initially or on follow-up to have high-risk or worrisome features after liver transplant. In this series, a single patient underwent resection with no finding of malignancy. Of the three patients not undergoing resection, pancreatic malignancy was not found as a cause of death at the end of follow-up. These small series emphasize the recommendation that resection in liver transplant patients may have limited potential benefit. Without high-risk or worrisome features and an anticipated prolonged survival from other medical comorbidities, continued observation is warranted rather than upfront resection.

## *Chronic Pancreatitis*

The overall incidence of chronic pancreatitis in the setting of cirrhosis has been reported to be as low as 3.8%. This reflects the different underlying pathophysiological mechanisms responsible for chronic pancreatitis than that of the cirrhosis. In this rare setting of concomitant chronic pancreatitis, the role of surgical intervention remains palliative as it is in the noncirrhotic population. Other therapies in the management of chronic pancreatitis are aimed at either minimizing the progression of the chronic pancreatitis or ameliorating the systemic effects of the disease. The impact of combined cirrhosis and chronic pancreatitis is yet to be studied due to the overall rarity of the disease. Furthermore, there is not a well-defined population of patients who have completed liver transplantation with chronic pancreatitis requiring surgical therapy to make strong evidence-based recommendations at the present time.

## Medical Therapies for Chronic Pancreatitis

As the primary and most important management principle for chronic pancreatitis, medical management of the disease has multiple approaches. First, management of these patients should aim to identify the underlying cause of the chronic pancreatitis before proceeding with interventional therapies. As alcohol is the most common etiology for chronic pancreatitis in the United States, a thorough history for substance abuse is necessary. Lifestyle modifications play a critical role in decreasing the progression and control of pain symptoms for these patients. More importantly, any patient with concurrent underlying cirrhosis or prior liver transplant would be strongly encouraged to avoid any use of alcohol, tobacco, or illicit substance which could negatively impact both organ systems. Abstinence from alcohol alone has been demonstrated to decrease overall pain measures in up 50% of patients, although this is oftentimes not the only pain therapy required.

Other medical therapies which are important in these patients are the diagnosis and control of exocrine pancreatic insufficiency. As has been demonstrated in post-pancreatoduodenectomy patients, the development of exocrine pancreatic insufficiency can be independently responsible for progression of hepatic insufficiency. Correction of the insufficiency resolves around adequate dosing of pancreatic enzyme replacement therapy, with a typical dosing guide of 25–75,000 units per meal and 10–25,000 units per snack as an initial therapy. Monitoring for weight stabilization, resolution of steatorrhea, or normalization of fecal elastase are all appropriate measures suggested to demonstrate adequacy of treatment. In those patients who have developed hepatic insufficiency due to exocrine pancreatic insufficiency, treatment with enzyme replacement therapy has been shown to lead to significant improvement and prevention of progression of liver disease. Therefore, in the cirrhotic and prior liver transplant population who are found to have chronic pancreatitis, identification and prompt intervention are important treatment goals.

Pain management in those patients with chronic pancreatitis remains the most important aspect of their care. As is the case of patients without cirrhosis, this population should be managed in a step-up approach to pain medications. Nonnarcotic agents are initially started for control and titrated up, and eventually the addition of narcotic agents as needed for reasonable pain control. In the setting of frequent bleeding events, the use of nonsteroidal agents could be associated with increased risk for bleeding, and therefore these agents should be avoided. A potentially beneficial strategy in the pain management of these patients is the use of a differential nerve blockade and subsequent celiac plexus nerve blockade, if visceral pain is identified. Furthermore, if central pain is observed, the use of neuromodulator agents can be used to better control the central pain component of the disease.

## Interventional Therapies for Chronic Pancreatitis

Of the interventional therapies available for chronic pancreatitis, the use of endo-scopic therapies has potentially a greater role in the setting of cirrhosis, particularly those with Child's B or other high-risk factors. Although the durability for endo-scopic therapies to either dilate an isolated obstructive lesion or perform extracor-poreal lithotripsy is limited in series evaluating normal patients with chronic pancreatitis, those patients with cirrhosis should be directed through an endoscopic approach, except in the setting of a Child's A patient without other high-risk fea-tures including portal hypertension. In this selected group of patients, the use of well-selected surgical therapies may be appropriate. Surgical interventions for these patients should be chosen with the intent to avoid large pancreatectomy procedures with prolonged anesthesia requirements to limit unnecessary surgical complications and potential hepatic decompensation.

Procedures which may be appropriate and performed with limited morbidity and mortality in this population consist predominately of drainage procedures. In gen-eral, the use of drainage cystjejunostomy for isolated symptomatic pancreatic pseu-docysts or lateral pancreatojejunostomy for well-defined main pancreatic duct proximal obstructive lesions can likely be performed with a low anticipated surgical complication rate. In the setting of portal hypertension, however, decompressive pancreatojejunostomy is contraindicated due to the development of collateral veins and a significant risk for bleeding in the Roux limb. Depending upon the medical status of a patient, the palliation achieved with these procedures can be significant and durable in relation to the anticipated overall survival of the patient. In general, the use of large resective procedures such as pancreatoduodenectomy should be avoided, given the elevated risk for complications in this population, unless there is an inability to differentiate chronic pancreatitis from pancreatic ductal adenocarcinoma.

## Conclusions

Pancreatic disease is a frequent finding in patients with cirrhosis and prior liver transplantation. A variety of challenges facing surgeons in selecting appropriate therapies for these patients require extrapolation of evidence predominately from noncirrhotic and nonimmunocompromised patients. As is the recommendation for the management of pancreatic surgery across the globe, this patient population should be centralized to centers with expertise in both the management of pancre-atic surgical disease and liver failure or transplantation. In conclusion, we believe that reasonable outcomes can be expected for pancreas-specific disease in the set-ting of cirrhosis or prior liver transplantation in high-volume centers when appropri-ately selected for either surgery or other therapies.

# Recommended References

1. Busquets J, Pelaez N, Gil M, et al. Is pancreaticoduodenectomy a safe procedure in the cirrhotic patient? Cir Esp. 2016;94:385–91.
2. Darstein F, Konig C, Hoppe-Lotichius M, et al. Impact of pancreatic comorbidities in patients with end-stage liver disease on outcome after liver transplantation. Eur J Intern Med. 2014;25:281–5.
3. El Nakeeb A, Sultan AM, Salah T, et al. Impact of cirrhosis on surgical outcome after pancreaticoduodenectomy. World J Gastroenterol. 2013;19:7129–37.
4. Fuks D, Sabbagh C, Yzet T, Delcenserie R, Chatelain D, Regimbeau JM. Cirrhosis should not be considered as an absolute contraindication for pancreatoduodenectomy. Hepatogastroenterology. 2012;59:881–3.
5. Girometti R, Intini SG, Cereser L, et al. Incidental pancreatic cysts: a frequent finding in liver-transplanted patients as assessed by 3D T2-weighted turbo spin echo magnetic resonance cholangiopancreatography. JOP. 2009;10:507–14.
6. Lennon AM, Victor D, Zaheer A, et al. Liver transplant patients have a risk of progression similar to that of sporadic patients with branch duct intraductal papillary mucinous neoplasms. Liver Transpl. 2014;20:1462–7.
7. Macinga P, Kautznerova D, Fronek J, Trunecka P, Spicak J, Hucl T. Pancreatic cystic lesions in liver transplant recipients: prevalence and outcome. Pancreatology. 2016;3:S105.
8. Mejia J, Sucandy I, Steel J, et al. Indications and outcomes of pancreatic surgery after liver transplantation. Clin Transplant. 2014;28:330–6.
9. Ngamruengphong S, Seeger KM, McCrone LM, et al. Prevalence and outcomes of cystic lesion of the pancreas in immunosuppressed patients with solid organ transplantation. Dig Liver Dis. 2015;47:417–22.
10. Regimbeau JM, Rebibo L, Dokmak S, et al. The short- and long-term outcomes of pancreaticoduodenectomy for cancer in Child A patients are acceptable: a patient-control study from the Surgical French Association report for pancreatic surgery. J Surg Oncol. 2015;111:776–83.
11. Stauffer JA, Steers JL, Bonatti H, et al. Liver transplantation and pancreatic resection: a single-center experience and a review of the literature. Liver Transpl. 2009;15:1728–37.

# Chapter 12
# Hepatic Surgery in Patients with Cirrhosis: Mitigating Risk

## Feasibility, Concerns, and Outcomes

**Susanne Warner and Yuman Fong**

## Introduction

While the exact prevalence of cirrhosis worldwide is unknown, it is suspected that up to 1% of the world's population may have some degree of histological cirrhosis [1]. In the United States, alcoholism is the most common etiology, followed by chronic viral hepatitis (C or B), and finally nonalcoholic fatty liver disease (NAFLD). Worldwide, viral hepatitis remains the predominant cause of cirrhosis [1]. Patients with chronic liver disease are a heterogeneous group, ranging from asymptomatic to severely decompensated, and as such they present unique clinical challenges. Perhaps, nowhere is this more obvious than in the perioperative setting. Patients with liver disease experience poor wound healing, malnutrition, coagulopathy, chronic immunosuppression, and poor hepatic regenerative capacity. Thus, they are known to have substantially higher perioperative risks following liver resection and even other general surgeries. While liver resections in cirrhotic patients were historically a prohibitively morbid pursuit, innovations in liver surgery and anesthesia techniques in the last 20 years have made aggressive surgical management a possibility in the management of cirrhotics with malignancy. Moreover, in the era of curative medical treatment for hepatitis, more and more resections will likely become medically appropriate. This chapter will review appropriate indications, risk stratification and modification, preoperative preparation, and postoperative management and outcomes for cirrhotic patients requiring liver resection.

S. Warner, MD • Y. Fong, MD (✉)
Department of Surgery, City of Hope National Medical Center,
1500 East Duarte Road, Duarte, CA 91010, USA
e-mail: yfong@coh.org

© Springer International Publishing AG 2017
B. Eghtesad, J. Fung (eds.), *Surgical Procedures on the Cirrhotic Patient*,
DOI 10.1007/978-3-319-52396-5_12

# Common Diagnoses and Indications for Surgical Intervention

## Hepatocellular Carcinoma

Most liver resections in patients with chronic liver disease are necessitated by hepatocellular carcinoma (HCC). Up to 20% of patients with cirrhosis will develop HCC [1]. However, a healthy debate surrounds who should be a candidate for transplantation and when along the course of their liver and oncological diseases this should occur. Guidelines developed by the Barcelona Clinic for Liver Cancer (BCLC) have been adopted by the European Association for the Study of Liver (EASL) and the American Association for the Study of Liver Diseases (AASLD) as the optimal staging system and treatment algorithms for HCC [2, 3]. HCCs are categorized into stages 0, A, B, C, and D based on a combination of tumor characteristics and patient cirrhosis and performance status. Stage 0 and A both contain algorithms, wherein resection is an appropriate option provided the patient is not a candidate for transplantation. Roayaie et al. established that resection of HCC ≤2 cm is safe and demonstrated similar survival to Eastern studies, but noted cirrhosis and platelet count <150/nL were associated with less favorable outcomes [2]. Current EASL and AASLD guidelines recommend liver resection as primary treatment for HCC for patients with small single tumors, Child's A liver function, absence of clinically significant portal hypertension, good performance status, and of course no extrahepatic disease or invasion of portal or hepatic veins [4].

Those eligible for transplant must usually fall within Milan criteria (single lesion ≤5 cm or up to three separate lesions with none larger than 3 cm, no evidence of vascular invasion, no regional nodal or distant extrahepatic metastases) [5] or within the UCSF criteria (same for nodal and metastatic status, but size is single tumor ≤6.5 cm or up to three tumors ≤4.5 cm, with total sum ≤8 cm) [6]. For those meeting transplant criteria but having severe liver disease (uncompensated Child's B or C), enrollment at a transplant center will confer the best long-term survival [7]. While they are listed for transplant, bridging therapies like ablation or transcatheter arterial chemoablation (TACE) can be employed. For patients with borderline or unresectable lesions for whom transplant is not an option, liver-directed therapies can be utilized for palliation.

## Colorectal Mets

In addition to the high risk of HCC development, patients with cirrhosis are at higher risk for colorectal cancer. It should be noted that while cirrhosis is considered by some authors to be protective against metastases, colorectal liver metastases (CRLM) are still common in cirrhotics and warrant resection when clinically appropriate in terms of lesion resectability and patient liver disease status [8–11]. Unfortunately, cirrhosis can preclude safe use of some aggressive treatment strategies such as hepatic intra-arterial infusions as well as staged resections for bilobar disease if more than 60% of functional liver parenchyma will need to be removed.

## Cholangiocarcinoma

Intrahepatic and hilar cholangiocarcinoma (iCCA and hCCA), especially in the setting of primary sclerosing cholangitis, can also present interesting management challenges. Resection is reserved for Child's A cirrhotics at most centers. The Mayo Clinic criteria for transplantation in those with hCCA are in use at many specialty centers, and patients who meet the strict criteria should be referred to a center. The protocol mandates that tumors be ≤3 cm, without evidence of intra- or extrahepatic metastases. Patients meeting the criteria undergo neoadjuvant therapy, including up to 4500 cGy of external beam radiation administered concomitantly with 5-FU, followed by 2–3000 cGy transcatheter irradiation with iridium and capecitabine until transplantation. Prior to transplantation, patients undergo exploratory staging laparoscopy. Any evidence of regional lymph node metastases, peritoneal metastases, or local advancement preclude transplantation [12].

Patients with resectable iCCA or hCCA should undergo resection. Those with borderline resectable lesions can receive regional therapies like TACE while they receive neoadjuvant treatments as a bridge to resection. Those with unresectable disease or prohibitive liver disease can have TACE or y90 radioembolization for local control with the understanding that these are palliative measures.

## Benign Disease

Benign hepatic lesions such as fibrous nodular hyperplasia (FNH) and giant hemangioma are very rare indications for hepatic surgery in cirrhotics, but if and when they occur, resection is only generally considered in the setting of debilitating symptoms. In patients with cirrhosis, hepatic adenoma and hepatocellular carcinoma can be difficult to differentiate. In general, arterially enhancing lesions in cirrhotics resembling hepatic adenoma should be very carefully examined to ensure HCC is not missed.

## Surgical Procedures and Liver-Directed Therapies: Guidelines and Suggestions for Use

### Resection Versus Ablation for HCC

Outside of Milan criteria, and very early HCC, most authors agree that resection portends the best long-term oncological outcomes for HCC >3 cm in patients with Child's A or B cirrhosis, with platelets >100/nL. Controversy surrounds management of early singular HCC as to whether ablation or resection should be first line. Cho et al. performed a Markov model analysis comparing primary RFA followed by hepatic resection in cases of initial local failure with RFA alone and resection alone [13]. They found similar outcomes in the RFA plus resection group and the resection-alone group, and slightly worse outcomes in the RFA-alone group. Other authors have also shown similar outcomes of RFA versus resection and have advocated ablation as first line for single early HCC, reserving surgery for salvage cases [14]. One dominant large retrospective study detailing experience with surgical resection with very early HCC showed respective 3-year and 5-year survivals of 84% and 66% [15]. This series included noncirrhotics; so, it should be noted that recurrence rates are higher in cirrhotics, and long-term survival is commensurately lower [2]. Additional features that confer inferior survival include microvascular invasion on histology, cirrhosis, platelets <150/nL (a surrogate marker for severity of portal hypertension), presence of satellite lesions, and inadequate resection margin [2, 16]. Generally speaking, the authors advocate for surgical resection when feasible and use percutaneous ablation for tumors smaller than 5 cm who are not good surgical candidates. Ablation can also be employed as part of a management strategy for patients with multiple tumors who may need a resection of a dominant nodule but ablation of smaller nodules to preserve liver parenchyma. The authors prefer to use microwave ablation.

## Resection Versus Transplantation for HCC

The EASL HCC treatment algorithm based on the BCLC guidelines is the current standard of care (Fig. 12.1) [4, 17]. Some groups employ resection as first line, with transplantation reserved for salvage treatment for early HCC, whereas others

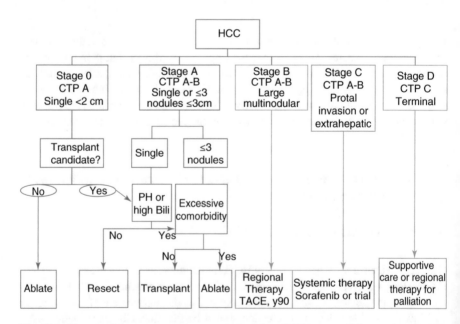

**Fig. 12.1** Hepatocellular carcinoma treatment algorithm. *HCC* hepatocellular carcinoma, *CTP* Child-Turcotte-Pugh, *TACE* transarterial chemoembolization, *PH* portal hypertension, *Bili* bilirubin; Orange outline indicates palliative treatments only

transplant first. Fuks et al. retrospectively compared resection followed by salvage transplantation versus first-line transplantation in 330 potential transplant recipients with early HCC. The study demonstrated that salvage transplantation allows excellent 5-year survival, similar to those undergoing transplant as a first-line therapy (around 70%); however, recurrence outside of Milan criteria occurred in 22% of those in the resection-first group [18]. The debate continues, and treatment algorithms for this gray area tend to vary by institution. Generally speaking, patients inside Milan (or UCSF) criteria should be managed at a transplant center, but otherwise, some combination of resection and ablation is typically employed in addition to the treatment of underlying cause of cirrhosis.

## Colorectal Liver Metastases

While older guidelines suggested that resection for CRLM should be limited to those with four or fewer lesions, and unilobar disease, surgeons are now able to safely pursue resection in both lobes in patients with more substantial numbers of lesions, provided that adequate inflow, outflow, and liver remnant volume is preserved. One study of 484 patients demonstrated that although large numbers of metastases portend poor outcomes, those with eight or more lesions still demonstrated 24% 5-year survivals [19]. Several large-scale studies have looked at ablation versus resection as first-line and second-line therapies for CRLM and have concluded that recurrence rates are unacceptably higher in the ablation group [20–22]. Thus, currently, even small singular resectable CRLM are resected preferentially even in cirrhotics. Of course, those with poorly compensated Child's B cirrhosis, or Child's C patients are not resection candidates. In these patients, percutaneous ablation is used for local control.

## Anatomical Versus Parenchymal Sparing Resections

For any of the indications above, partial liver resections in Child's A cirrhotics (or with MELD <9) with only mild portal hypertension must leave at least 40% of the previous liver volume behind in order to ensure adequate postoperative liver function [23]. Necessary functional liver remnant volume numbers are less clearly defined, but decidedly larger for those patients with more severe liver disease. Thus, parenchymal sparing techniques are preferred to preserve liver function for those with chronic liver disease (CLD) and portal hypertension. This helps enhance postoperative liver function and preserves parenchyma in case additional procedures are needed in the future. When it comes to HCC, several large-scale studies have demonstrated that survival following liver resection depends on the severity of cirrhosis and tumor features rather than anatomical versus nonanatomical resection [24, 25].

# Risk Stratification

Several scores have been developed to grade medical well-being and mortality risks in cirrhotic patients. The Child-Turcotte-Pugh (CTP) classification assigns points to five factors associated with cirrhosis (encephalopathy, ascites, bilirubin, albumin, and international normalized ratio) and assigns a class A, B, or C based on point range. The Model for End-Stage Liver Disease (MELD) uses bilirubin, INR, and creatinine to calculate disease severity. These have been validated in perioperative settings as well to correlate certain scores with perioperative mortality rates [26]. MELD ≥9 portends less favorable operative mortality [27]. The Mayo Clinic has evaluated the contribution of additional features including American Society of Anesthesiologists (ASA) score, etiology of hepatitis (viral vs. alcohol or cholestatic), and patient age in order to calculate scores for individual patients and determine perioperative mortality risk [26]. While these scores fail to take into account major risk factors like portal hypertension, they are very helpful in having honest discussions with patients and their families.

Additional features of clinically significant portal hypertension can be taken into account if the risk scores are falsely low. Surrogate markers for clinically significant portal hypertension include but are not limited to thrombocytopenia (platelets < 100/nL), splenomegaly, endoscopic visualization or cross-sectional imaging showing varices or excessive venous collaterals, clinical signs of collateralization such as caput medusa, and substantial hemorrhoids. That being said, portal hypertension alone should not be considered a contraindication for hepatic resection in cirrhotics [28]. But it should be used as a warning sign that perhaps extent of liver disease has been underestimated. Case-matched controlled studies have demonstrated that MELD score and extent of hepatectomy are the best predictors of perioperative mortality, regardless of the presence or absence of portal hypertension [28].

# Risk Modification

Etiology of cirrhosis in patients anticipating liver resection determines preoperative risk modification priorities. In patients undergoing resection for CCA or CRLM, cholestatic or intrinsic hepatic dysfunction can occur as a result of mechanical biliary obstruction or as a result of chemotoxicity from a variety of regimens. Adequate wait times from chemotherapy until surgery can allay the severity of hepatic toxicity. Thus, if there is evidence of chemotherapy-associated steatohepatitis, the authors prefer to wait 6–8 weeks until operative intervention rather than standard 3–4 weeks from last dose of chemotherapy. These recommendations are of course dependent upon patient status and regimens used. For those patients with viral hepatitis-induced cirrhosis, viral load can be associated with recurrence of HCC. Thus, the authors recommend close coordination with a skilled hepatologist, and treatment of

Hepatitis C with new curative agents or with older supportive care therapies is necessary to decrease viral load prior to operative intervention.

Operative planning always involves consideration of the extent of resection. Patients with insufficient liver remnant volume to sustain normal liver function are at high risk for postoperative liver failure. In patients with normal liver, a future liver remnant can be 20–25% of preresection liver volume. However, in patients with hepatic failure or cirrhosis, that number is closer to 30–40%. Some authors have set a numerical value of 250 mL/m² as the minimum liver remnant volume for patients with chronic hepatitis and cirrhosis [29].

Postoperative liver failure (POLF) is perhaps the most significant potential postoperative complication. Risk factors for postoperative liver failure are listed in Table 12.1 [30]. Liver regeneration after major hepatic resection is blunted in patients with cirrhosis or chronic hepatitis [29]. Careful preoperative planning, use of parenchymal sparing techniques, and ablative procedures when resection is impossible can substantially decrease the risk of POLF. Postoperative vigilance in preventing and treating infection and thromboembolic complications can also help avoid POLF. Nutritional status is a modifiable risk factor for poor postoperative outcomes. A large majority of patients with advanced liver disease are malnourished, secondary to defects in protein metabolism [31]. A growing body of literature supports perioperative care pathways that include preoperative nutritional supplementation, with emphasis on protein intake in order to help optimize this risk factor.

Coagulopathy can occur via many different mechanisms in liver failure. All coagulation factors with the exception of von Willebrand factor are produced in the liver. Thus, derangement in hepatic function can directly and indirectly effect coagulopathy. Cholestasis and malnutrition can result in vitamin K malabsorption. Portal hypertension resulting in hypersplenism can facilitate platelet trapping and peripheral thrombocytopenia. Thus, supplementation with vitamin K, fresh frozen plasma, and platelets can be helpful in the emergent preoperative setting or in patients with postoperative coagulopathy. However, if an elective resection patient is requiring coagulation factor supplementation, the operation is very likely to cause the patient harm and should therefore be considered very carefully. It is important to note that coagulopathy secondary to chronic liver disease does not protect against venous thromboembolism (VTE) in hospitalized

**Table 12.1** Risk factors and modifications for postoperative liver failure

| Nonmodifiable risk factors | Modifiable risk factors |
| --- | --- |
| Age > 70 | Hepatitis |
| Male | Excessive intraoperative blood loss |
| Fibrosis | Need for blood transfusion |
| Preoperative chemotherapy | Prolonged ischemia time |
| Steatosis | Prolonged operative time |
| Diabetes | Preoperative hypoalbuminemia |
| Portal hypertension | Cholestasis |

patients with chronic liver disease [32]. Thus, standard perioperative VTE prophylaxis should still be considered.

## Surgical Technique

When possible, and particularly in patients with no prior abdominal operations and peripheral liver lesions, minimally invasive surgical techniques should be employed. Use of laparoscopic techniques for resection or ablation has become the standard of care for small (<5 cm) peripheral lesions [33]. Several groups have proven that minimally invasive surgery is safe in patients with mild liver disease [34].

Anticipating and preparing for problems that can arise when operating on cirrhotics is half the battle of a successful resection. Close communication with the anesthesia team in the perioperative setting is critical. We do not recommend use of a central line, but do require two large bore IVs as well as an arterial line in cases where high blood loss is possible. It is critical that central venous pressure (CVP) be maintained at or below 5 mmHg until parenchymal transection is complete [35–37]. Restrictive transfusion policies can also be of benefit, and these along with blood product resuscitation protocols should be established with anesthesia colleagues in advance of the surgery [38]. Some of the more challenging aspects of surgery in cirrhotics and ways to combat them are listed in Table 12.2. Generally, surgeons should be prepared for robust collateral veins in unexpected locations with the propensity toward vigorous bleeding secondary to increased portal pressure. The more prominent collaterals are often visible on preoperative imaging. However, meticulous dissection techniques should be employed at all points of dissection in order to avoid vascular injury.

Regarding abdominal entry, standard port placements for left and right robotic and laparoscopic hepatectomies have been described at length [39, 40]. When comparing open with laparoscopic resections in a case-matched study of patients with CLD, one group found that major complications were observable but not significantly more common in the open group, while there was no difference in

**Table 12.2** Technical modifications for surgery in cirrhotics

| Problem | Solution |
| --- | --- |
| Bleeding | Medical optimization |
| | Meticulous dissection |
| | Adequate preoperative imaging |
| | Expect collaterals—preop embolization prn |
| Difficult mobilization | Hand assist |
| | Positioning—use suspensory ligaments and gravity |
| Postoperative ascites | Preoperative optimization |
| | Postoperative dieresis |
| | Adequate liver remnant |

margin status or long-term survival [34]. For open procedures, the authors generally prefer a so-called inverse L-shaped incision with the option to carry the incision to the left and make a so-called mercedes incision if needed. In cirrhotic patients, great care must be taken to ligate or preserve if possible any recanalized umbilical veins.

In terms of parenchymal transection, some authors advocate use of ultrasonic dissector combined with bipolar electrocautery in cirrhotics [41]. While others note that a less tedious method involves precoagulation and a combination of vascular sealing devices and staplers for larger vessels [42]. In practice, laparoscopically, the authors utilize cautery to enter Glisson's capsule, and then the laparoscopic LigaSure is used for crush-clamp, sealing, and cutting (Covidien, Minneapolis, MN), with intermittent use of staplers as needed for larger vessels for the vast majority of patients. If a liver is particularly fibrotic, crush-clamp techniques are not as useful and can result in excessive trauma. In these instances, a combination of blunt and thermal dissection techniques is utilized, and a harmonic endoshear device is utilized. The laparoscopic argon beam coagulator is used to obtain hemostasis and biliary stasis from the cut liver's edge. Of note, both laparoscopically and robotically, Weck clips are utilized rather than metal ones in order to facilitate continued use of vessel-sealing devices. Robotically, the authors utilize similar technique, except that we are able to employ the robotic vessel sealer and stapler tools for added flexibility. For open hepatic resections, the authors employ a combination of crush-clamp and impact LigaSure (Covidien, Minneapolis, MN) for parenchymal transection. Larger vessels are divided with a stapler. When suturing for bleeding, the authors encourage use of silk material, as it does not melt when in contact with thermal cautery or other thermal vascular control agents.

With regard to hilar vascular occlusion (aka the Pringle maneuver), some authors recommend little to no vascular clamping in cirrhotics. Most acknowledge that some cases mandate use of vascular occlusion but that the time should be limited in patients with cirrhosis again to optimize postoperative liver function. Use of intermittent versus continuous clamping has been analyzed by many different authors who have reached disparate conclusions. However, the general consensus is that in terms of morbidity and mortality, there is no difference between the two techniques [37, 43]. That being said, few studies have looked at this issue specifically in cirrhotics.

The authors do not use drains following liver resection as they have been shown in multiple studies to result in increased infectious complications [44]. This remains true in resections of cirrhotics [45]. Should an infected biloma develop postoperatively, our preference is to perform interventional radiology-guided drainage. There is minimal controversy in the literature regarding drain placement following minor resections of noncirrhotic livers; however, there exists some disagreement in the data when cirrhotics with demonstrable preoperative portal hypertension [46]. The authors reserve drain placement for extremely rare occasions such as hepaticojejunostomy creation to tenuous secondary or tertiary radicles.

## Outcomes

Increased rates of postoperative morbidity following liver resections in cirrhotics are typically attributed more to poor patient protoplasm than to surgical technique. Cirrhotics have more comorbidities and are at higher risk for POLF and thereby postoperative mortality, more especially following major hepatectomy [42, 47]. POLF is an insidious problem that can result in a frustrating and terrifying march toward postoperative mortality. Because POLF following resection for malignancy can inherently not be remedied with liver transplantation, identification of patients at risk for such a course, and then making every effort to maintain perfusion and biliary continuity in the liver remnant, is critical. Several systems have been developed to identify patients who are on a course toward POLF, the most prominent of which are the so-called 50–50 criteria and the International Study Group of Liver Surgery (ISGLS) criteria [30, 47]. The 50–50 criteria state that patients with bilirubin >50 µmol/L and prothrombin time <50% (INR > 1.7) on postoperative day (POD) 5 have a mortality risk exceeding 50% after hepatectomy [47]. Subsequent prospective validation of the 50–50 criteria has verified this and adds that patients meeting 50–50 criteria on POD 3 are also at high risk for mortality [48]. The ISGLS also utilizes liver function derangements on POD 5 as a guide and further classifies POLF into grades A, B, and C. Risk factors for postoperative mortality taking all comers include meeting the 50–50 criteria, age over 65 years, and presence of severe hepatic fibrosis [47]. Table 12.3 summarizes the two predominant POLF systems.

Additional complications following liver resection in those with CLD include ascites which can result in poor wound healing and should be managed aggressively with restrictive fluid resuscitation strategies and liberal use of diuretics [49]. Not surprisingly, infectious complications following any abdominal surgery are significantly increased in those with CLD, particularly in the setting of portal hypertension [50, 51]. More specifically, infectious complications are very closely associated

**Table 12.3** Postoperative liver failure

| System | Criteria | Intervention |
|--------|----------|--------------|
| 50–50 criteria | Bilirubin >50 µmol/L and PT <50% (INR >1.7) on POD 5 yield mortality >50% | Investigate for portal thrombus and other infectious complications |
| ISGLS | Increased INR and hyperbilirubinemia on POD 5 ISGLS A—mild lab derangement from preop ISGLS B—abnormal postop course may require ICU transfer ISGLS C—severe hepatic dysfunction resulting in ≥1 organ system support | No intervention Noninvasive intervention (i.e., Ffp, albumin, diuresis, noninvasive ventilation) Invasive intervention (i.e., hemodialysis, intubation, extracorporeal liver support, vasoactive drugs, glucose infusion) |

*ISGLS* International Study Group of Liver Surgery, *FFP* fresh frozen plasma, *INR* international normalized ratio, *PT* prothrombin time, *POD* postoperative day with those experiencing severe postoperative hepatic dysfunction [52]. Whether one causes the other remains unclear, but clinical vigilance postoperatively to both support hepatic function and combat any brewing infections is critical to enhancing postoperative outcomes.

## Conclusion

Identification of the extent of perioperative risk is essential to effective operative preparation both for the patient and the surgeon. Medical optimization of the underlying causes and effects of cirrhosis should be undertaken where possible. Because of the potential for life-threatening perioperative complications, decision-making in regards to appropriate interventions for cirrhotics can be difficult. However, with a team of experienced surgeons, competent hepatologists, and anesthesiologists, patients with well-compensated chronic liver disease can safely undergo liver resections when indicated.

## References

1. Schuppan D, Afdhal NH. Liver cirrhosis. Lancet. 2008;371(9615):838–51.
2. Roayaie S, Obeidat K, Sposito C, et al. Resection of hepatocellular cancer </=2 cm: results from two Western centers. Hepatology. 2013;57(4):1426–35.
3. Forner A, Reig ME, de Lope CR, Bruix J. Current strategy for staging and treatment: the BCLC update and future prospects. Semin Liver Dis. 2010;30(1):61–74.
4. Llovet JM, Bru C, Bruix J. Prognosis of hepatocellular carcinoma: the BCLC staging classification. Semin Liver Dis. 1999;19(3):329–38.
5. Mazzaferro V, Regalia E, Doci R, et al. Liver transplantation for the treatment of small hepatocellular carcinomas in patients with cirrhosis. N Engl J Med. 1996;334(11):693–9.
6. Yao FY, Ferrell L, Bass NM, et al. Liver transplantation for hepatocellular carcinoma: expansion of the tumor size limits does not adversely impact survival. Hepatology. 2001;33(6):1394–403.
7. Iwatsuki S, Starzl TE, Sheahan DG, et al. Hepatic resection versus transplantation for hepatocellular carcinoma. Ann Surg. 1991;214(3):221–8; discussion 228–9.
8. Cai B, Liao K, Song XQ, Wei WY, Zhuang Y, Zhang S. Patients with chronically diseased livers have lower incidence of colorectal liver metastases: a meta-analysis. PLoS One. 2014;9(9):e108618.
9. Sorensen HT, Mellemkjaer L, Jepsen P, et al. Risk of cancer in patients hospitalized with fatty liver: a Danish cohort study. J Clin Gastroenterol. 2003;36(4):356–9.
10. Sorensen HT, Friis S, Olsen JH, et al. Risk of liver and other types of cancer in patients with cirrhosis: a nationwide cohort study in Denmark. Hepatology. 1998;28(4):921–5.
11. Dahl E, Rumessen J, Gluud LL. Systematic review with meta-analyses of studies on the association between cirrhosis and liver metastases. Hepatol Res Off J Jpn Soc Hepatol. 2011;41(7):618–25.
12. Rosen CB, Heimbach JK, Gores GJ. Surgery for cholangiocarcinoma: the role of liver transplantation. HPB (Oxford). 2008;10(3):186–9.
13. Cho YK, Kim JK, Kim WT, Chung JW. Hepatic resection versus radiofrequency ablation for very early stage hepatocellular carcinoma: a Markov model analysis. Hepatology. 2010;51(4):1284–90.

14. Livraghi T, Meloni F, Di Stasi M, et al. Sustained complete response and complications rates after radiofrequency ablation of very early hepatocellular carcinoma in cirrhosis: Is resection still the treatment of choice? Hepatology. 2008;47(1):82–9.
15. Ikai I, Arii S, Kojiro M, et al. Reevaluation of prognostic factors for survival after liver resection in patients with hepatocellular carcinoma in a Japanese nationwide survey. Cancer. 2004;101(4):796–802.
16. Lee JI, Lee JW, Kim YS, Choi YA, Jeon YS, Cho SG. Analysis of survival in very early hepatocellular carcinoma after resection. J Clin Gastroenterol. 2011;45(4):366–71.
17. European Association For The Study Of The L, European Organisation For R, Treatment Of C. EASL-EORTC clinical practice guidelines: management of hepatocellular carcinoma. J Hepatol. 2012;56(4):908–943.
18. Fuks D, Dokmak S, Paradis V, Diouf M, Durand F, Belghiti J. Benefit of initial resection of hepatocellular carcinoma followed by transplantation in case of recurrence: an intention-to-treat analysis. Hepatology. 2012;55(1):132–40.
19. Malik HZ, Hamady ZZ, Adair R, et al. Prognostic influence of multiple hepatic metastases from colorectal cancer. Eur J Surg Oncol: J Eur Soc Surg Oncol Br Assoc Surg Oncol. 2007;33(4):468–73.
20. Abdalla EK, Vauthey JN, Ellis LM, et al. Recurrence and outcomes following hepatic resection, radiofrequency ablation, and combined resection/ablation for colorectal liver metastases. Ann Surg. 2004;239(6):818–25 ; discussion 825–7.
21. Ko S, Jo H, Yun S, Park E, Kim S, Seo HI. Comparative analysis of radiofrequency ablation and resection for resectable colorectal liver metastases. World J Gastroenterol. 2014;20(2):525–31.
22. Park IJ, Kim HC, Yu CS, Kim PN, Won HJ, Kim JC. Radiofrequency ablation for metachronous liver metastasis from colorectal cancer after curative surgery. Ann Surg Oncol. 2008;15(1):227–32.
23. Vauthey JN, Chaoui A, Do KA, et al. Standardized measurement of the future liver remnant prior to extended liver resection: methodology and clinical associations. Surgery. 2000;127(5):512–9.
24. Dahiya D, Wu TJ, Lee CF, Chan KM, Lee WC, Chen MF. Minor versus major hepatic resection for small hepatocellular carcinoma (HCC) in cirrhotic patients: a 20-year experience. Surgery. 2010;147(5):676–85.
25. Tang YH, Wen TF, Chen X. Anatomic versus non-anatomic liver resection for hepatocellular carcinoma: a systematic review. Hepato-Gastroenterology. 2013;60(128):2019–25.
26. Schroeder RA. Predictive indices of morbidity and mortality after liver resection. Ann Surg. 2006;244(4):637.
27. Teh SH, Christein J, Donohue J, et al. Hepatic resection of hepatocellular carcinoma in patients with cirrhosis: model of end-stage liver disease (MELD) score predicts perioperative mortality. J Gastrointest Surg 2005;9(9):1207–15; discussion 1215.
28. Cucchetti A, Ercolani G, Vivarelli M, et al. Is portal hypertension a contraindication to hepatic resection? Ann Surg. 2009;250(6):922–8.
29. Nagasue N, Yukaya H, Ogawa Y, Kohno H, Nakamura T. Human liver regeneration after major hepatic resection. A study of normal liver and livers with chronic hepatitis and cirrhosis. Ann Surg. 1987;206(1):30–9.
30. Rahbari NN, Garden OJ, Padbury R, et al. Posthepatectomy liver failure: a definition and grading by the International Study Group of Liver Surgery (ISGLS). Surgery. 2011;149(5):713–24.
31. Lautz HU, Selberg O, Korber J, Burger M, Muller MJ. Protein-calorie malnutrition in liver cirrhosis. Clin Investig. 1992;70(6):478–86.
32. Dabbagh O, Oza A, Prakash S, Sunna R, Saettele TM. Coagulopathy does not protect against venous thromboembolism in hospitalized patients with chronic liver disease. Chest. 2010;137(5):1145–9.

33. Buell JF, Cherqui D, Geller DA, et al. The international position on laparoscopic liver surgery: the Louisville Statement, 2008. Ann Surg. 2009;250(5):825–30.
34. Truant S, Bouras AF, Hebbar M, et al. Laparoscopic resection vs. open liver resection for peripheral hepatocellular carcinoma in patients with chronic liver disease: a case-matched study. Surg Endosc. 2011;25(11):3668–77.
35. Jones RL, Qian YM, Chan KM, Yim AP. Characterization of a prostanoid EP3-receptor in guinea-pig aorta: partial agonist action of the non-prostanoid ONO-AP-324. Br J Pharmacol. 1998;125(6):1288–96.
36. Yang Y, Zhao LH, Fu SY, et al. Selective hepatic vascular exclusion versus pringle maneuver in partial hepatectomy for liver hemangioma compressing or involving the major hepatic veins. Am Surg. 2014;80(3):236–40.
37. Chouillard EK, Gumbs AA, Cherqui D. Vascular clamping in liver surgery: physiology, indications and techniques. Ann Surg Innov Res. 2010;4:2.
38. Villanueva C, Colomo A, Bosch A, et al. Transfusion strategies for acute upper gastrointestinal bleeding. N Engl J Med. 2013;368(1):11–21.
39. Soubrane O, Schwarz L, Cauchy F, et al. A conceptual technique for laparoscopic right hepatectomy based on facts and oncologic principles: the caudal approach. Ann Surg. 2015;261(6):1226–31.
40. Leung U, Fong Y. Robotic liver surgery. Hepatobil Surg Nutr. 2014;3(5):288–94.
41. Cherqui D, Laurent A, Tayar C, et al. Laparoscopic liver resection for peripheral hepatocellular carcinoma in patients with chronic liver disease: midterm results and perspectives. Ann Surg. 2006;243(4):499–506.
42. Worhunsky DJ, Dua MM, Tran TB, et al. Laparoscopic hepatectomy in cirrhotics: safe if you adjust technique. Surg Endosc. 2016;30:4307–14.
43. Capussotti L, Nuzzo G, Polastri R, Giuliante F, Muratore A, Giovannini I. Continuous versus intermittent portal triad clamping during hepatectomy in cirrhosis. Results of a prospective, randomized clinical trial. Hepato-Gastroenterology. 2003;50(52):1073–7.
44. Fong Y, Brennan MF, Brown K, Heffeman N, Blumgart LH. Drainage is unnecessary after elective liver resection. Am J Surg. 1996;171(1):158–62.
45. Liu CL, Fan ST, Lo CM, et al. Abdominal drainage after hepatic resection is contraindicated in patients with chronic liver diseases. Ann Surg. 2004;239(2):194–201.
46. Fuster J, Llovet JM, Garcia-Valdecasas JC, et al. Abdominal drainage after liver resection for hepatocellular carcinoma in cirrhotic patients: a randomized controlled study. Hepato-Gastroenterology. 2004;51(56):536–40.
47. Balzan S, Belghiti J, Farges O, et al. The "50-50 criteria" on postoperative day 5: an accurate predictor of liver failure and death after hepatectomy. Ann Surg. 2005;242(6):824–9.
48. Paugam-Burtz C, Janny S, Delefosse D, et al. Prospective validation of the "fifty-fifty" criteria as an early and accurate predictor of death after liver resection in intensive care unit patients. Ann Surg. 2009;249(1):124–8.
49. Hackl C, Schlitt HJ, Renner P, Lang SA. Liver surgery in cirrhosis and portal hypertension. World J Gastroenterol. 2016;22(9):2725.
50. de Goede B, Klitsie PJ, Hagen SM, et al. Meta-analysis of laparoscopic versus open cholecystectomy for patients with liver cirrhosis and symptomatic cholecystolithiasis. Br J Surg. 2013;100(2):209–16.
51. Pessaux P, Msika S, Atalla D, Hay JM, Flamant Y, French Association for Surgical R. Risk factors for postoperative infectious complications in noncolorectal abdominal surgery: a multivariate analysis based on a prospective multicenter study of 4718 patients. Arch Surg. 2003;138(3):314–24.
52. Schindl MJ, Redhead DN, Fearon KC, et al. The value of residual liver volume as a predictor of hepatic dysfunction and infection after major liver resection. Gut. 2005;54(2):289–96.

# Chapter 13
# Hernia Repair in Cirrhotic Patients: Type, Timing, and Procedure of Choice

Ivy N. Haskins and Michael J. Rosen

## Introduction

Chronic liver disease (CLD) is a common entity, affecting approximately 4.5–9.5% of the general population worldwide [1]. It is the tenth leading cause of death in the United States [2].

Despite these facts, the true incidence of CLD remains unknown and is likely higher than the current estimates [1, 2]. The cause of the discrepancy between the real and perceived prevalence of CLD is multifold but can largely be attributed to the fact that upward of 40% of patients with advanced liver disease are asymptomatic, and therefore, undiagnosed [1, 3, 4].

Chronic liver disease, and in particular liver disease in the presence of cirrhosis and ascites, carries a poor prognosis [1–7]. The presence of ascites is associated with a poor quality of life, increased risk of spontaneous abdominal infections, and renal failure [5]. For these reasons, in addition to the presumed perioperative decompensation in this patient population, the repair of abdominal wall and groin hernias in these patients has traditionally been managed by a "watch and see strategy" [5–9]. Nevertheless, recent studies have challenged this management strategy [8, 9]. In this chapter, we will discuss the pathophysiology of abdominal wall and groin hernias, the timing of hernia repair, and the surgical approach to hernia repair in patients with CLD.

I.N. Haskins, MD • M.J. Rosen, MD, FACS (✉)
Comprehensive Hernia Center, Digestive Disease and Surgery Institute,
9500 Euclid Avenue, A-100, Cleveland, OH 44195, USA
e-mail: ihaskins@gwu.edu; rosenm@ccf.org

© Springer International Publishing AG 2017
B. Eghtesad, J. Fung (eds.), *Surgical Procedures on the Cirrhotic Patient*,
DOI 10.1007/978-3-319-52396-5_13

## Pathophysiology of Abdominal Wall Hernias in Patients with Chronic Liver Disease

There is a distinct difference in the propensity for abdominal wall and groin hernia development between those patients with CLD only and those patients with CLD associated with ascites. In those patients with chronic liver disease and/or cirrhosis only, the prevalence of abdominal wall and groin hernias is similar to that seen in the general population. However, for patients with CLD plus ascites, the prevalence of abdominal wall and inguinal hernias is estimated to be 20% [5, 7–11].

In order to understand how patients with CLD develop abdominal wall and groin hernias, it is important to first understand the pathophysiology of ascites formation. Ascites, by definition, is the pathologic accumulation of extracellular fluid which is stored in the peritoneal cavity [12, 13]. The formation of ascites is dependent on the presence of portal hypertension and, in fact, cannot occur in its absence [13]. As portal hypertension progresses, the splanchnic arterial system vasodilates past the capacity that can be mitigated with an increase in cardiac output, ultimately leading to a decrease in systemic vascular resistance [12, 13]. Decreased systemic vascular resistance activates the renin-angiotensin-aldosterone system, which leads to increased sodium retention, subsequent increased water reabsorption, and the accumulation of ascites [12]. Furthermore, due to altered and often ineffective protein synthesis in the setting of chronic liver disease, the presence of ascites is further supported by an increase in capillary permeability and decreased oncotic pressure [13].

It is well-established that factors that increase intra-abdominal pressure make patients susceptible to abdominal wall and groin hernia formation [5, 14–17]. Therefore, it should come as no surprise that the prevalence of abdominal wall and groin hernias in patients with ascites is higher than that of the general population. The most common location for hernia formation in these patients is at the umbilicus. In addition to increased intra-abdominal pressure from ascites and weakening of the abdominal wall fascia from loss of protein synthesis and subsequent malnutrition, patients with portal hypertension also have a dilated umbilical vein as part of their collateral vascular system which leads to enlargement of the preexisting supraumbilical fascial opening and thus an increase in umbilical hernia formation [8, 9].

## Timing of Abdominal Wall and Inguinal Hernia Repair

The optimal timing for hernia repair in patients with advanced liver disease remains elusive. Historically, a "wait and see" approach has been used in this patient population due to higher rates of morbidity and mortality [6–8, 11]. But, this strategy may actually lead to worse patient outcomes. Nonelective cases in the general population often carry an increased risk of perioperative morbidity and mortality and this same pattern has recently been observed in patients with CLD [6–12].

To date, there are no prospective studies that address the timing of hernia repair in patients with liver disease. However, we will detail the results of more recent case series and retrospective chart reviews that we think provide substantial evidence for a paradigm shift in the timing of surgical repair of abdominal and groin hernias in this patient population. This topic will likely remain highly debated for years to come, but we strongly recommend an aggressive attempt at optimization of these patients to allow elective surgical repair of their hernia.

McKay et al., in 2009, used a literature search and a survey sent to hepatobiliary surgeons in Canada to conclude that early repair of umbilical hernias in patients with cirrhosis and ascites is safe [6]. The results of the survey showed that the severity of liver disease (as reflected in the Child-Turcotte-Pugh core), albumin level, and control of ascites impacted the decision to proceed with elective umbilical hernia repair [6]. The Child-Turcotte-Pugh score consists of five variables that are used to gauge the severity and prognosis of patients with chronic liver disease as reflected in a three-tiered system with "A" being the least severe disease and "C" being the most advanced [16]. According to this study, most surgeons would repair an asymptomatic umbilical hernia in patients with Child's A disease but would only repair an umbilical hernia in a patient with Child's B or C disease if complications (i.e., strangulation) were present or as a concomitant procedure when controlling for ascites. We generally agree with the practice of an aggressive surgical approach for patients with minor liver disease to allow for hernia repair before it becomes increasingly complex or a patient's liver disease progresses. However, the patient with advanced liver disease remains a significant challenge. It is our contention that these patients need a multidisciplinary approach with a hepatology specialist in order to try all measures possible to optimize liver disease and ascites control to allow a safe and elective hernia repair or consideration of liver transplantation prior to presenting with an emergency related to their hernia disease.

In a retrospective chart review performed by Andraus et al. in 2015, they found that patients with CLD who underwent emergency hernia repair were 10.8 times more likely to experience perioperative morbidity and mortality than those patients who underwent a planned, elective hernia repair [7]. This study reproduced the findings published by Marsman et al. in 2007 that showed that patients who underwent elective umbilical hernia repair did better perioperatively compared to those patients who were originally treated with "watchful waiting" [8]. In fact, in the group of patients who were originally managed nonoperatively, almost 80% required hospital admission for hernia incarceration, nearly 50% required an emergency operation, and 15% of this cohort died from hernia-related complications [8].

Questions regarding the use of mesh in this patient population and the feasibility of hernia repair in patients with more advanced liver disease were answered by Eker et al. in 2011. In their study, 30 patients diagnosed with liver cirrhosis and ascites were followed prospectively and outcomes following elective umbilical hernia repair were collected. Eighty percent of the patients had a Child's Score B or C and the average model for end-stage liver disease (MELD) score was 12 [9]. The MELD score was developed in response to criticism regarding the clinical utility of the Child-Turcotte-Pugh score. The Child-Turcotte-Pugh score and the MELD score are often used together to prioritize liver transplantation [18]. Prophylaxis for spontaneous bacterial peritonitis is recommended at a MELD score of 12 or greater and liver transplantation is recommended at a MELD score of 19 or greater [18].

The findings from the Eker et al. study have helped to shape our clinical practice with respect to abdominal wall hernia repair. Specifically, 10 of the 30 patients underwent umbilical hernia repair with mesh and had no postoperative wound or mesh-related complications [9]. Additionally, there were no surgery-related mortalities in this study [9]. This study shows the importance of a multidisciplinary team approach to the treatment of liver patients with concomitant hernias. If patients can be successfully optimized, standard hernia repair techniques seem appropriate.

Finally, there remains a paucity of literature that discusses the repair of inguinal hernias in this patient population. Nevertheless, the findings from two case reports detailing the approach to inguinal hernia repair in patients with chronic liver disease seem to correlate well with the approach to abdominal wall hernia repair in this patient population. Specifically, Hur et al. and Hurst et al. both support elective repair of inguinal hernias without a major increase in perioperative morbidity or mortality as compared to a "watch and see" strategy [11, 19].

Our surgical approach to abdominal wall and groin hernias in this patient population will be discussed in more detail in the next section. What remains to be answered regarding the timing of surgery is the safety and feasibility of performing a hernia repair at the time of procedure for control of ascites, such as transjugular intrahepatic portosystemic shunt (TIPS) or temporary peritoneal dialysis catheter placement for drainage of ascites [5]. Previous studies have shown that these procedures are often performed when a patient is not a candidate for liver transplantation [7, 10, 20]. Nevertheless, these procedures also carry a risk of perioperative morbidity and mortality which must be taken into consideration when choosing the timing of hernia repair. Additionally, if ascites cannot be controlled prior to urgent or semielective hernia repair, we often place a tunneled intraperitoneal drain to divert the ascites away from the incision and mesh to allow healing to occur. This is removed several weeks later based on the extent of healing of the hernia repair.

## Surgical Approach to Abdominal Wall Hernias in Patients with Chronic Liver Disease

As stated in the previous sections, patients with chronic liver disease comprise a high-risk surgical patient population with limited information guiding surgical approach to abdominal wall hernia repair. Most of the information that will be detailed in this section is our experience with these patients, including the timing, indications, and type of hernia repair performed. What is most important to take away from this section is that surgical planning should not be performed in isolation. Rather, the use of a multidisciplinary team, including hepatology, general surgery, and transplant surgery, will help facilitate preoperative optimization of this patient population and minimize the potential for hepatic decompensation postoperatively.

The important considerations when evaluating patients with CLD in the surgery clinic is the extent of the patient's disease, as evidenced by the presence or absence of portal hypertension and ascites. Figure 13.1 details the care pathway that we commonly use when deciding the surgical approach to these patients. Each step will be further detailed below.

## *Presence of Portal Hypertension*

In the absence of portal hypertension, we have found that patients with liver disease respond similarly to the stress of general anesthesia and surgery as other patients with abdominal wall hernias. In these patients, our surgical approach is consistent with our standard of care, which is a retromuscular hernia repair with permanent mesh for larger defects (>10 cm in width) and laparoscopic repair for smaller defects (<10 cm in width).

Our surgical technique has been previously described and will not be detailed here [21, 22]. However, the type of mesh used during these repairs is important and will be discussed briefly. Historically, general surgeons have been hesitant to use permanent mesh in patients with chronic liver disease due to the risk of potential coinfection should the patient develop spontaneous bacterial peritonitis at any point postoperatively. Nevertheless, there are no studies that have supported this belief [23]. Furthermore, the proposed benefits of biologic mesh utilization, including increased resistance to infection and long-term durability, have not held true [24].

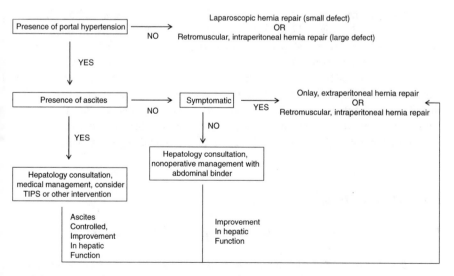

**Fig. 13.1** Surgical care pathway for abdominal wall hernias in patients with chronic liver disease

Because of the high-risk nature of these patients, all precautions should be taken to provide for a durable, long-term hernia repair. Current literature supports permanent large pore synthetic mesh in this regard, which is why we prefer to use this type of mesh in these patients. In addition, placing the mesh extraperitoneally can facilitate less adhesiolysis during future liver transplantation,

In the presence of portal hypertension, the degree of hepatic dysfunction is important. If esophageal or intra-abdominal varices or thrombocytopenia are present, the extent of hepatic dysfunction is almost certainly severe. For these patients, delineating the presence of symptoms as well as overlying skin changes such as dermal thinning is important to determining appropriate management. In the absence of obstructive symptoms or skin changes, patients should be treated with an abdominal binder and referral to a hepatologist for management of their portal hypertension. On the other hand, patients with obstructive symptoms or worrisome skin findings require surgical intervention.

The surgical approach to symptomatic patients with portal hypertension varies based on the degree of portal hypertension. For patients with new-onset portal hypertension without associated varices or thrombocytopenia, a retromuscular repair with permanent mesh is often performed. On the other hand, for patients with more advanced disease, an onlay, extraperitoneal approach with permanent mesh is used. This approach requires less manipulation of intra-abdominal tissues than our standard retromuscular approach, which therefore reduces the risk of surgical hemorrhage or postoperative liver decompensation in these higher-risk patients.

## Presence of Ascites

As previously mentioned, the development of ascites cannot occur without the presence of portal hypertension [12]. This means that patients with ascites are inherently at a higher risk for surgery than patients with portal hypertension alone. The option for surgical intervention in patients with ascites, therefore, is rarely discussed during the first clinical visit. Rather, these patients are referred to a hepatologist for medical management of their liver disease through the use of a beta-blocker, a salt-restricted diet, and aldosterone antagonists. Once patients with portal hypertension or portal hypertension with ascites are medically optimized in the opinion of a hepatologist, these patients are considered for surgery based on the extent of their remaining symptoms.

## Special Considerations

### Patients with Refractory Disease Despite Medical Management

There are a small number of patients who will have refractory, severe disease despite specialized care by a hepatologist. If these patients progress to develop symptoms associated with their abdominal wall hernia or they develop overlying skin changes, it is best to proceed with an elective abdominal wall hernia repair. The option for a longer-term subcutaneous drain, placement of a peritoneal dialysis catheter for drainage of ascites, or the concomitant performance of an ascites-controlling procedure such as a TIPS during abdominal wall hernia repair should be discussed in detail with the patient. Patients with uncontrolled ascites at the time of operation have a higher risk of liver decompensation, mesh infection, hernia recurrence, and death, all of which should be discussed with the patient preoperatively [6]. These patients should only be managed in a center with a multidisciplinary team that is equipped to handle and address the potential morbidity in these patients.

**Patients Undergoing Liver Transplantation**

Patients with a symptomatic abdominal hernia who are approaching liver transplantation should undergo primary hernia repair at the time of liver transplantation if at all possible. After successful transplantation, symptoms of portal hypertension and ascites will have been addressed, allowing for ideal circumstances under which to proceed with definitive hernia repair in the future. Furthermore, all patients with incidental or asymptomatic hernias found at the time of liver transplantation should also undergo primary repair. This is because previous studies have found that the risk of hernia incarceration is highest after liver transplantation due to resolution of ascites [8].

# Surgical Approach to Groin Hernias in Patients with Chronic Liver Disease

Similar to our approach to abdominal wall hernias in patients with CLD, our approach to groin hernias in this patient population is based largely on our own experience. Although these patients remain a high-risk population, the risk of inguinal hernia surgery is significantly lower than that of abdominal wall surgery as inguinal hernias can be repaired without the use of a general anesthetic. Therefore, we recommend the repair of all groin hernias in this patient population. It has been our experience that the laparoscopic approach to inguinal hernia repair in patients with CLD is taught with an increased risk of hemorrhage in the retroperitoneum and does not afford similar benefits such as earlier return to work as seen in patients without CLD. We therefore recommend an open primary tissue repair for inguinal hernias if the defect is small or a Lichtenstein repair with only mesh if the defect is large.

# Conclusions

Patients with chronic liver disease are at high-risk of developing abdominal wall and groin hernias. Despite its frequency, the ideal approach to hernia repair in this patient population remains unknown. In order to minimize the risk of perioperative decompensation, a multidisciplinary approach for the management of a patient's chronic liver disease, perioperative optimization, and surgical repair on an elective basis should be employed.

# References

1. Lim YS, Kim R. The global impact of hepatic fibrosis and end-stage liver disease. Clin Liver Dis. 2008;12(4):733–46.
2. Kim WR, Brown RS, Terrault NA, et al. Burden of liver disease in the United States: summary of a workshop. Hepatology. 2002;36:227–42.
3. Falagas ME, Vardakas KZ, Vergidis PI. Under-diagnosis of common chronic diseases prevalence and impact on human health. Int J Clin Pract. 2007;61:1569–79.
4. Friedman SL. Liver fibrosis-from bench to bedside. J Hepatol. 2003;38:S38–53.
5. Park JK, Lee SH, Yoon WJ, et al. Evaluation of hernia repair operations in Child-Turcotte-Pugh class C cirrhosis and refractory ascites. J Gastroenterol Hepatol. 2007;22(3):377–82.
6. McKay A, Dixon E, Bathe O, et al. Umbilical hernia repair in the presence of cirrhosis and ascites: results of a surgery and review of the literature. Hernia. 2009;13:461–8.
7. Andraus W, Pinheiro RS, Lai Q, et al. Abdominal wall hernia in cirrhotic patients: emergency surgery results in higher morbidity and mortality. BMC Surg. 2015;15:65–71.
8. Marsman HA, Heisterkamp J, Halm JA, et al. Management in patients with liver cirrhosis and an umbilical hernia. Surgery. 2007;142(3):372–5.
9. Eker HH, van Ramshorst GH, de Goede B, et al. A prospective study on elective umbilical hernia repair in patients with liver cirrhosis and ascites. Surgery. 2011;150(3):542–6.
10. Carbonell AM, Wolge LG, DeMaria EJ. Poor outcomes in cirrhosis-associated hernia repair: a nationwide cohort study of 32,033 patients. Hernia. 2005;9:353–7.
11. Hur YH, Kim JC, Kim SK, et al. Inguinal hernia repair in patients with liver cirrhosis accompanied by ascites. J Korean Surg Soc. 2011;80(6):420–5.
12. Sola E, Gines P. Renal and circulatory dysfunction in cirrhosis: current management and future perspectives. J Hepatol. 2010;53(6):1135–45.
13. Such J, Runyon BA. Pathogenesis of ascites in patients with cirrhosis. In: UpToDate, Lindor KD, editor, Waltham. Accessed 5 May 2016.
14. Anthony T, Bergen PC, Kim LT, et al. Factors affecting recurrence following incisional herniorrhaphy. World J Surg. 2000;24:95–101.
15. Froylich D, Segal M, Weinstein A, et al. Laparoscopic versus open ventral hernia repair in obese patients: a long-term follow-up. Surg Endosc. 2016;30(2):670–5.
16. Rosen MJ, Aydogdu K, Grafmiller K, et al. A multidisciplinary approach to medical weight loss prior to complex abdominal wall reconstruction: is it feasible? J Gastrointest Surg. 2015;19(8):1399–406.
17. Velkovic R, Protic M, Gluhovic A, et al. Prospective clinical trial of factors predicting the early development of incisional hernia after midline laparotomy. J Am Coll Surg. 2010;210(2):210–9.
18. Singal AK, Kamath PS. Model for end-stage liver disease. J Clin Exp Hepatol. 2013;3(1):50–60.
19. Hurst RD, Butker BN, Soybel DI, et al. Management of groin hernias in patients with ascites. Ann Surg. 1992;216(6):696–700.
20. Fagan SP, Awad AA, Berger DH. Management of complicated umbilical hernias in patients with end-stage liver disease and refractory ascites. Surgery. 2004;135(6):679–82.
21. Krpata DM, Blatnik JA, Novitsky YW, et al. Posterior and open anterior components separations: a comparative analysis. Am J Surg. 2012;203(3):318–22.

22. Novitsky YW, Elliott HL, Orenstein SB, et al. Transversus abdominis muscle release: a novel approach to posterior component separation during abdominal wall reconstruction. Am J Surg. 2012;204(5):709–16.
23. Ammar SA. Management of complicated hernias in cirrhotic patients using permanent mesh: randomized clinical trial. Hernia. 2010;14(1):35–8.
24. Rosen MJ, Krpata DM, Ermlich B, et al. A 5-year clinical experience with single-staged repairs of infection and contaminated abdominal wall defects utilizing biologic mesh. Ann Surg. 2013;257(6):991–6.

# Chapter 14
# Bariatric Surgery in Patients with Cirrhosis

Zubaidah Nor Hanipah, Linden Karas, and Philip R. Schauer

## Obesity and Nonalcoholic Fatty Liver Disease

Obesity is a worldwide epidemic and its prevalence is rising in the United States; one-third of the adults in the USA are obese. Further, obesity has strong associations with metabolic disorders such as type 2 diabetes (T2D), hypertension, hyperlipidemia, and fatty liver disease.

The prevalence of nonalcoholic fatty liver disease (NAFLD) is increasing along with the prevalence of obesity; between 84% and 96% of patients with obesity have NAFLD and 25–55% have nonalcoholic steatohepatitis (NASH) [1]. NASH is a histological diagnosis characterized by the presence of steatosis found in greater than 5% of hepatocytes, hepatocellular ballooning, and lobular inflammation [2]. Up to 15–20% of patients with biopsy-proven NASH will progress to cirrhosis [3]. Currently, the most common indication for liver transplant is hepatitis C virus infection [4], but with increasing obesity rates globally, NASH could soon become the leading cause of liver transplantation worldwide.

In addition to liver related morbidity and mortality, patients with NAFLD have a higher risk of cardiovascular disease (CVD) and mortality [5]. A recent meta-analysis that included 16 studies and 34,043 patients showed that patients with NAFLD have a higher risk of fatal and nonfatal CVD events when compared to patients without NAFLD (odds ratio [OR] 1.64, 95% confidence interval [CI] 1.26–2.13) [6]. Also, Adam et al. [7] reported on causes of mortality in a cohort of 420 patients with NAFLD with a mean follow-up of 7.6 years. The total overall mortality, cardiovascular (CV) mortality, and liver disease associated mortality was 7.6%, 3.6%, and 1.7%, respectively. Similar findings were reported by Jepsten et al. [8] and Ekstedt et al. [9]: the CV mortality rate in the NAFLD patients was 11% and

Z.N. Hanipah, MD • L. Karas, MD • P.R. Schauer, MD (✉)
Bariatric and Metabolic Institute, M61, Cleveland Clinic,
9500 Euclid Avenue, Cleveland, OH 44195, USA
e-mail: shauep@ccg.org; http://weightloss.clevelandclinic.org

© Springer International Publishing AG 2017
B. Eghtesad, J. Fung (eds.), *Surgical Procedures on the Cirrhotic Patient*,
DOI 10.1007/978-3-319-52396-5_14

12.4%, respectively, in those studies. It is clear that patients with NAFLD are more likely to die from CVD than liver disease; thus, treatment strategy should be prioritized accordingly.

## Bariatric Surgery

Bariatric surgery has evolved since the 1950s and has been proven to be the most effective and long-lasting mode of treatment for severe obesity. Furthermore, it has consistently been shown to resolve both metabolic and other comorbidities related to obesity. The laparoscopic approach to bariatric surgery started in the early 1990s, and today most bariatric procedures (>95%) are performed laparoscopically throughout the world. The laparoscopic technique is associated with a significant decrease in postoperative morbidity, mortality, recovery time, and cost when compared to prior open techniques [10]. In the USA, a total of 196,000 bariatric procedures were performed in 2015. Sleeve gastrectomy (SG) is the most common (53.8%), followed by Roux-en-Y gastric bypass (RYGB), 23.1%, laparoscopic adjustable gastric banding (LAGB), 5.7%, and biliopancreatic diversion with or without duodenal switch (BPD ± DS), 0.6% (Fig. 14.1, [11]). SG and RYGB together are the most popular procedure (77%), while LAGB has become less popular due to poor long-term results. BPD is the least often performed procedure due to the significant risk of nutritional deficiencies (3–18%) [12, 13]. Outcomes of bariatric surgery in terms of resolving and improving comorbidities and reducing long-term mortality are well documented (Fig. 14.2, [10]).

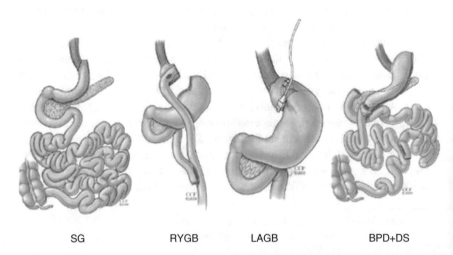

SG                    RYGB              LAGB                    BPD+DS

**Fig. 14.1** Common bariatric procedures. Reprinted with permission, Cleveland Clinic Center for Medical Art & Photography © 2006-2016. All Rights Reserved

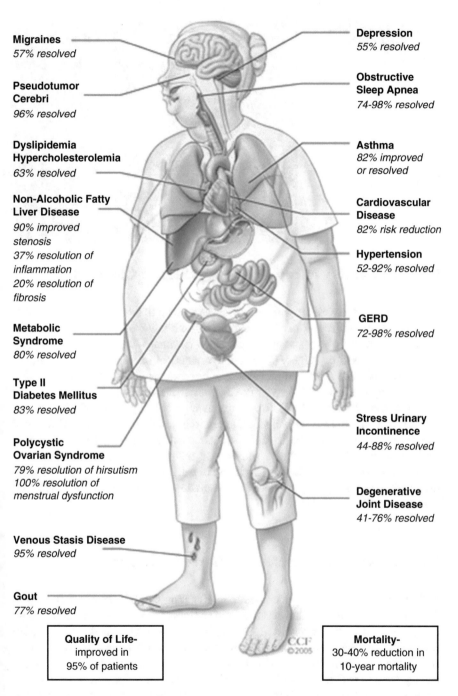

**Migraines**
*57% resolved*

**Pseudotumor Cerebri**
*96% resolved*

**Dyslipidemia Hypercholesterolemia**
*63% resolved*

**Non-Alcoholic Fatty Liver Disease**
*90% improved stenosis*
*37% resolution of inflammation*
*20% resolution of fibrosis*

**Metabolic Syndrome**
*80% resolved*

**Type II Diabetes Mellitus**
*83% resolved*

**Polycystic Ovarian Syndrome**
*79% resolution of hirsutism*
*100% resolution of menstrual dysfunction*

**Venous Stasis Disease**
*95% resolved*

**Gout**
*77% resolved*

**Depression**
*55% resolved*

**Obstructive Sleep Apnea**
*74-98% resolved*

**Asthma**
*82% improved or resolved*

**Cardiovascular Disease**
*82% risk reduction*

**Hypertension**
*52-92% resolved*

**GERD**
*72-98% resolved*

**Stress Urinary Incontinence**
*44-88% resolved*

**Degenerative Joint Disease**
*41-76% resolved*

**Quality of Life-**
improved in
95% of patients

**Mortality-**
30-40% reduction in
10-year mortality

**Fig. 14.2** Outcome of bariatric surgery in obesity-related comorbidities. Reprinted with permission, Cleveland Clinic Center for Medical Art & Photography © 2006–2016. All Rights Reserved

**Fig. 14.3** Bariatric patient
with cirrhosis after liver
biopsy

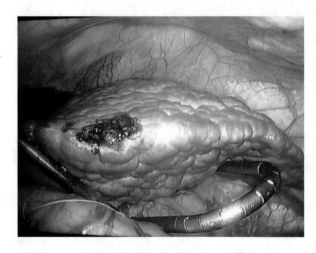

## Bariatric Surgery in Patients with NASH and Cirrhosis

Bariatric surgery in patients with cirrhosis was thought to be contraindicated due to
the potential excessive risk of complications and mortality. More recently, however,
studies involving cirrhotic patients have shown reasonable and lower rates of complication after bariatric surgery (see section on safety of bariatric surgery in patients
with cirrhosis). The estimated prevalence of cirrhotic patients undergoing bariatric
surgery is approximately 2%, with the diagnosis usually made incidentally at the
time of surgery [14] (Fig. 14.3). Recent trends suggest that patients with known cirrhosis are being referred for bariatric surgery to improve both liver and CV-related
outcomes. Patients with obesity and cirrhosis may benefit from bariatric surgery
through both weight loss and resolution of metabolic comorbidities [15, 16].
Furthermore, surgically induced weight loss in patients with end-stage liver disease
may enable them to qualify for liver transplantation based on the preoperative BMI
requirement (BMI < 35 kg/m$^2$).

## Weight Loss Improvement After Bariatric Surgery

Bariatric surgery is the only therapeutic intervention that has been proven to produce clinically significant and sustained weight loss for over 5 years in the severely
obese. Typically, surgery results in 20 and 50 kg of weight loss and a 10–15 kg/m$^2$
BMI reduction. Weight loss varies between the bariatric procedures. In the SOS trial
[17] of the long-term effects of bariatric surgery compared with nonsurgical weight
management in patients with a BMI >34 kg/m$^2$, the mean weight loss after 10 years
for gastric band plication, vertical banded gastroplasty, and gastric bypass was
14 kg, 16 kg, and 25 kg, respectively. The mean changes of body weight after 10,
15, and 20 years were −17%, −16%, and −18% in bariatric surgical groups as

compared to control group; 1%, −1%, and −1%, respectively. A meta-analysis by Buchwald et al. [18] showed that overall excess weight loss was 55.9% after bariatric surgery.

Weight loss in cirrhotic patients is comparable to noncirrhotic patients who underwent bariatric surgery (Child Pugh A or B; reported by Dallal et al. [19], 30 patients and Shimizu et al. [15], 23 patients). The 1-year excess weight loss was 62% and 67.4%, respectively.

## Changes in Liver Histology After Bariatric Surgery

Studies involving bariatric patients with NASH have shown significant improvement in liver function studies, steatosis, inflammation, and fibrosis after surgery [5–7]. Rabl et al. [20] in a systematic review reported that NASH improved histologically after bariatric surgery irrespective of procedure type (Table 14.1). Mattar et al. [21] showed that there was a significant improvement in liver steatosis (from 88% to 8%, $p < 0.001$), inflammation (from 23% to 2%), and fibrosis (from 31% to 13%). Inflammation and fibrosis resolved in 37% and 20% of patients, respectively, corresponding to an improvement of 82% in grade and 39% in stage of liver disease ($p < 0.001$). Weight loss after bariatric surgery results in a reduction of visceral fat and an increase in insulin sensitivity, which is a major drive of histological improvement of NAFLD [2].

## Cirrhosis Improvement After Bariatric Surgery

Due to the infrequency of bariatric surgery performed in patients with frank cirrhosis, data on histological changes in cirrhosis after bariatric surgery are limited. However, in this systemic review, Rabl et al. [20] showed that in patients with NASH and advanced liver disease, all the histological components of cirrhosis including steatosis, inflammation, and fibrosis generally improved with bariatric procedures, especially RYGB. Kral et al. [22] showed that after BPD in patients

**Table 14.1** Liver histological changes following bariatric surgery

| Bariatric procedures | Number of studies | Total number of patients | Histology changes in NASH post bariatric surgery |
|---|---|---|---|
| RYGB | 12 | 576 | Significant and consistent improvement |
| LAGB | 2 | 441 | Improvement/no change |
| BPD | 2 | 182 | Mostly improvement, worsening in some patients with fibrosis |
| VBG (vertical band gastroplasty) | 4 | 303 | Mostly improvement |

with cirrhosis ($n = 11/14$, with pre- and postoperative biopsy), steatosis, inflammation, and fibrosis all improved significantly. However, in this study there were three patients without fibrosis at baseline who developed cirrhosis on follow-up. Whether bariatric surgery definitely results in histological improvement in frank cirrhosis requires further study.

## Resolution of T2D After Bariatric Surgery

The prevalence of T2D in patients with severe obesity and cirrhosis is 70–80% [15, 19]. Bariatric surgery has shown significant improvement and sometimes resolution of T2D in both observational and randomized control trials (RCTs). A recent systemic review involving 73 studies with 19,543 patients showed 73% remission/improvement for T2D at a mean follow-up of 57.8 months [23]. Buchwald et al. [18] showed that diabetic patients had an overall 78.1% rate of complete resolution and an 86.6% rate of improvement in T2D. At 2 years, BPD-DS has the best T2D resolution (95.9%), followed by gastric bypass (70.9%), and gastric band (58.3%). In the STAMPEDE trial, Schauer et al. [24] showed that at 3 years after bariatric surgery versus intensive medical therapy, glycated hemoglobin level of 6.0% or less was achieved by 38% in the gastric bypass group, 24% in the sleeve gastrectomy group, and 5% in the medical-therapy group ($p < 0.001$). Shimizu et al. [15] reported 85.7% improvement in T2D with remission rate of 66.7% in the cirrhotic patients who underwent bariatric procedures (RYGB, SG, and LAGB).

## CV Risk Reduction After Bariatric Surgery

Bariatric surgery has also shown improvement in obesity-related comorbidities such as hypertension, hyperlipidemia and CVD. The SOS trial [17] showed significantly decreased rates of myocardial infarction, stroke, CV mortality and all causes of CV risk, and cancer in women after bariatric surgery. Bolen et al. [25] showed 53% resolution or improvement in hypercholesterolemia in 5 years and Sugerman et al. [26] showed 66% of resolution or improvement in hypertension in 7 years. In a systematic review of CV outcomes after bariatric surgery, Vest et al. [23] showed that there was improvement and resolution of hypertension (63%) and hyperlipidemia (65%), and reduction in all-cause mortality compared to nonoperative controls. The study also showed evidence of left ventricular hypertrophy regression and improvement in diastolic function post bariatric surgery. In patients with advanced liver disease and NASH, Mattar et al. showed that bariatric surgery resulted in improvements in all metabolic conditions including diabetes, hypertension, and dyslipidemia [21]. In 23 patients with cirrhosis, Shimizu et al. [15] reported improvement of hypertension and dyslipidemia at rates of 88.9% and 66.7%, respectively, following bariatric surgery.

## Safety of Bariatric Surgery in Patients with Cirrhosis

Patients with cirrhosis undergoing major abdominal surgery have a greater than tenfold higher mortality risk (9%) than patients without cirrhosis [27]. For this reason, the safety of bariatric surgery in cirrhotic patients has raised concern. Mosko et al. [28] conducted a study involving the Nationwide Inpatient Sample (NIS) Database from 1998 to 2007 and demonstrated that the mortality rate of bariatric surgery for patients without cirrhosis, decompensated cirrhosis and decompensated cirrhosis was 0.3%, 0.9%, and 16.3%, respectively. High-volume centers (>100 cases/year) compared to medium volume (50–100 cases/year) and lower volume (<50 cases/year) centers have significantly lower mortality rates (0.2%, 0.4%, and 0.7%, respectively) suggesting that bariatric surgery in cirrhotic patients should be performed in high volume centers.

A recent systemic review (11 studies including 122 patients) of patients with Child Pugh A cirrhosis who underwent bariatric surgery demonstrated major morbidity and mortality rates much lower than expected: 21.3% and 1.6%, respectively. Postsurgical liver decompensation was seen in only 6.6%, and the delayed mortality rate (>30 days) was only 2.5% [16]. Despite the greater risk of bariatric surgery in cirrhotic patients, both Dallal et al. [19] and Shimizu et al. [15] reported no postsurgical (1–3 years follow up) liver decompensation or related mortality in their series. These studies suggest that bariatric surgery in cirrhotic patients (Child Pugh A) is relatively safe with an overall benefit in terms of weight loss, metabolic improvement, and CV risk reduction. Outcomes of patients with more advanced cirrhosis (Child–Pugh B and C) are not well documented. Appropriate perioperative management of the cirrhotic patient with a multidisciplinary team approach is likely a key factor in achieving low complication rates in this population.

## Complications

Complications following bariatric surgery are often influenced by preexisting risk factors and illness. Cirrhotic patients have higher morbidity and rates of postoperative complications compared to the general population. Jan et al. [16] showed that cirrhotic patients who underwent "restrictive" procedures (LAGB and SG) had less complications and mortality than those having malabsorptive procedures (RYGB and BPD) (Table 14.2). This study also reported that delayed mortality was observed, albeit rarely, in the RYGB and BPD groups due to liver decompensation and fulminant hepatic failure. Liver decompensation in cirrhotic patients postbariatric surgery may be related to malnutrition and malabsorption resulting from these procedures. The relative increase in risk of the malabsorptive procedures must be balanced with the relatively less effective weight loss and metabolic improvement observed with the "restrictive" procedures.

**Table 14.2** Bariatric surgery morbidity and mortality in cirrhotic patients in a systemic review of 122 patients in 9 studies [16]

| Bariatric procedure | Complication (%) | Liver decompensation (%) | Mortality (%) |
|---|---|---|---|
| LAGB ($n = 15$) | 20 | 0 | 0 |
| SG ($n = 41$) | 14.6 | 12.5 | 0 |
| RYGB ($n = 51$) | 31.3 | 3.92 | 2 |
| BPD ($n = 15$) | 13.3 | 13.3 | 20 |

Other common postoperative complications include infection, bleeding, and venous thromboembolism (VTE). Infection can include wound infections, intra-abdominal abscesses, catheter-related infections, pneumonia, and surgical site infections. Cirrhotic patients with ascites have a higher risk of wound infections and breakdown. Therefore, prophylactic antibiotic such as a cephalosporin is recommended. Cirrhotic patients are often coagulopathic and demonstrate platelet dysfunction that can result in intra-abdominal bleeding. Therefore, careful tissue handling and hemostasis are essential and the usage of anticoagulants is recommended with caution.

Finally, the incidence of VTE is higher in obese patients and it is one of the main causes of mortality after bariatric surgery. More than 80% of these episodes of VTE occur after discharge [29]. Prophylactic perioperative VTE prophylaxis, as well as extended VTE prophylaxis in high risk surgical patients is recommended with caution. There is no standard guideline regarding type, dose and duration of VTE prophylaxis available for bariatric patients with cirrhosis but the American Society for Metabolic and Bariatric Surgery (ASMBS) [30] has recommended the following general recommendations for patients undergoing bariatric surgery; Mechanical VTE prophylaxis such as sequential compression devices or elastic compression stockings, and early ambulation are recommended in all bariatric surgical patients. Chemoprophylaxis is recommended for patients undergoing bariatric surgery provided there is no significant increased risk for major bleeding.

## Patient Selection

General indications for bariatric surgery are based on the NIH Consensus Conference of 1991 [31]. More recently, international guidelines for patients with diabetes and metabolic disease suggest that bariatric surgery or metabolic surgery also be considered for patients with inadequately controlled T2D diabetes and a BMI as low as 30 kg/m$^2$ (27.5 kg/m$^2$ for high-risk populations such as Asians) [32]. A multidisciplinary team approach plays an important role in the care of obese patients, as does family and social support. There is no published clinical practice guideline for bariatric surgery in cirrhotic patients; the data available is only based on a few clinical studies. For patients with Child–Pugh B and C cirrhosis, any major surgical procedure carries a higher perioperative risk and mortality. Notable to this textbook on surgery in patients with cirrhosis, with the exception of liver transplantation, bariatric, and metabolic surgery, is the only surgery that may actually improve cirrhosis.

Indications for bariatric surgery:

- BMI ≥ 40 kg/m² or BMI ≥ 35 kg/m² with significant obesity-related comorbidities or (New) BMI 30–34 kg/m² with uncontrolled T2D [32]
- The patient must be psychologically stable

Relative Contraindications for bariatric surgery:

- Inability to understand the procedure, its risks and benefits
- Inability or unwillingness to change lifestyle postoperatively
- Addiction to drugs or alcohol
- Psychological instability

Bariatric Procedure Selection for Cirrhotic Patients
The choice of which type of bariatric procedure is appropriate for each cirrhotic patient is based on the criteria below:

- Child–Pugh Scoring (A/B/C);
- Presence and severity of portal hypertension (mild/moderate/severe);
- And endoscopic evidence of portal gastropathy, varices, and gastroesophageal reflux disease (GERD)

Cirrhotic patients with Child–Pugh score A or B may be appropriate candidates for bariatric surgery after proper assessment and multidisciplinary evaluation. Studies have shown that these patients in general have reasonable risk and benefit after bariatric procedures and resolution of NASH [16]. LAGB, SG, RYGB, and BPD (ascending operative risk, respectively) are all options depending on the liver function and presence of portal hypertension. Adequate data to compare risks and benefits of these operations in patients with cirrhosis does not exist presently.

Portal hypertension is defined by the presence of thrombocytopenia, ascites, endoscopic evidence of varices and portal gastropathy. Grading of portal hypertension is as below:

- Mild: <8 mmHg
- Moderate: 8–10 mmHg
- Severe: >12 mmHg

Patients with mild portal hypertension can benefit from bariatric surgery. Any bariatric operation should be performed with caution because these patients have a higher likelihood of having gastric varices which may induce major bleeding. In cirrhotic patients with moderate portal hypertension, very little outcome data exists to make strong recommendations except consider the lower risk procedures. Bariatric surgery is relatively contraindicated in patients with severe portal hypertension as they are at an extremely high risk for bleeding. However, in patients with preserved liver function, transjugular intrahepatic porto-systemic shunt (TIPS) placement can reduce portal pressure making it safer to perform surgery [33]. Shimizu et al. [15] demonstrated successful SG after TIPS procedure in cirrhotic patients. However, these patients should be jointly managed by hepatologist and transplant surgeon for optimal outcomes.

Up to 2% of bariatric surgical patients are incidentally diagnosed with cirrhosis at the time of surgery [14]. If this situation arises, we recommend that the surgeon should look for intraoperative evidence of portal hypertension such as ascites, varices or large dilated perigastric veins. If the patient has evidence of portal hypertension, a reasonable option is to perform a liver biopsy (if safe and feasible) and abandon the bariatric procedure until further assessment. If cirrhosis is diagnosed intraoperatively and there are no signs of portal hypertension, several studies suggest that bariatric procedures (LAGB, SG, RYGB) can be performed relatively with low complications rates and benefit to the patient [15, 16, 19, 22].

In summary, Fig. 14.4 shows the flow chart on selection of bariatric procedures in cirrhotic patients.

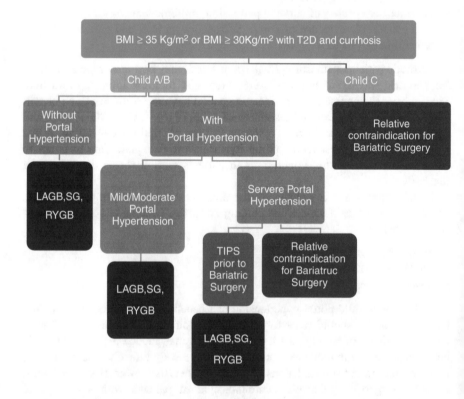

**Fig. 14.4** Flow chart on selection of bariatric procedures in cirrhotic patients

**Table 14.3**  Preoperative evaluation for bariatric surgery

| | |
|---|---|
| Complete history Physical examination | • Causes for obesity, related comorbidities and the treatment (history of portal hypertension complications and bleeding tendencies), history of blood transfusion and hepatitis infection, past surgical history, diet history, weight loss history and commitment to lose weight<br>• Weight, height, BMI, signs of liver failure (Child–Pugh scoring) |
| Blood investigations | • Complete blood count/platelet, prothrombin time/INR, blood type, liver and renal function tests, hepatitis screening, fasting blood glucose and lipid panel, urine analysis |
| Nutritional assessment | • Appropriate clinical nutritional evaluation (RD), nutrient screening with iron studies, $B_{12}$ and folic acid and 25-vitamin D levels |
| Cardiopulmonary assessment | • CXR, ECG, sleep apnea screening (± confirmatory polysomnography)<br>• In patients with cardiac disease or pulmonary hypertension: echocardiogram and proceed<br>• In patients with intrinsic lung disease or disordered sleep patterns: ABG, formal pulmonary evaluation<br>• In patients with risk of VTE: DVT evaluation needed |
| Endocrine assessment | • Prediabetic or diabetic:<br>  HbA1c level<br>  Optimization of glycemic control: (including HbA1c $\leq$ 7%, fasting blood sugar $\leq$110 mg/dL, 2-h postprandial blood glucose of $\leq$140 mg/dL)<br>  In long standing diabetic patients: HbA1c 7–8% (if feasible)<br>• Thyroid disease: thyroid function test (TSH)<br>• Patient suspected with androgen with polycyctic ovarian syndrome:<br>• Total or bioavailable testosterone, DHEAS, $D4$-androstenedione<br>• Cushing's syndrome:<br>• 1 mg overnight dexamethasone test, 24-h urinary free cortisol, 11 p.m. salivary cortisol |
| GI assessment | • Ultrasound or computed tomography of hepatobiliary system (presence of liver cirrhosis, ascites, splenomegaly, intra-abdominal varices, gallstone)<br>• Portal hypertension (portal pressure measurement, role of TIPS)<br>• Upper endoscopy (esophageal or gastric varices, portal gastropathy, GERD)<br>  Helicobacter pylori screening in high prevalence areas |
| Psychosocial-behavioral assessment | • Evaluation of environmental, familial and behavioral factors<br>• In suspected patients with psychiatric illness or substance abuse:<br>• Formal mental health evaluation |
| Medical documentation and informed consent | • Reason for bariatric surgery and complication of bariatric procedures in cirrhotic patients<br>• Options available if incidental cirrhosis intra-operatively<br>• Intra-operative liver biopsy |
| Preoperative weight loss | • Counsel patient prior to surgery |
| Counseling | • Childbearing women: Pregnancy and contraceptive<br>• Smokers: stop smoking at least 6 weeks prior to surgery<br>• Stop alcohol consumption |
| Cancer screening | • Verified by primary care physician<br>• Screening for breast, colorectal, endometrium, cervix and prostate cancers |

**Table 14.4** Intraoperative care in cirrhotic patients

| Port placement | • Beware of abdominal wall varices |
|---|---|
| Liver retraction | • Liver lobes are heavy and cirrhotic- watch out for bleeding and liver injury |
| Liver biopsy | • Percutaneous biopsy under laparoscopic guidance with cauterization using 16–18 gauge needle |
| Presence of gastric varices | • Caution for all bariatric procedures due to increased bleeding risk |
| Presence of ascites | • Perioperative antibiotic prophylaxis for gram-negative bacteria to prevent spontaneous bacterial peritonitis |
| Bleeding tendencies | • Prone to bleeding due to vitamin K coagulation factor derangement and thrombocytopenia<br>• Extra precaution in tissue handling during dissection and retraction to prevent bleeding<br>• Anticipate hemostatic problems: use of hemostatic agents hemoclips, cautery, ligation of bleeding vessel |
| VTE chemoprophylaxis | • Caution in usage of intraoperative anticoagulant especially if patient has bleeding tendencies or thrombocytopenia |

**Table 14.5** Early postoperative care

| Cardiopulmonary care | • High risk of MI: At least 24 H telemetry monitoring<br>• Pulmonary toilet, incentive spirometry<br>• Early CPAP if required<br>• DVT prophylaxis, encourage ambulation<br>• If unstable: consider leak or VTE |
|---|---|
| Hydration | • Maintain adequate hydration (depends on the liver and renal function) |
| Healthy eating education | • Protocol derived stage meal progression<br>• Caution in protein intake in cirrhotic patients |
| Monitoring | • Blood glucose levels monitoring<br>• Watch out for hypoglycemic symptoms<br>• Caution on opioids usage due to mental status deterioration, respiratory compromise, impaired gut function<br>• Watch out for delirium or encephalopathy (avoid precipitating factors) |
| Pressure sore prevention | • Early ambulation<br>• Adequate padding at pressure points<br>• If suspected rhabdomyolysis: check for creatine kinase level |
| Medications | • 1- 2 adult multivitamin-mineral supplements containing iron, 1200 to 1500 mg/d of calcium citrate, and a vitamin B-complex preparation |

**Table 14.6**  Follow-up care

| Follow-up visit (depends on the condition of patients and type of bariatric surgery) | • 1/3/6/12 months<br>  – 1st month: LAGB, SG, RYGB,BPD ± DS<br>  – 2nd month: LAGB<br>  – 3rd month: SG, RYGB, BPD ± DS<br>  – 6th month: SG, RYGB, BPD ± DS<br>  – 12th month (annually once stable): SG, RYGB |
|---|---|
| Monitoring | • Weight loss trend<br>• Nutritional assessment<br>• Psychological assessment (if support group needed)<br>• Evidence of postoperative complications<br>• Physical activity |
| Evaluation and adjustment | • Need for antihypertensive, anti-diabetic and lipid medications |
| Avoid | • Nonsteroidal anti-inflammatory drugs due to bleeding, ulcers |
| Prophylactic medication | • For gout and gallstone in appropriate patients |
| Investigations to be monitored | • SMA-21, CBC/platelet with each visit (and iron at baseline and after as needed)<br>• Lipid profile every 6–12 months based on risk and therapy<br>• Thiamine evaluation with specific findings<br>• 24-h urinary calcium excretion at 6 months and then annually<br>• $B_{12}$ (annually; MMA and HCV optional) then 3–6 months if supplemented)<br>• Folic acid (RBC folic acid optional)<br>• Bone density (DXA) at 2 years<br>• In malabsorptive surgery:<br>  – iron studies, 25-vitamin D, intact parathyroid hormone<br>  – vitamin A (initially and 6–12 months thereafter)<br>  – copper, zinc, and selenium evaluation with specific finding |
| Surveillance upper endoscopy | • In patients with cirrhosis with portal hypertension (for variceal assessment) |

## Perioperative Management

Preoperative evaluation of bariatric patients includes a complete medical history, psychological history, nutritional assessment, physical examination, and investigations to assess surgical risk. Further screening tests and a more detailed assessment involving a multidisciplinary team are advisable in patients with known or suspected cirrhosis. Perioperative care of these patients is summarized in Tables 14.3, 14.4, 14.5, and 14.6, based on ASMBS perioperative guidelines for bariatric surgery [34] and an update on abdominal surgery for patients with cirrhosis [35].

## Conclusion

Obesity and NASH have been increasing globally leading to higher incidences of liver cirrhosis. Bariatric surgery is an effective long-term treatment of obesity and its associated comorbidities. Many studies show that NASH has significant histological improvement after bariatric surgery, and therefore, surgery has a role in preventing progression of NAFLD. Although bariatric surgery carries higher perioperative risks in cirrhotic patients than in the general population, morbidity, and mortality rates after bariatric surgery are less than expected in well-compensated cirrhotic patients. The overall outcomes in patients with Child Pugh A and B are good in terms of weight loss, metabolic improvement, and CV risk reduction.

Thorough preoperative evaluation and management with a multidisciplinary approach involving an experienced bariatric surgeon, bariatric physician, hepatologist, liver transplant surgeon, cardiologist, anesthesiologist, radiologist, psychologist, and dietician can yield very good outcomes in cirrhotic patients. Preoperative counseling specific to the risks associated with liver disease is advised.

## References

1. Clark JM. The epidemiology of nonalcoholic fatty liver disease in adults. J Clin Gastroenterol. 2006;40:S5–10.
2. Stephen S, Baranova A, Younossi ZM. Nonalcoholic fatty liver disease and bariatric surgery. Expert Rev Gastroenterol Hepatol. 2012;6(2):163–71.
3. Sanyal AJ. NASH: a global health problem. Hepatol Res. 2011;41(7):670–4.
4. Koehler E, Watt K, Charlton M. Fatty liver and liver transplantation. Clin Liver Dis. 2009;13(4):621–30.
5. Targher G, Arcaro G. Non-alcoholic fatty liver disease and increased risk of cardiovascular disease. Atherosclerosis. 2007;191(2):235–40.
6. Targher G, Byrne CD, Lonardo A, Zoppini G, Barbui C. Nonalcoholic fatty liver disease and risk of incident cardiovascular disease: a meta-analysis of observational studies. J Hepatol. 2016;65:589–600.

7. Adams LA, Lymp JF, Sauver JS, Sanderson SO, Lindor KD, Feldstein A, Angulo P. The natural history of nonalcoholic fatty liver disease: a population-based cohort study. Gastroenterology. 2005;129(1):113–21.

8. Jepsen P, Vilstrup H, Mellemkjaer L, Thulstrup AM, Olsen JH, Baron JA, Sørensen HT. Prognosis of patients with a diagnosis of fatty liver–a registry-based cohort study. Hepato-Gastroenterology. 2002;50(54):2101–4.

9. Ekstedt M, Franzén LE, Mathiesen UL, Thorelius L, Holmqvist M, Bodemar G, Kechagias S. Long-term follow-up of patients with NAFLD and elevated liver enzymes. Hepatology. 2006;44(4):865–73.

10. Brethauer SA, Chand B, Schauer PR. Risks and benefits of bariatric surgery: current evidence. Cleve Clin J Med. 2006;73(11):993.

11. Ponce J, DeMaria EJ, Nguyen NT, Hutter M, Sudan R, Morton JM. American Society for Metabolic and Bariatric Surgery estimation of bariatric surgery procedures in 2015 and surgeon workforce in the United States. Surg Obes Relat Dis. 2016;12:1637–9.

12. Scopinaro N. Thirty-five years of biliopancreatic diversion: notes on gastrointestinal physiology to complete the published information useful for a better understanding and clinical use of the operation. Obes Surg. 2012;22(3):427–32.

13. Sethi M, Chau E, Youn A, Jiang Y, Fielding G, Ren-Fielding C. Long-term outcomes after biliopancreatic diversion with and without duodenal switch: 2-, 5-, and 10-year data. Surg Obes Relat Dis. 2016;12:1697–705.

14. Brolin RE, Bradley LJ, Taliwal RV. Unsuspected cirrhosis discovered during elective obesity operations. Arch Surg. 1998;133(1):84–8.

15. Shimizu H, Phuong V, Maia M, Kroh M, Chand B, Schauer PR, Brethauer SA. Bariatric surgery in patients with liver cirrhosis. Surg Obes Relat Dis. 2013;9(1):1–6.

16. Jan A, Narwaria M, Mahawar KK. A systematic review of bariatric surgery in patients with liver cirrhosis. Obes Surg. 2015;25(8):1518–26.

17. Sjöström L, Peltonen M, Jacobson P, Sjöström CD, Karason K, Wedel H, Ahlin S, Anveden Å, Bengtsson C, Bergmark G, Bouchard C. Bariatric surgery and long-term cardiovascular events. JAMA. 2012;307(1):56–65.

18. Buchwald H, Estok R, Fahrbach K, Banel D, Jensen MD, Pories WJ, Bantle JP, Sledge I. Weight and type 2 diabetes after bariatric surgery: systematic review and meta-analysis. Am J Med. 2009;122(3):248–56.

19. Dallal RM, Mattar SG, Lord JL, Watson AR, Cottam DR, Eid GM, Hamad G, Rabinovitz M, Schauer PR. Results of laparoscopic gastric bypass in patients with cirrhosis. Obes Surg. 2004;14(1):47–53.

20. Rabl C, Campos GM. The impact of bariatric surgery on nonalcoholic steatohepatitis. Sem Liver Dis. 2012;32(01):80–91. Thieme Medical Publishers

21. Mattar SG, Velcu LM, Rabinovitz M, Demetris AJ, Krasinskas AM, Barinas-Mitchell E, Eid GM, Ramanathan R, Taylor DS, Schauer PR. Surgically-induced weight loss significantly improves nonalcoholic fatty liver disease and the metabolic syndrome. Ann Surg. 2005;242(4):610–20.

22. Kral JG, Thung SN, Biron S, Hould FS, Lebel S, Marceau S, Simard S, Marceau P. Effects of surgical treatment of the metabolic syndrome on liver fibrosis and cirrhosis. Surgery. 2004;135(1):48–58.

23. Vest AR, Heneghan HM, Agarwal S, Schauer PR, Young JB. Bariatric surgery and cardiovascular outcomes: a systematic review. Heart. 2012;98:1763–77.

24. Schauer PR, Bhatt DL, Kirwan JP, et al.; STAMPEDE Investigators. Bariatric surgery versus intensive medical therapy for diabetes–3-year outcomes. N Engl J Med. 2014;370:2002–13.

25. Bolen SD, Chang HY, Weiner JP, Richards TM, Shore AD, Goodwin SM, Johns RA, Magnuson TH, Clark JM. Clinical outcomes after bariatric surgery: a five-year matched cohort analysis in seven US states. Obes Surg. 2012;22(5):749–63.

26. Sugerman HJ, Wolfe LG, Sica DA, Clore JN. Diabetes and hypertension in severe obesity and effects of gastric bypass-induced weight loss. Ann Surg. 2003;237(6):751–8.

27. Neeff H, Mariaskin D, Spangenberg HC, Hopt UT, Makowiec F. Perioperative mortality after non-hepatic general surgery in patients with liver cirrhosis: an analysis of 138 operations in the 2000s using Child and MELD scores. J Gastrointest Surg. 2011;15(1):1–1.
28. Mosko JD, Nguyen GC. Increased perioperative mortality following bariatric surgery among patients with cirrhosis. Clin Gastroenterol Hepatol. 2011;9(10):897–901.
29. Aminian A, Andalib A, Khorgami Z, Cetin D, Burguera B, Bartholomew J, Brethauer SA, Schauer PR. Who should get extended thromboprophylaxis after bariatric surgery?: A risk assessment tool to guide indications for post-discharge pharmacoprophylaxis. Ann Surg. 2017;265(1):143–150.
30. The American Society for Metabolic and Bariatric Surgery Clinical Issues Committee. ASMBS updated position statement on prophylactic measures to reduce the risk of venous thromboembolism in bariatric surgery patients. Surg Obes Relat Dis. 2013;9(4):493–7.
31. Consensus Development Conference Panel. NIH conference. Gastrointestinal surgery for severe obesity. Ann Intern Med. 1991;115:956–61.
32. Rubino F, Nathan DM, Eckel RH, Schauer PR, Alberti KG, Zimmet PZ, Del Prato S, Ji L, Sadikot SM, Herman WH, Amiel SA. Metabolic surgery in the treatment algorithm for type 2 diabetes: a joint statement by international diabetes organizations. Diabetes Care. 2016;39(6):861–77.
33. Kim JJ, Dasika NL, Yu E, Fontana RJ. Cirrhotic patients with a transjugular intrahepatic porto-systemic shunt undergoing major extrahepatic surgery. J Clin Gastroenterol. 2009;43(6):574–9.
34. Mechanick JI, Youdim A, Jones DB, Garvey WT, Hurley DL, McMahon MM, Heinberg LJ, Kushner R, Adams TD, Shikora S, Dixon JB. Clinical practice guidelines for the perioperative nutritional, metabolic, and nonsurgical support of the bariatric surgery patient—2013 update: cosponsored by American Association of Clinical Endocrinologists, The Obesity Society, and American Society for Metabolic & Bariatric Surgery. Obesity. 2013;21(S1):S1–27.
35. Lopez-Delgado JC, Ballus J, Esteve F, Betancur-Zambrano NL, Corral-Velez V, Mañez R, Betbese AJ, Roncal JA, Javierre C. Outcomes of abdominal surgery in patients with liver cirrhosis. World J Gastroenterol. 2016;22(9):2657.

# Chapter 15
# Colorectal Surgery in Cirrhotics

Maysoon Gamaleldin and Luca Stocchi

## Introduction

Cirrhosis carries a heavy burden on both patients and the health system at large with respect to morbidity, mortality and costs, particularly if surgery becomes necessary. Keys to minimize morbidity and mortality associated with colorectal surgery in the presence of cirrhosis are preoperative patient optimization and appropriate indications for surgery, by tailoring the best possible operation to the individual patient tolerance for risk. This chapter presents an overview of preoperative medical optimization, the role of predictive models and preoperative transjugular intrahepatic portosystemic shunt (TIPS) in colorectal surgery, and the reported outcomes of surgery for inflammatory bowel disease and colorectal cancer.

## Preoperative Optimization

Preoperative medical management of cirrhosis is the initial step to reduce perioperative risk. In general, intravenous fluids should be restricted and diuretics can be useful to either prevent the onset of ascites or control existing ascites. Electrolyte imbalances should be corrected and potassium-sparing diuretics can minimize the severity of hypokalemia in this patient population. Coagulation parameters and platelet counts should be assessed and any coagulopathy associated with cirrhosis should be corrected preoperatively. For example, the administration of vitamin K

The authors have no conflicts of interest or financial ties relevant to the current submission.

M. Gamaleldin, MD • L. Stocchi, MD, FACS (✉)
Department of Colorectal Surgery, Digestive Disease Institute, Cleveland Clinic,
9500 Euclid Ave. A-30, Cleveland, OH 44195, USA
e-mail: stocchl@ccf.org

© Springer International Publishing AG 2017
B. Eghtesad, J. Fung (eds.), *Surgical Procedures on the Cirrhotic Patient*,
DOI 10.1007/978-3-319-52396-5_15

with or without added fresh frozen plasma can reduce the International Normalized Ratio (INR) to 1.5 or less in preparation for surgery. With respect to platelet dysfunction, a preoperative plated transfusion, typically administered immediately before surgery, should be considered only when the platelet count is less than 50,000/mm³, while a milder degree of thrombocytopenia is generally just monitored. Patients with known portal hypertension should also undergo preoperative upper endoscopy to band or clip possible esophageal or gastric varices and reduce the risk of postoperative variceal bleeding. Often times patients with cirrhosis are malnourished and nutritional optimization including salt restriction and abstinence from alcohol can be beneficial, if time allows. Patients with ongoing encephalopathy are of particular concern, considering their high risk of perioperative mortality. When surgery is inevitable, correctable causes of encephalopathy such as infections or bleeding should be treated if possible to decrease perioperative risk. The additional use of lactulose to improve encephalopathy by promoting ammonia excretion remains controversial.

## Perioperative Risk of Colorectal Surgery Associated with Cirrhosis and Predictive Models

The relationship between severity of cirrhosis and mortality has been known for a long time. For example, in an earlier study on patients with documented cirrhosis undergoing a variety of colorectal operations between 1971 and 1984, the overall in-hospital mortality was 24% but all patients with preoperative encephalopathy died postoperatively and preoperative ascites, lower serum levels of hemoglobin and albumin were also significantly associated with postoperative mortality [1]. In a more recent study from the National Inpatient Sample (NIS), which included the assessment of postoperative outcomes of colectomy in over 4,700 patients with cirrhosis and over 1,300 with cirrhosis and portal hypertension, the inpatient mortality was almost four times higher among patients with earlier stage cirrhosis (hazard ratio, HR 3.7), while portal hypertension was associated with a HR of 14.3. Not surprisingly, cirrhosis was also associated with longer hospital stay and higher total hospital charges by a percentage exceeding 40% [2]. Table 15.1 summarizes the outcomes of cirrhotic patients undergoing colorectal surgery. The substantial mortality associated with cirrhosis has prompted the development of predictive models for postoperative mortality risk stratification. The two most important to date are the Child–Pugh or Child–Turcotte–Pugh (CTP) [11] score and the Model of End Stage Liver Disease (MELD) Score [12]. The CTP score was initially proposed in 1964 to measure the severity of liver disease in patients with portal hypertension undergoing surgery. It included two continuous variables, albumin and bilirubin, and three discrete variables, namely encephalopathy, nutritional status, and ascites [11]. In 1973 Pugh, when assessing the association between severity of liver disease and outcomes of esophageal transection for bleeding esophageal varices, modified the score where the nutritional status was replaced by prothrombin time [13].

**Table 15.1** Outcomes after colorectal surgery in patients with cirrhosis

| Author | Year | Study design | Diagnosis | Patient number | Overall morbidity rate (%) | Overall mortality rate (%) | Anastomotic leak rate (%) |
|--------|------|--------------|-----------|----------------|----------------------------|----------------------------|----------------------------|
| Metcalf [1] | 1984 | Retrospective, single-institution | Mixed | 54 | 48 | 41 | 19[a] |
| Wind [3] | 1994 | Retrospective, single-institution | Mixed | 84 | 51 | 23 | 7 |
| Gervaz [4] | 2003 | Retrospective, single-institution | Colorectal cancer | 72 | 46 | 13 | 3 |
| Martinez [5] | 2004 | Retrospective, single-institution | Mixed | 17 | 29 | 0 | 0 |
| Meunier [6] | 2008 | Retrospective, single-institution | Mixed | 41 | 77 | 26 | 18 |
| Nguyen [7] | 2009 | Administrative database | Mixed | 4042 | 43–55[b] | 18 | N/A |
| Ghaferi [8] | 2010 | Administrative database | Mixed | 1565 | 50 | 22 | N/A |
| Montomoli [9] | 2013 | Nationwide Cohort | Colorectal cancer | 158 | N/A | 13 | N/A |
| Sabbagh [10] | 2016 | Case-Matched, single-institution | Colorectal cancer | 40 | 83 | 23 | 18 |

[a]Reported as "intrabdominal sepsis".
[b]Morbidity rates reported separately for patients with cirrhosis and cirrhosis associated with portal hypertension
Ghaferi used the definition of "chronic liver disease" instead of cirrhosis (see text).

Earlier assessments of the relationship between CTP scores and mortality after a variety of abdominal operations indicated a proportional relationship between increased CTP score and mortality rates, which was approximately 10% for CTP A class, 31–31% for CTP B class, and 76–82% for CTP C class [14, 15]. However, subsequent assessments of CTP when specifically tested in colorectal surgery have been less consistent. In at least two single-institutional reports, CTP score was not statistically associated with mortality, nor the absolute mortality rates were highest among CTP C patients [4, 6], which might depend on patient selection and the greater impact of other relevant factors on postoperative outcomes. For example, in a series on 41 such patients, CTP was not significantly associated with either post-operative morbidity or mortality. The only independent factor significantly associated with mortality was the onset of postoperative infection, while preoperative ascites was the only factor independently associated with postoperative morbidity [6]. Although widely used to evaluate the severity of cirrhosis, the CTP score also carries significant inherent limitations. Two of the variables are very subjective, namely encephalopathy and ascites, and can also be affected by the use of diuretics and lactulose. In addition, all variables in CTP are weighted equally in the construction of the ultimate score. The MELD score should ideally be the alternative predictive model addressing such limitations. It is a mathematical formula based on the values of serum creatinine, bilirubin, and International Normalized Ratio (INR). The MELD score was initially developed as a statistical model predicting survival in patients undergoing TIPS [16], but was later prospectively validated as a predictive model for patients awaiting orthotopic liver transplantation (OLT) [12], and has subsequently become widely used as a predictive model of surgical risk associated with nontransplant surgery [17].

The MELD score has been shown to predict 1-year and 5-year mortality in a large cohort of cirrhotic patients having a variety of underlying liver disease etiologies and severity [18] and has also been specifically tested on patients undergoing colorectal surgery included in large administrative databases. In a study on over 10,000 patients included in the National Surgical Quality Improvement Program (NSQIP) database, almost 70% of the patients undergoing colorectal surgery had a MELD score of less than 10, which was associated with a perioperative mortality of 2.9%. However, an increased crude MELD score in the whole study population was associated with a substantially increased perioperative mortality. For example, a MELD score between 10 and 14 was associated with a perioperative mortality of almost 10%, while a MELD score between 15 and 19 was associated with a mortality rate exceeding 20%. The authors constructed multivariate regression models on the predicted probability of death, including a number of other relevant variables, stratified by the MELD score. When applying such models to elective procedures, the risk of death increased by 0.5% with each point increase in the MELD score up to 20, after which the risk of death increased by 1% for each additional score point increase. Even more direct was the association between mortality and MELD score following emergent procedures, in which the predicted morality increased by 1% with each MELD score point increase, up to a score of 15, after which each point score increase resulted in a 2% increase in the probability of death. As the authors suggested, while perhaps less sophisticated than other established models to predict perioperative mortality, the MELD score can be easily calculated and practically used to discuss with patients the risk of surgery [19]. It is notable that this study was not limited to patients with known liver disease.

When specifically looking at the adverse outcomes in patients with chronic liver disease, Ghaferi et al. examined 30,927 NSQIP patients undergoing colorectal resections, 1,565 of whom had chronic liver disease. The definition of chronic liver disease used was based on clinical findings indicative of liver dysfunction, namely ascites, esophageal varices and serum total bilirubin greater than 2 mg/dL. The MELD score was used for further risk stratification in the patient cohort thus defined. Patients with chronic liver disease had almost a 6.5-fold increased risk of mortality following colorectal operations. In particular, the mortality among patients without chronic liver disease was 3.2% versus 21.5% among those with chronic liver disease. The same group was also associated with a significantly increased risk of major complications by a relative risk factor of 2.72, based on the absolute percentages of

41.9% among patients with chronic liver disease vs. 15.4% among patients without liver disease. Mortality following major complications (failure to rescue rate) was also markedly increased among patients with chronic liver disease (relative risk 2.27, 34.2%, vs. 15.1%). Stratification of chronic liver disease patients by MELD score demonstrated a significantly higher rate of complications, failure to rescue and mortality in patients with chronic liver disease having a MELD score of 15 or greater compared with patients having a MELD score of less than 15 [8]. This threshold is close to the MELD score cutoff of 14, which has been proposed as a more accurate equivalent of the CTP C class as a predictor of very high risk status after intrabdominal surgery [20].

There is no conclusive evidence indicating the superiority of one predictive score over the other among cirrhotic patients undergoing surgery or other interventional procedures [21]. At this time either score should therefore be considered acceptable for risk stratification and to facilitate the preoperative discussion of patient prognosis.

# Preoperative Transjugular Intrahepatic Portosystemic Shunt Placement

TIPS is a minimally invasive procedure, which accomplishes a diversion of the portal system blood flow into the hepatic veins. TIPS has been proposed as a method to correct portal hypertension and allow extrahepatic abdominal surgery in patients initially deemed inoperable due to their liver disease. In their seminal paper, Azoulay et al. reported on seven patients undergoing preoperative TIPS, also referred to as "neoadjuvant TIPS", followed by a waiting period ranging from 1 to 5 months before abdominal surgery, during which the mean venous pressure gradient successfully decreased from 18 to 9 mmHg. Three out of the seven patients underwent colorectal surgery procedures (left hemicolectomy in two, Hartmann's reversal in one), complicated by one death secondary to liver failure, 36 days after colonic resection [22]. More recently, Menahem et al. reported successful placement of TIPS in eight patients, 1–9 weeks prior to colorectal surgery (three with right colectomy, two with left colectomy, and three with procotectomy), which also resulted in a significant reduction of the hepatic portal venous pressure. There were two postoperative deaths, which occurred in the two patients with the highest pre-TIPS MELD scores [23]. A number of reports, generally including only few selected patients, have confirmed the feasibility of preoperative TIPS before colorectal surgery (Table 15.2). However, not all studies concur in supporting the preoperative use of TIPS to optimize patients undergoing extrahepatic surgery. In particular, Vinet et al. analyzed 18 patients, 10 of whom underwent colectomy, who received preoperative TIPS placement followed by elective extrahepatic surgery after a median interval of $72 \pm 21$ days. Patients undergoing preoperative TIPS placement were case-matched with a control group of 17 cirrhotic patients who underwent surgery without TIPS placement based on age, etiology of cirrhosis, indications for surgery, type of surgery and coagulation parameters. While the CTP score was

Table 15.2 Studies on preoperative placement of TIPS prior to colorectal surgery

| Author | Year | Study design | Patient number | Operations performed | TIPS–surgery interval | Perioperative morbidity n (%) | Perioperative mortality, n (%) |
|--------|------|--------------|----------------|----------------------|------------------------|-------------------------------|---------------------------------|
| Azoulay [22] | 2001 | Retrospective | 3 | Left Hemicolectomy (2) Hartmann's Reversal (1) | 1–5 months[a] | 1(33) | 1(33) |
| Vinet [24] | 2006 | Case-matched | 18 | Colectomy | 72 ± 21 days[b] (mean) | 13[b](72) | 2[b](11) |
| Kim [25] | 2009 | Retrospective | 3 | Subtotal Colectomy (2) Total Colectomy (1) | 33,12 and 46 days | 2 (67) | 0 |
| Menahem [23] | 2014 | Retrospective | 8 | Right hemicolectomy (2) Left hemicolectomy (3) Proctectomy (3) | 1–9 weeks | 6(75) | 2(25) |
| Kochar [26] | 2014 | Retrospective Case Control | 9 | Colectomy for UC with PSC | 2.3 months (median) | 8 (89) | 1 (11) |

[a]Interval based on eight procedures as a whole, including the three colorectal operations
[b]Data based on colectomy and other procedures, namely antrectomy (n = 5), pancreatectomy (n = 1), small bowel resection (n = 1), and nephrectomy (n = 1)

significantly higher in the TIPS group (7.7 versus 6.2), no significant differences were observed with respect to operative blood loss, postoperative complications, duration of hospitalization, 30-day and 1-year mortality. A Cox proportional hazard model failed to demonstrate that either CTP score or TIPS placement had any significant association with survival. While the present study cautioning against the routine use of preoperative TIPS includes a relatively large number of patients, it is important to point out that despite the case-matched design, the CTP score was significantly decreased among patients who did not receive preoperative TIPS. In addition, the portal hepatic pressure gradient was not measured in all patients so that it is possible that portal hypertension was less severe in the control group. With a relatively limited number of events, even a multivariate analysis could fail to account for important differences in the severity of baseline cirrhosis between the two groups, favoring the control group [24]. The use of preoperative TIPS has also been reported among patient undergoing surgery for ulcerative colitis (UC). In a retrospective study on 50 patients with primary sclerosing cholangitis (PSC) requiring surgery for synchronous UC, 13 patients receiving preoperative TIPS were compared with the remaining 37. Duration of UC at the time of surgery, preoperative medical management, or indications for colectomy were similar between the two groups. Not surprisingly, the study group was associated with a significantly more severe liver disease and in particular increased MELD scores, longer aPTT, lower hemoglobin and platelet levels, and decreased mean albumin serum levels. Postoperative mortality only occurred in one patient treated with preoperative TIPS and overall morbidity was statistically comparable, albeit quite common (100% vs. 88% in the TIPS vs. control group, respectively). Patients undergoing preoperative TIPS suffered significantly increased rates of wound infection, wound dehiscence, blood transfusion, and experienced longer hospital stay (8 vs. 5 days, $p = 0.041$) and increased readmission rates (57% vs. 19%, $p = 0.032$). A total of 95% of the patients in the control group ultimately achieved restoration of the intestinal continuity compared with only 43% after preoperative TIPS. This study once more underscores the selection bias for preoperative TIPS toward patients with more severe disease, so that it is difficult to conclusively attribute any increase in postoperative complications mainly to the baseline disease severity or whether preoperative TIPS placement may have played an additional role [27].

## Surgery for Inflammatory Bowel Disease

In an analysis from the Nationwide Inpatient Sample from 1988 to 2006 to determine the frequency of chronic liver disease among patients with IBD and their in-hospital outcomes, the age-adjusted rate of chronic liver disease among hospitalized patients with IBD increased from 4.35 per 100,000 persons during the period between 1988 and 2001 to 7.45 per 100,000 persons in the period between 2004 and 2006. Not surprisingly, the presence of cirrhosis was a significant factor associated with mortality, even among patients receiving medical treatment without undergoing surgery. In particular, there was more than a twofold increase in mortality in patients with concomitant IBD and liver disease compared to other patients with IBD. Not surprisingly, the most common etiology of chronic liver disease was PSC, with over 50% of the cases among patients with UC and 26.5% among patients with Crohn's disease [28]. PSC is a progressive disease associated with the development of cholestasis, which predisposes to an increased risk of cholangiocarcinoma and ultimately leads to end-stage liver disease. Patients with UC have a 2.5–10% risk of synchronous PSC [29–31], while up to 90% of PSC patients have underlying UC [32–36]. The association between Crohn's disease and PSC is less well studied, but at least one study reported that the prevalence of PSC among patients with Crohn's disease was 3.4% [37], while the prevalence of Crohn's disease among PSC patients has been estimated at 16% [38]. With respect to implications for the colon and rectum, PSC is also associated with an increased risk of colorectal dysplasia, progression to colorectal cancer, and pouchitis among patients undergoing ileal pouch-anal anastomosis (IPAA) for UC. In a study comparing 65 patients with PSC and IBD undergoing restorative proctocolectomy vs. 260 IBD patients without associated PSC undergoing the same operation, Gorgun and colleagues identified an increased incidence of cancer and dysplasia in the resected specimen among patients with concurrent PSC, an increased risk of postoperative pelvic sepsis and a higher long-term mortality (35% versus 4%, $p < 0.001$) after a mean follow-up of 68 months, which in the majority of cases was related to liver disease. The 5-year survival in the synchronous PSC group was also significantly decreased, while no significant differences were noted in functional and quality of life results between the two groups. These findings indicate that despite the inherently increased risks, patients with UC and synchronous PSC do benefit from IPAA [39].

The coexistence of PSC and UC can result in a variety of clinical scenarios, depending on their respective severity. When both conditions are in their early stages there is no need for immediate surgery. When instead UC is quiescent, while PSC is more rapidly progressing, OLT may be indicated without any synchronous or sequential colorectal procedures. At the opposite end of the spectrum could be a patient who has UC unresponsive to medical management without evidence of PSC progression. In this case a total proctocolectomy is indicated, generally associated with immediate or staged reconstruction of the intestinal continuity with IPAA. A less common alternative, in cases of contraindication to IPAA or patient preference, is total proctocolectomy with end ileostomy. In this regard, there is a particular caveat associated with end ileostomy among patients with PSC, which is the development of stomal varices due to PSC-associated portal hypertension. Kartheuser et al. reported on 72 patients with UC associated with PSC, of whom 32 having an end ileostomy were compared with 40 patients undergoing IPAA. Eight patients out of 32 developed ileostomy varices and bleeding versus none in the IPAA group [40]. While most patients generally prefer IPAA to avoid a permanent stoma, it is important that the risk of stomal varices associated with PSC is discussed whenever an end ileostomy is considered.

When both PSC and UC require surgical treatment, it has been proposed that OLT could be performed along with a synchronous total abdominal colectomy, followed by delayed completion proctectomy and IPAA once the patient general condition improves. This particular option has been reported in rare cases [41] and in most instances liver and inflammatory bowel disease have been addressed separately. There is evidence indicating that the ultimate outcomes of OLT for PSC are independent from the presence of UC or the results of its own surgical treatments. In a study on 79 patients undergoing OLT for PSC, 27 patients undergoing OLT for PSC associated with UC not requiring surgery were compared with 30 patients undergoing OLT for PSC not associated with UC and with a third group of 22 patients who underwent both OLT for PSC and IPAA for UC. Within the latter group, 9 patients underwent initial IPAA followed by OLT, while 13 patients had OLT and then IPAA. There were no statistical differences among the study groups in either patient or graft survivals. No specific factors were found to be associated with bacteremia or intra-abdominal abscesses on multivariate analysis [42]. These findings resemble a different, previous report on patients receiving both IPAA and OLT indicating stable outcomes over a median of 3.6 years in 32 patients, regardless of their specific treatment sequence (13 had OLT first, 19 had initial IPAA) [27]. These studies indicate that there is no predetermined best combination or sequence of OLT and IPAA and the specific surgical approach should be established on an individual basis, depending on the severity of the respective conditions.

## Peristomal Varices

Peristomal varices are a particular complication of portal hypertension, described since 1968 [43]. Bleeding can originate from local trauma, for example from manipulation of the stoma appliance, or erosion of a submucosal varix [44]. Local treatment options include application of epinephrine-soaked gauze, suture ligation and/or cauterization of the varices, sclerotherapy, endovascular coil embolization, and mucocutaneous disconnection with reconstruction of the ostomy using the same aperture. The goal of mucocutaneous disconnection is to divide the portosystemic communications around the stoma in the subcutaneous tissue of the abdominal wall. While recognizing the risk of recurrence, proponents of mucocutaneous disconnection have argued that this relatively minor procedure carried under local anesthesia can be repeated during follow-up as needed [45]. Subsequent reports have questioned the effectiveness of mucocutaneous disconnection, mainly due to risk of recurrent bleeding, which is common complication of local procedures in general [46]. More extensive stoma revisions or stoma relocations are other surgical options, which, however, carry their own risk of substantial perioperative morbidity. The most consistent and definitive treatment of peristomal varices requires correction of the underlying portal hypertension, which can be accomplished through a surgical portosystemic shunt, OLT or TIPS. Surgical portosystemic shunt is associated with significant mortality and morbidity and is uncommonly performed at this time. Liver transplantation is effective but not always possible, particularly to address ongoing bleeding in a timely fashion. On the other hand, TIPS has been reported as effective treatment of peristomal varices since 1994 [47, 48]. Even after TIPS placement recurrent stomal bleeding can occur, which can depend on stent dysfunction or a lower threshold in the portal pressure gradient resulting in peristomal variceal bleeding.

## Surgery for Colorectal Cancer

While colorectal cancer and cirrhosis could coexist simply because of their individual prevalence, there is data actually indicating that there is an 1.5 to twofold increased incidence of colon cancer in patients with cirrhosis [49, 50]. In a nationwide cohort study on the entire Danish population, including almost 40,000 patients undergoing surgery for colorectal cancer, the 30-day mortality among patients without cirrhosis was 8.7%, while it was 24.1% in patients with cirrhosis. In particular, the mortality among cirrhotic patients electively admitted was 17.2%, while it was 35.6% in case of acute admission. After adjustment for relevant comorbidities, the presence of cirrhosis increased the overall postoperative mortality by a RR of 2.59 [9].

One single institutional study has assessed the complex relationship between underlying cirrhosis and colorectal cancer in the determination of long-term prognosis. Gervaz et al. examined 72 patients undergoing surgery for colorectal cancer. CTP class was the most important factor associated with 5-year overall survival rates. In particular, Child's A patients were associated with a significantly longer 5-year overall survival compared with in Child's classes B and C combined (52% vs. 23%, $p = 0.008$). Unlike Child class, tumor stage was not predictive of survival in this study population and actually node-negative patients had a worse survival rate than stage III patients [4]. This study points out that the decisions regarding management of colorectal cancer in this particular patient population should be tempered by the knowledge on the status and natural history of cirrhosis, which are the critical factors affecting overall survival. In a more recent series, Sabbagh et al. compared 40 patients with cirrhosis (25 with Child A disease and 15 with Child B disease) undergoing resection for colorectal cancer with 80 noncirrhotic controls who were case-matched in a 1:2 ratio based on age, gender, tumor site, and TNM stage (50 matched with Child A patients and 30 with Child B patients). Postoperative complications were not significantly more frequent in Child A patients when compared to controls, unlike patients with Child B cirrhosis, who suffered a significantly increased postoperative morbidity rate when compared with controls. On a percentage basis, Child B patients experienced a 28% anastomotic leak rate and a 20% liver failure rate. Fifty-five percent of the cirrhotic patients for whom chemotherapy was indicated underwent chemotherapy compared with 65% of the control group, a difference that was not statistically significant. Overall survival was significantly worse in the cirrhotic patients, while disease-free survival and cancer-specific survival were statistically comparable between the two groups. In particular the 3-year overall survival was 71% among Child A patients compared with 92% in the case-matched noncirrhotic counterparts, while the 3-year overall survival was 69% in the Child B group compared with 100% in the matched controls. [10] As pointed out by the authors and unlike previous data [51], this series reported good tolerance of chemotherapy by cirrhotic patients, which might depend on accurate treatment selection. These data indicate that the presence of cirrhosis is not an absolute contraindication to surgery or chemotherapy and severity of cirrhosis in the individual patient should be the most critical factor in guiding decisions on management.

## Anastomotic Leak and Stoma Diversion

The occurrence of anastomotic leaks in patients with cirrhosis is particularly worrisome because of the potential to precipitate liver failure and lead to infected ascites, both of which are particularly difficult to manage in the postoperative setting. Unfortunately, large administrative databases typically lack detailed information on this specific complication. The evidence on the incidence and consequences of anastomotic leakage remains therefore confined to single-institution, relatively small retrospective series. The anastomotic leak rate after colorectal surgery in cirrhotic patients ranges between 0 and 19% (Table 15.1). It is notable that the only series without reported anastomotic leaks is also the only series describing the systematic use of laparoscopic colorectal surgery in selected patients with cirrhosis [5]. Gervaz and colleagues reported a 3% anastomotic leak rate without any resulting death, which according to the authors indicated that "colonic anastomosis is safe in cirrhotic patients" [4], thus reversing the results of an earlier publication from the same institution in which 5 out of 54 patients undergoing colorectal surgery developed an anastomotic leakage, ultimately leading to death [1]. Other series, also including contemporary data, have instead confirmed the difficulty in rescuing a cirrhotic patient developing anastomotic leakage, reporting a mortality rate following anastomotic leaks ranging from 60% to 100% [3, 6, 23]. While impressive on a percentage basis, it is important to point out that the data mentioned above relies on single-digit event numbers. Despite the significant concerns associated with the possible adverse consequences of an anastomotic leak, there is insufficient data to assess the potential advantages associated with more widespread use of nonrestorative procedures or the creation of an additional stoma diversion to at least minimize the morbidity associated with anastomotic complications. This is not surprising, considering that the ileostomy aperture may become an additional avenue for ascetic fluid leakage and other substantial stoma-related complications. Future studies will need to clarify this dilemma and delineate possible indications for elective stoma creation.

## Conclusions

Colorectal surgery in the presence of cirrhosis is a realistic scenario considering the prevalence of chronic liver disease and the frequency of colorectal resections for both benign disease and malignancy. Patients with cirrhosis have a substantially increased perioperative risk, which can be more precisely assessed by using formal predictive models. When such risk is high, as in the case of advanced cirrhosis associated with portal hypertension, a preoperative TIPS placement may have a role in reducing perioperative mortality when used combined with medical optimization. Accurate patient selection is also important to obtain satisfactory postoperative outcomes, which have been reported in a relatively small studies conducted by single institutions for both benign and malignant diseases. Future efforts should focus at further improving patient selection and perioperative management to reduce the still considerable morbidity and mortality.

# References

1. Metcalf AMT, Dozois RR, Wolff BG, Beart Jr RW. The surgical risk of colectomy in patients with cirrhosis. Dis Colon Rectum. 1987;30:529–31.
2. Csikesz NG, Nguyen LN, Tseng JF, Shah SA. Nationwide volume and mortality after elective surgery in cirrhotic patients. J Am Coll Surg. 2009;208:96–103.
3. Wind P, Teixeira A, Parc R. La chirurgie colo-rectale chez le cirrhotique, Gillet M. La chirurgie digestive chez le cirrhotique. Paris: Springer; 1994. p. 81–90.
4. Gervaz P, Pak-art R, Nivatvongs S, Wolff BG, Larson D, Ringel S. Colorectal adenocarcinoma in cirrhotic patients. J Am Coll Surg. 2003;196:874–9.
5. Martínez J, Rivas H, Delgado S, Castells A, Pique J, Lacy A. Laparoscopic-assited colectomy in patients with liver cirrhosis. Surg Endosc Other Intervent Techn. 2004;18:1071–4.
6. Meunier K, Mucci S, Quentin V, Azoulay R, Arnaud J, Hamy A. Colorectal surgery in cirrhotic patients: assessment of operative morbidity and mortality. Dis Colon Rectum. 2008;51: 1225–31.
7. Nguyen GC, Correia AJ, Thuluvath PJ. The impact of cirrhosis and portal hypertension on mortality following colorectal surgery: a nationwide, population-based study. Dis Colon Rectum. 2009;52:1367–74.
8. Ghaferi AA, Mathur AK, Sonnenday CJ, Dimick JB. Adverse outcomes in patients with chronic liver disease undergoing colorectal surgery. Ann Surg. 2010;252:345–50.
9. Montomoli J, Erichsen R, Christiansen CF, Ulrichsen SP, Pedersen L, Nilsson T, et al. Liver disease and 30-day mortality after colorectal cancer surgery: a Danish population-based cohort study. BMC Gastroenterol. 2013;13:1.
10. Sabbagh C, Chatelain D, Nguyen-Khac E, Rebibo L, Joly J, Regimbeau J. Management of colorectal cancer in patients with cirrhosis: a retrospective, case-matched study of short-and long-term outcomes. Dig Liver Dis. 2016;48(4):429–34.
11. Child CG, Turcotte JG. Surgery and portal hypertension. Major Probl Clin Surg. 1964;1:1–85.
12. Wiesner R, Edwards E, Freeman R, Harper A, Kim R, Kamath P, et al. Model for end-stage liver disease (MELD) and allocation of donor livers. Gastroenterology. 2003;124:91–6.
13. Pugh R, Murray-Lyon I, Dawson J, Pietroni M, Williams R. Transection of the oesophagus for bleeding oesophageal varices. Br J Surg. 1973;60:646–9.
14. Garrison RN, Cryer HM, Howard DA, Polk Jr HC. Clarification of risk factors for abdominal operations in patients with hepatic cirrhosis. Ann Surg. 1984;199:648–55.
15. Mansour A, Watson W, Shayani V, Pickleman J. Abdominal operations in patients with cirrhosis: still a major surgical challenge. Surgery. 1997;122:730–6.
16. Malinchoc M, Kamath PS, Gordon FD, Peine CJ, Rank J, Ter Borg PC. A model to predict poor survival in patients undergoing transjugular intrahepatic portosystemic shunts. Hepatology. 2000;31:864–71.

17. Northup PG, Wanamaker RC, Lee VD, Adams RB, Berg CL. Model for End-Stage Liver Disease (MELD) predicts nontransplant surgical mortality in patients with cirrhosis. Ann Surg. 2005;242:244–51.
18. Said A, Williams J, Holden J, Remington P, Gangnon R, Musat A, et al. Model for end stage liver disease score predicts mortality across a broad spectrum of liver disease. J Hepatol. 2004;40:897–903.
19. Hedrick TL, Swenson BR, Friel CM. Model for End-stage Liver Disease (MELD) in predicting postoperative mortality of patients undergoing colorectal surgery. Am Surg. 2013;79:347–52.
20. Befeler AS, Palmer DE, Hoffman M, Longo W, Solomon H, Di Bisceglie AM. The safety of intra-abdominal surgery in patients with cirrhosis: model for end-stage liver disease score is superior to Child-Turcotte-Pugh classification in predicting outcome. Arch Surg. 2005;140:650–4.
21. Peng Y, Qi X, Guo X. Child-Pugh versus MELD score for the assessment of prognosis in liver cirrhosis: a systematic review and meta-analysis of observational studies. Medicine (Baltimore). 2016;95:e2877.
22. Azoulay D, Buabse F, Damiano I, Smail A, Ichai P, Dannaoui M, et al. Neoadjuvant transjugular intrahepatic portosystemic shunt: a solution for extrahepatic abdominal operation in cirrhotic patients with severe portal hypertension. J Am Coll Surg. 2001;193:46–51.
23. Menahem B, Lubrano J, Desjouis A, Lepennec V, Lebreton G, Alves A. Transjugular intrahepatic portosystemic shunt placement increases feasibility of colorectal surgery in cirrhotic patients with severe portal hypertension. Dig Liver Dis. 2015;47:81–4.
24. Vinet E, Perreault P, Bouchard L, Bernard D, Wassef R, Richard C, et al. Transjugular intrahepatic portosystemic shunt before abdominal surgery in cirrhotic patients: a retrospective, comparative study. Can J Gastroenterol Hepatol. 2006;20:401–4.
25. Kim JJ, Dasika NL, Yu E, Fontana RJ. Cirrhotic patients with a transjugular intrahepatic portosystemic shunt undergoing major extrahepatic surgery. J Clin Gastroenterol. 2009;43:574–9.
26. Kochhar G, Navaneethan U, Parungao JM, Hartman J, Gupta R, Lopez R, et al. Impact of transjugular intrahepatic portosystemic shunt on post-colectomy complications in patients with ulcerative colitis and primary sclerosing cholangitis. Gastroenterol Rep (Oxf). 2015;3:228–33.
27. Mathis K, Dozois E, Larson D, Cima R, Sarmiento J, Wolff B, et al. Ileal pouch–anal anastomosis and liver transplantation for ulcerative colitis complicated by primary sclerosing cholangitis. Br J Surg. 2008;95:882–6.
28. Nguyen DL, Bechtold ML, Jamal MM. National trends and inpatient outcomes of inflammatory bowel disease patients with concomitant chronic liver disease. Scand J Gastroenterol. 2014;49:1091–5.
29. Boberg K, Aadland E, Jahnsen J, Raknerud N, Stiris M, Bell H. Incidence and prevalence of primary biliary cirrhosis, primary sclerosing cholangitis, and autoimmune hepatitis in a Norwegian population. Scand J Gastroenterol. 1998;33:99–103.
30. Olsson R, Danielsson Å, Järnerot G, Lindström E, Lööf L, Rolny P, et al. Prevalence of primary sclerosing cholangitis in patients with ulcerative colitis. Gastroenterology. 1991;100:1319–23.
31. O'Toole A, Alakkari A, Keegan D, Doherty G, Mulcahy H, O'Donoghue D. Primary sclerosing cholangitis and disease distribution in inflammatory bowel disease. Clin Gastroenterol Hepatol. 2012;10:439–41.
32. Bambha K, Kim WR, Talwalkar J, Torgerson H, Benson JT, Therneau TM, et al. Incidence, clinical spectrum, and outcomes of primary sclerosing cholangitis in a United States community. Gastroenterology. 2003;125:1364–9.
33. Escorsell A, Parés A, Rodés J, Solís-Herruzo JA, Miras M, de la Morena E. Epidemiology of primary sclerosing cholangitis in Spain. J Hepatol. 1994;21:787–91.
34. Tung BY, Brentnall TA, Kowdley KV, Emond M, Kimmey MB, Stevens AC, Rubin CE, Haggitt RC. Diagnosis and prevalence of ulcerative colitis in patients with sclerosing cholangitis (abstract) Hepatology. 1996;24:169A.

35. Loftus Jr EV, Harewood GC, Loftus CG, Tremaine WJ, Harmsen WS, Zinsmeister AR, et al. PSC-IBD: a unique form of inflammatory bowel disease associated with primary sclerosing cholangitis. Gut. 2005;54:91–6.
36. Sano H, Nakazawa T, Ando T, Hayashi K, Naitoh I, Okumura F, et al. Clinical characteristics of inflammatory bowel disease associated with primary sclerosing cholangitis. J Hepato-Biliary-Pancreat Sci. 2011;18:154–61.
37. Rasmussen H, Fallingborg J, Mortensen P, Vyberg M, Tage-Jensen U, Rasmussen S. Hepatobiliary dysfunction and primary sclerosing cholangitis in patients with Crohn's disease. Scand J Gastroenterol. 1997;32:604–10.
38. de Vries AB, Janse M, Blokzijl H, Weersma RK. Distinctive inflammatory bowel disease phenotype in primary sclerosing cholangitis. World J Gastroenterol. 2015;21:1956–71.
39. Gorgun E, Remzi FH, Manilich E, Preen M, Shen B, Fazio VW. Surgical outcome in patients with primary sclerosing cholangitis undergoing ileal pouch–anal anastomosis: A case-control study. Surgery. 2005;138:631–9.
40. Kartheuser, Alex H., et al. Comparison of surgical treatment of ulcerative colitis associated with primary sclerosing cholangitis: ileal pouch-anal anastomosis versus Brooke ileostomy. Mayo Clinic Proceedings. Vol. 71. No. 8. Elsevier, 1996.
41. Poritz LS, Koltun WA. Surgical management of ulcerative colitis in the presence of primary sclerosing cholangitis. Dis Colon Rectum. 2003;46:173–8.
42. Obusez EC, Lian L, Shao Z, Navaneethan U, O'Shea R, Kiran RP, et al. Impact of ileal pouch-anal anastomosis on the surgical outcome of orthotopic liver transplantation for primary sclerosing cholangitis. J Crohn's Colitis. 2013;7:230–8.
43. Resnick RH, Ishihara A, Chalmers TC, Schimmel EM. A controlled trial of colon bypass in chronic hepatic encephalopathy. Gastroenterology. 1968;54:1057–69.
44. Conte JV, Arcomano TA, Naficy MA, Holt RW. Treatment of bleeding stomal varices. Dis Colon Rectum. 1990;33:308–14.
45. Beck DE, Fazio VW, Grundfest-Broniatowski S. Surgical management of bleeding stomal varices. Dis Colon Rectum. 1988;31:343–6.
46. Spier BJ, Fayyad AA, Lucey MR, Johnson EA, Wojtowycz M, Rikkers L, et al. Bleeding stomal varices: case series and systematic review of the literature. Clin Gastroenterol Hepatol. 2008;6:346–52.
47. Lagier E, Rousseau H, Maquin P, Olives J, Le Tallec C, Vinel J. Treatment of bleeding stomal varices using transjugular intrahepatic portosystemic shunt. J Pediatr Gastroenterol Nutr. 1994;18:501–3.
48. Kochar N, Tripathi D, McAvoy N, Ireland H, Redhead D, Hayes P. Bleeding ectopic varices in cirrhosis: the role of transjugular intrahepatic portosystemic stent shunts. Aliment Pharmacol Ther. 2008;28:294–303.
49. Sørensen HT, Friis S, Olsen JH, Thulstrup AM, Mellemkjær L, Linet M, et al. Risk of liver and other types of cancer in patients with cirrhosis: a nationwide cohort study in Denmark. Hepatology. 1998;28:921–5.
50. Goldacre MJ, Wotton CJ, Yeates D, Seagroatt V, Collier J. Liver cirrhosis, other liver diseases, pancreatitis and subsequent cancer: record linkage study. Eur J Gastroenterol Hepatol. 2008;20:384–92.
51. Madbouly KM, Hussein AM, Zeid A. Colorectal cancer surgery in portal hypertensive patients: does adjuvant oxaliplatin affect prognosis? Dis Colon Rectum. 2013;56:577–85.

# Chapter 16
# Urologic Procedures in Patients with Cirrhosis

Peter A. Caputo and Jihad H. Kaouk

## Introduction

Surgery has recently become more commonplace in patients with liver cirrhosis, likely due to the improved survival of patients with cirrhosis over the past few decades [1]. Cirrhotic patients more commonly require surgical intervention for liver procedures, abdominal wall hernia, cholelithiasis, and peptic ulcer disease; however, urologic issues such as urinary calculus disease and genitourinary malignancy may also arise and require surgical intervention. The patient with liver cirrhosis is at increased risk for a host of life-threatening perioperative complications including infection, encephalopathy, bleeding, intractable ascites, liver decompensation, and multiorgan failure. There is a marked increase in surgical morbidity and mortality in patients with liver cirrhosis undergoing all types of surgery. Here we will address some of the specific considerations to be undertaken during urologic surgical procedures.

## Preoperative Assessment and Preparations

Patients with mild to moderate liver disease are frequently asymptomatic. Further, patients are oftentimes unaware of the presence or severity of their liver dysfunction and will not report this on routine history questioning. Thus, preoperative questioning aimed to elucidate liver dysfunction should be performed, specifically regarding prior diagnoses of hepatitis as well as thorough review of systems inquiring about the presence of pruritus, excessive bleeding, abnormal abdominal distention, and

P.A. Caputo, MD • J.H. Kaouk, MD, FACS (✉)
Center for Robotic and Advanced Laparoscopic Surgery,
Glickman Urologic Institute, Cleveland Clinic, Cleveland, OH, USA

© Springer International Publishing AG 2017                                    215
B. Eghtesad, J. Fung (eds.), *Surgical Procedures on the Cirrhotic Patient*,
DOI 10.1007/978-3-319-52396-5_16

inadvertent weight gain. Physical exam findings that suggest liver dysfunction include jaundice, scleral icterus, abdominal fluid wave, caput medusae, clubbing, spider angiomata, and palmar erythema.

Upon identification of the cirrhotic patient, the clinician can make an accurate assessment of the surgical morbidity and mortality using combination of both the Child–Pugh classification and the Model for End-Stage Liver Disease score [2]. Most urologic surgery is possible in well-compensated chronic liver disease patients; however, very little is possible in those with decompensated cirrhosis. For this reason, preoperative risk assessment is of utmost importance for those with liver disease.

It is important when planning retroperitoneal surgery one has a good knowledge of portosystemic collateral drainage that may exists in the retroperitoneum of cirrhosis patients. Apart from the classical collateral pathways, such as the left gastric, short gastric, recanalized umbilical, paraumbilical, and superior rectal veins, there exist nonclassical collateral pathways from the left gastric veins through the inferior phrenic and adrenal vein eventually reaching the left renal vein and into systemic circulation [3, 4]. Contrasted cross-sectional imaging of the abdomen is paramount in evaluating such patients for surgical planning.

# Endoscopic Surgery in Patients with Cirrhosis

## Urolithiasis

Cirrhotic patients are at increased risk for the development of calcium oxalate urinary calculi. This is attributed to the presence of multiple concurrent calculogenic states such as hyperoxaluria, malnutrition, intravascular volume depletion, and poor performance status [5]. Due to this, urolithiasis is among the most common surgical dilemmas encountered by an urologist in cirrhotic patients.

A study by Pattaras et al. presented data on a small series of 16 patients requiring 23 endoscopic surgeries for urolithiasis for patients with a diagnosis of liver cirrhosis. The cirrhosis in this series was significant enough the patients had previously been evaluated for liver transplant. The patients underwent both ureteroscopy and percutaneous nephrolithotripsy. The authors report a 26.1% complication rate, a 26.1% postoperative transfusion rate, and one mortality [5].

## Benign Prostatic Hyperplasia

Lower urinary tract symptoms affect over half the population of aging men. Likewise about 30% of cirrhotic men will experience lower urinary tract symptoms [6]. Although the most bothersome lower urinary tract symptoms experienced by men with cirrhosis are largely attributed to diuretic use there are some who experience obstructive urinary symptoms. A Danish population-based study identified patients with the diagnosis of cirrhosis based on ICD codes that had then undergone transurethral resection of the prostate. They report a 30-day mortality rate of 6.7% in those men with cirrhosis following transurethral resection of the prostate [7]. It should be noted that transurethral resection of the prostate is an elective surgery to improve the patients quality of life through the relief of urinary tract symptoms. The undertaking of this procedure in the cirrhotic population should be done only in select cases and when nonsurgical options have proven unsuccessful.

## Surgery for Urologic Malignancy in Patients with Cirrhosis

### Renal Cell Carcinoma

Cirrhotic patients with renal tumors are ideal candidates for active surveillance or minimally invasive treatment options such as thermal ablation. However, active surveillance and thermal ablation for renal tumors are indeed limited by tumor size and location. When conservative measures fail more invasive surgical options may become necessary. Also a unique dilemma arises in which a cirrhotic patient being evaluated for liver transplant is found to have a renal neoplasm and for whom extirpative surgery would render the patient eligible for transplant. Laparoscopic radical and partial nephrectomy have been shown to be a feasible treatment option for renal neoplasms in cirrhotic patients with reported rates of complications up to 30% all of which were hemorrhagic complications [8, 9]. It should be noted that these reports in the urologic literature are sparse and are case series with relatively small numbers of patients treated.

### Urothelial Carcinoma

Liver cirrhosis is not only a risk factor for hepatocellular carcinoma but also for nonhepatic carcinoma, particularly those associated with tobacco use [10]. Urothelial carcinoma usually presents with hematuria. The presence of liver cirrhosis may lead to more pronounced hematuria. Radical cystectomy is already a procedure that carries a high risk of morbidity and mortality. Severe bleeding has been reported in patients with urinary diversion created from intestinal segments in cirrhotic patients. The bleeding is found to be from intestinal segment variceal hemorrhage requiring TIPS procedure [11, 12]. Urothelial carcinoma should be treated via endoscopic means when possible in patients with cirrhosis.

## Laparoscopic and Robotic Surgical Approach

Cirrhosis is not an absolute contraindication to laparoscopic surgery. Multiple series have shown that laparoscopy is not only safe but actually provides many advantages over open surgery in carefully selected cirrhotic patients [13]. Minimally invasive laparoscopic and robotic approaches should be considered in patients with liver cirrhosis.

# References

1. Friedman LS. Surgery in the patient with liver disease. Trans Am Clin Climatol Assoc. 2010; 121:192–204; discussion 205.
2. O'Leary JG, Friedman LS. Predicting surgical risk in patients with cirrhosis: from art to science. Gastroenterology. 2007;132(4):1609–11.
3. Moll R, von Ludinghausen MH, Lackner K, Landwehr P. Collateral pathways in portal hypertension. Surg Radiol Anat. 1990;12(2):127–33.
4. Widrich WC, Srinivasan M, Semine MC, Robbins AH. Collateral pathways of the left gastric vein in portal hypertension. AJR Am J Roentgenol. 1984;142(2):375–82.
5. Pattaras JG, Ogan K, Martinez E, Nieh P. Endourological management of urolithiasis in hepatically compromised patients. J Urol. 2008;179(3):976–80.
6. Margreiter M, Heinisch BB, Schwarzer R, Klatte T, Shariat SF, Ferlitsch A. Lower urinary tract symptoms in patients with liver cirrhosis. World J Urol. 2015;33(3):315–21.
7. Nielsen SS, Thulstrup AM, Lund L, Vilstrup H, Sorensen HT. Postoperative mortality in patients with liver cirrhosis undergoing transurethral resection of the prostate: a Danish nationwide cohort study. BJU Int. 2001;87(3):183–6.
8. Johnston 3rd WK, Montgomery JS, Wolf Jr JS. Retroperitoneoscopic radical and partial nephrectomy in the patient with cirrhosis. J Urol. 2005;173(4):1094–7.
9. Hayn MH, Averch TD, Jackman SV. Transperitoneal laparoscopic radical and partial nephrectomy in patients with cirrhosis: report of three cases. Can J Urol. 2009;16(4):4770–3.
10. Sorensen HT, Friis S, Olsen JH, Thulstrup AM, Mellemkjaer L, Linet M, et al. Risk of liver and other types of cancer in patients with cirrhosis: a nationwide cohort study in Denmark. Hepatology. 1998;28(4):921–5.
11. Chavez DR, Snyder PM, Juravsky LI, Heaney JA. Recurrent ileal conduit hemorrhage in an elderly cirrhotic man. J Urol. 1994;152(3):951–3.
12. Carrafiello G, Lagana D, Giorgianni A, Lumia D, Mangini M, Paragone E, et al. Bleeding from peristomal varices in a cirrhotic patient with ileal conduit: treatment with transjugular intrahepatic portocaval shunt (TIPS). Emerg Radiol. 2007;13(6):341–3.
13. Cobb WS, Heniford BT, Burns JM, Carbonell AM, Matthews BD, Kercher KW. Cirrhosis is not a contraindication to laparoscopic surgery. Surg Endosc. 2005;19(3):418–23.

# Chapter 17
# Kidney Transplantation in Cirrhotic Patients

Antonios Arvelakis, Sander Florman, and Ron Shapiro

## Introduction

Kidney transplantation in cirrhotic patients represents an area of some controversy. The high morbidity and mortality associated with major surgery in cirrhotic patients has led many programs to exclude cirrhotic patients from kidney transplantation. In the majority of cases, cirrhotic patients with end-stage renal disease are listed for a combined kidney and liver transplant. With the advent of the MELD system, the number of combined liver/kidney transplants increased by 300% [1]. However, there are a large number of patients who do not have a high enough MELD score to qualify for a liver/kidney offer. These are the cirrhotic patients with normal liver function tests and INR who are on dialysis; they automatically receive a MELD of 21 because of dialysis, but the sad reality is that this score cannot give them a liver offer in most regions. Unfortunately, the mortality of these patients on dialysis is very high, with a median survival of 11 months [2]. This has raised the question of whether these patients would benefit from a kidney transplant alone as opposed to waiting on the list for a combined liver/kidney transplant. Multiple studies have been carried out on kidney transplantation in patients with end-stage liver disease, mainly but not exclusively on hepatitis C–infected patients, and have addressed multiple end points such as patient survival with and without kidney transplantation, graft survival, incidence of liver decompensation, and worsening of hepatitis C. The results, although in some settings controversial and conflicting, suggest that kidney transplantation in cirrhotic patients is justifiable and should be done in certain circumstances and with certain indications.

A. Arvelakis (✉) • S. Florman • R. Shapiro
Recanati/Miller Transplantation Institute, The Mount Sinai Hospital,
One Gustave L. Levy Place, Box 1104, New York, NY 10029-6574, USA
e-mail: antonios.arvelakis@mountsinai.org

© Springer International Publishing AG 2017
B. Eghtesad, J. Fung (eds.), *Surgical Procedures on the Cirrhotic Patient*,
DOI 10.1007/978-3-319-52396-5_17

# Overview

Chronic liver disease is not uncommon among patients with end-stage renal disease. In the majority of cases the etiology is hepatitis C. Studies on hemodialysis patients have shown that the incidence of chronic hepatitis C infection is higher in this group than in the general population [3]. The number of years on hemodialysis and the number of blood products received seem to correlate with the infection risk. In developed countries, advanced methods of detecting hepatitis C infected products and the increased use of erythropoiesis stimulating factors instead of transfusions have caused a decline in hepatitis C infection in hemodialysis patients, with a prevalence between 3% and 30% [4–8]; however this percentage remains higher in developing countries (6–80%) [9–11]. The incidence of cirrhosis among these patients is quite high, with reports of over 20% [12]. Other etiologies of liver cirrhosis can also be found among ESRD patients but with a much lower incidence than hepatitis C. In particular, Nonalcoholic steatohepatitis, a rapidly emerging etiology of chronic liver disease and cirrhosis in the western population has also been linked with ESRD. Interestingly, this correlation seems to be independent of the metabolic syndrome and traditional common risk factors such as diabetes [13, 14].

Major concerns about kidney transplantation in patients with chronic hepatitis C are the potential acceleration of the hepatitis C infection due to the immunosuppression treatment post transplant and eventual histological progression and decompensation of the liver disease [15, 16]. Some studies have shown a rising viral load after a kidney transplant, especially in patients with significant viremia at the time of transplantation; the hepatitis C-RNA levels after transplant have been shown to increase between 2-fold and 30-fold [17]. However, the impact of this increase on the liver histopathology and function is not clear. Few studies have performed serial liver biopsies after the kidney transplantation [18, 19]. Most of them showed several degrees of histological progression of Hepatitis C disease, especially in patients with worse histopathology pretransplant, but not persistently and without significant worsening of the liver function [20–23].

Regardless of the evolution of the hepatitis C infection and liver fibrosis the most important question is how hepatitis C affects survival after kidney transplantation. There are a large number of studies which evaluated the effects of Hepatitis C on patient and graft survival [12, 15, 24]. Most of the studies have shown that graft survival in hepatitis C positive recipients is lower than the Hepatitis C negative counterparts. Fabrizi et al. conducted a meta-analysis on observational studies and demonstrated a 1.56 Relative Risk of graft loss in Hepatitis C positive patients when compared to hepatitis C negative patients. The same study showed that hepatitis C positivity is an independent risk factor for graft loss [25]. In a more recent review of 18 studies Rostami et al. showed similar results with a Hazard Ratio of 1.5 for graft loss and also demonstrated that hepatitis C infection is an independent predictor of unfavorable graft outcome [26].

The reasons for inferior graft function in hepatitis C positive recipients are not fully understood, but certain mechanisms are possible. These patients can develop a de novo hepatitis C–related glomerulonephritis. This can be a cryoglobulinemic or noncryoglobulinemic membranoproliferative glomerulonephritis (MPGN) or membranous glomerulonephritis (MGN), and the pathogenesis seems to be the deposition of immune complexes containing viral RNA in the glomerulus [27]. Berthoux et al. [17] studied MPGN and MGN in renal transplant recipients and found that hepatitis C positivity was statistically higher in patients who developed these types of glomerulonephritis post transplant. In addition, hepatitis C infection increases the risk of interstitial fibrosis/tubular atrophy (IF/TA). Post-transplant glomerulopathy among hepatitis C recipients has a prevalence of IF/TA of up to 50% [27]. The mechanisms underlying this correlation are not fully understood; however, direct effect of the hepatitis C virus on the glomeruli or higher immunologic risk in hepatitis C patients are very likely. Rejection has also been considered a potential causative factor of graft loss in hepatitis C patients. However, the majority of studies have failed to demonstrate increased rate of rejection in this group. Corell et al. [28] showed a decreased prevalence of rejection in hepatitis C patients, while others have showed increased [29] or similar rates between the two groups [30]. Another possible explanation of the reduced graft survival in hepatitis C patients is the increased incidence of new onset diabetes after transplant (NODAT). It is well known that there is a correlation between hepatitis C infection and diabetes, because of insulin resistance caused by inhibitory actions of the virus on the insulin regulatory pathways of the liver [27, 31]. NODAT can negatively affect graft survival, but it is also an independent risk factor for lower patient survival.

The survival of hepatitis C infected patients after kidney transplantation has been extensively studied. Even though the results are not consistent in all the studies it has been shown that hepatitis C positive patients have lower survival post kidney transplant compared to hepatitis C negative patients [32]. Some studies did not show any difference in survival between the hepatitis C positive and hepatitis C negative groups until after the first 5 years post transplant [33]. In a retrospective study of 835 patients Mathuri et al. [33] found a decrease in patient survival after 10 years post transplant but no difference prior to 10 years. In the two largest meta-analyses of Fabrizi and Rostami the hazard ratio of death in the hepatitis C population was 1.79 and 1.69, respectively, vs. nonhepatitis C patients. The majority of deaths were due to cardiovascular causes, infection and liver related complications [15, 26]. It is known that hepatitis C patients have an increased risk of infection post transplant [34]. In many studies, hepatitis C has been shown to be an independent risk factor for blood stream infections. On the other hand, the increased incidence of NODAT in these patients may explain the higher rate of cardiovascular complications and death especially after 10 years. Finally, some increase in PTLD and myeloma has been observed in hepatitis C patients post transplant and may be contributing to the increased mortality [35]. However, despite the decreased survival of hepatitis C patients compared to the nonhepatitis C population, it is important to point out that there is a significant survival advantage within the hepatitis C group [36]. All the studies which compared the survival of hepatitis C patients with end-stage renal disease with and without a kidney transplant showed a significant benefit with transplantation [36, 37]. The mortality of hepatitis C patients on dialysis, especially when they have diabetes [37], is substantial, with a survival of less than 30% at 8 years [38]. Cirrhotic patients on dialysis have a 35% higher death rate than their noncirrhotic counterparts [2]. Roth et al. in a prospective study of 175 hepatitis C–positive patients listed for a kidney transplant showed that the mortality in the transplant group was significantly lower than staying on the waiting list, with a Hazard Ratio for death of 0.3 in favor of transplantation [34, 39]. So despite the lower patient and graft survival that the hepatitis C infected patients demonstrate after kidney transplantation in comparison to hepatitis C–negative patients, these differences are less important than the clear survival benefit in the hepatitis C population from a kidney transplantation vs. staying on dialysis. This survival benefit is comparable with the benefit observed after transplantation in the general population with ESRD [34].

Many researchers have investigated the factors that affect the mortality of patients with hepatitis C who receive a kidney transplant. One of the first studies was by Rao et al. who looked at the effect of liver fibrosis pretransplant on patient and graft survival post-transplant [22]. They demonstrated that the severity of liver histopathology was correlated with worse postransplant outcomes. Their study and other similar studies showed the importance of the liver biopsy in the evaluation of hepatitis C and other chronic liver disease patients who need a kidney transplant. Their suggestion was that advanced stages of fibrosis and histological evidence of cirrhosis should be a contraindication for a kidney transplant alone. More recent studies, however, showed that the severity of the liver histopathology is not the only predictor of post-transplant outcome. Maluf et al. demonstrated that worse liver histopathology (Knodel score > 6) is indeed a predictor of worse outcome after a kidney transplant with a mortality Hazard Ratio of 1.3, but it is not the only risk factor and not the strongest one either. In their multivariate analysis, they showed that apart from liver histology, deceased donor (HR: 17.9), previous kidney transplant (HR: 9.3) and pretransplant diabetes (HR: 4.7), are independent predictors of mortality post transplant [24]. Moreover, Campbel et al. in their cohort of 108 chronic hepatitis C patients with end-stage renal disease (18 of whom had cirrhosis) showed that the degree of liver fibrosis did not affect patient survival post transplant. The hazard ratio of death for cirrhotic patients post kidney transplant was 0.64 (P: 0.38). They also showed that diabetes mellitus was an independent factor of mortality post-transplant [32]. These studies supported that advanced fibrosis and cirrhosis in the pretransplant biopsy should not exclude patients from a kidney transplant, but they should be evaluated in the context of other comorbidities especially diabetes, previous transplantation and advanced age of the recipient. We must emphasize that the cirrhotic patients included in these studies were younger, with no portal hypertension and with well compensated cirrhosis. Any signs of portal hypertension or any decompensating episode such as encephalopathy, ascites or varices/upper GI bleeding were excluding factors. In the same context Paramesh et al. compared the 1 and 3 year patient and graft survival between cirrhotic and noncirrhotic hepatitis C patients who received a kidney transplant. They used HVPG measurements in all the cirrhotic patients and a portal pressure of less than 10 was the cut off for acceptance for transplantation. They found no statistically significant difference between the two groups in their post-transplant outcomes [40]. Advanced age and low albumin were two independent factors which affected negatively the survival in the cirrhotic group. Parsikia et al. in a similar retrospective study showed that when they transplanted hepatitis C well compensated cirrhotic patients with normal (<10) HVPG, normal PLT count, and normal albumin levels, their 1 and 3 year patient and graft survival were similar to their noncirrhotic counterparts [2]. Finally Chan et al. looked at cirrhotic patients with ESRD in the UNOS data base from 1987 to 2012 and demonstrated that well-compensated patients who received kidney transplantation had excellent survival and in some cases better than patients with combined liver/kidney transplants [1].

Separate consideration should be given to the patient population with decompensated liver cirrhosis and renal dysfunction. Up to 20% of hospitalized patients with decompensated liver cirrhosis have some degree of acute renal failure [41]. In these patients the renal failure is part of the extrahepatic manifestations of severe liver disease. The 3-month survival of these patients without a liver transplantation is very low, ranging between 20% and 40% [42]. The only option for these patients is a liver transplantation. As determined by ASTS/UNOS guidelines a kidney should be transplanted simultaneously with the liver in the following cases: (i) end-stage renal disease with cirrhosis and symptomatic portal hypertension or hepatic vein wedge pressure gradient ≥10 mm Hg, (ii) liver failure and chronic kidney disease with GFR ≤30 mL/min, (iii) acute kidney injury or hepatorenal syndrome with creatinine ≥2.0 mg/dL and dialysis ≥8 weeks, (iv) liver failure and chronic kidney disease with kidney biopsy demonstrating >30% glomerulosclerosis or 30% fibrosis [43].

## Conclusions

Kidney transplantation in patients with hepatitis C chronic liver disease is justifiable. It may not achieve the excellent patient and graft survival of the nonhepatitis C patients but it offers comparable results; most importantly hepatitis C patients on dialysis have a much higher mortality than the nonhepatitis C counterparts, and within this population kidney transplantation offers a markedly improved survival vs. staying on dialysis. We need to emphasize that all the studies on hepatitis C patients were conducted in the interferon era where a sustained virologic response before or after transplantation was achieved in a small percentage of patients. The new Protease inhibitors and the revolutionary second generation direct acting antivirals (DAAs) have made hepatitis C a curable disease today. Even though the pivotal studies on these medications did not include patients with compromised renal function [44], more and more literature is actively immerging showing that they can be used in that population [45] and even on patients on dialysis [11, 46, 47]. Also other studies have demonstrated the efficacy and safety of those medications in patients after kidney transplantation [48, 49]. A question that sometimes emerges is whether to treat a patient with hepatitis C before or after kidney transplantation. The treatment before may halt the progression of liver disease, but the patient loses the chance of a more expeditious transplantation with a hepatitis C–positive kidney. The treatment after transplantation seems to be a better option, as it is associated with nearly routine and complete eradication of the virus. Even though we do not have enough data at this point, we can safely assume that in hepatitis C patients, patient and graft survival will only improve. Regardless of the etiology of the liver disease, there is a proven correlation between the degree of the liver fibrosis/inflammation pretransplant and the outcomes after kidney transplant. That is why routine liver biopsy should be a part of the pretransplant evaluation of these patients. Patients with advanced fibrosis and fully developed cirrhosis can be candidates for kidney transplantation, under certain conditions. Absence of portal hypertension and liver decompensation (ascites, encephalopathy, esophageal varices, or variceal bleeding) is of paramount importance. An HVPG measured portal pressure of <10 is a prerequisite. Finally, the patients should ideally be free of other comorbidities such as advanced age, previous kidney transplantation, and diabetes. When these conditions are met, kidney transplantation in a cirrhotic patient with end-stage renal disease offers a substantial survival advantage compared to staying on dialysis.

# References

1. Chan EY, Bhattacharya R, Eswaran S, et al. Outcomes after combined liver-kidney transplant vs. kidney transplant followed by liver transplant. Clin Transpl. 2015;29(1):60–6. doi:10.1111/ctr.12484.
2. Parsikia A, Campos S, Khanmoradi K, et al. Equal 3-year outcomes for kidney transplantation alone in HCV-positive patients with cirrhosis. Int Surg. 2015;100(1):142–54. doi:10.9738/INTSURG-D-13-00231.1.
3. Morales JM, Fabrizi F. Hepatitis C and its impact on renal transplantation. Nat Rev Nephrol. 2015;11(3):172–82. doi:10.1038/nrneph.2015.5.
4. Chan TM, Lok AS, Cheng IK, Chan RT. Prevalence of hepatitis C virus infection in hemodialysis patients: a longitudinal study comparing the results of RNA and antibody assays. Hepatology. 1993;17(1):5–8. 0270-9139(93)90183-N [pii].
5. Finelli L, Miller JT, Tokars JI, Alter MJ, Arduino MJ. National surveillance of dialysis-associated diseases in the United States, 2002. Semin Dial. 2005;18(1):52–61. SDI18108 [pii].
6. Fissell RB, Bragg-Gresham JL, Woods JD, et al. Patterns of hepatitis C prevalence and seroconversion in hemodialysis units from three continents: The DOPPS. Kidney Int. 2004;65(6):2335–42. doi:10.1111/j.1523-1755.2004.00649.x.
7. Jadoul M, Poignet JL, Geddes C, et al. The changing epidemiology of hepatitis C virus (HCV) infection in haemodialysis: European multicentre study. Nephrol Dial Transplant. 2004;19(4):904–9. doi:10.1093/ndt/gfh012.
8. Pereira BJ, Levey AS. Hepatitis C virus infection in dialysis and renal transplantation. Kidney Int. 1997;51(4):981–99.
9. Covic A, Iancu L, Apetrei C, et al. Hepatitis virus infection in haemodialysis patients from moldavia. Nephrol Dial Transplant. 1999;14(1):40–5.
10. Hmaied F, Ben Mamou M, Saune-Sandres K, et al. Hepatitis C virus infection among dialysis patients in Tunisia: incidence and molecular evidence for nosocomial transmission. J Med Virol. 2006;78(2):185–91. doi:10.1002/jmv.20526.

11. Saxena AK, Panhotra BR. The impact of nurse understaffing on the transmission of hepatitis C virus in a hospital-based hemodialysis unit. Med Princ Pract. 2004;13(3):129–35. doi:10.1159/000076951.
12. Morales JM, Campistol JM, Dominguez-Gil B. Hepatitis C virus infection and kidney transplantation. Semin Nephrol. 2002;22(4):365–74. S0270929502500474 [pii].
13. Musso G, Gambino R, Tabibian JH, et al. Association of non-alcoholic fatty liver disease with chronic kidney disease: a systematic review and meta-analysis. PLoS Med. 2014;11(7):e1001680. doi:10.1371/journal.pmed.1001680.
14. Musso G, Gambino R, Cassader M, Pagano G. Meta-analysis: natural history of non-alcoholic fatty liver disease (NAFLD) and diagnostic accuracy of non-invasive tests for liver disease severity. Ann Med. 2011;43(8):617–49. doi:10.3109/07853890.2010.518623.
15. Fabrizi F, Poordad FF, Martin P. Hepatitis C infection and the patient with end-stage renal disease. Hepatology. 2002;36(1):3–10. S0270913902000009 [pii].
16. Patel V, Marsano L, Eng M. Decompensated cirrhosis after renal transplantation: a case report. Case Rep Transplant. 2011;2011:862567. doi:10.1155/2011/862567.
17. Berthoux F. Hepatitis C virus infection and disease in renal transplantation. Nephron. 1995;71(4):386–94.
18. Glicklich D, Thung SN, Kapoian T, Tellis V, Reinus JF. Comparison of clinical features and liver histology in hepatitis C-positive dialysis patients and renal transplant recipients. Am J Gastroenterol. 1999;94(1):159–63. S0002927098006698 [pii].
19. Perez RM, Ferreira AS, Medina-Pestana JO, et al. Is hepatitis C more aggressive in renal transplant patients than in patients with end-stage renal disease? J Clin Gastroenterol. 2006;40(5):444–8. 00004836-200605000-00016 [pii].
20. Hanafusa T, Ichikawa Y, Kishikawa H, et al. Retrospective study on the impact of hepatitis C virus infection on kidney transplant patients over 20 years. Transplantation. 1998;66(4):471–6.
21. Izopet J, Rostaing L, Sandres K, et al. Longitudinal analysis of hepatitis C virus replication and liver fibrosis progression in renal transplant recipients. J Infect Dis. 2000;181(3):852–8. JID991149 [pii].
22. Rao KV, Anderson WR, Kasiske BL, Dahl DC. Value of liver biopsy in the evaluation and management of chronic liver disease in renal transplant recipients. Am J Med. 1993;94(3):241–50. 0002-9343(93)90055-T [pii].
23. de Oliveira Uehara SN, Emori CT, da Silva Fucuta Pereira P, et al. Histological evolution of hepatitis C virus infection after renal transplantation. Clin Transpl. 2012;26(6):842–8. doi:10.1111/j.1399-0012.2012.01635.x.
24. Maluf DG, Fisher RA, King AL, et al. Hepatitis C virus infection and kidney transplantation: predictors of patient and graft survival. Transplantation. 2007;83(7):853–7. doi:10.1097/01.tp.0000259725.96694.0a.
25. Fabrizi F, Martin P, Dixit V, Bunnapradist S, Dulai G. Hepatitis C virus antibody status and survival after renal transplantation: meta-analysis of observational studies. Am J Transplant. 2005;5(6):1452–61. AJT864 [pii].
26. Rostami Z, Nourbala MH, Alavian SM, Bieraghdar F, Jahani Y, Einollahi B. The impact of hepatitis C virus infection on kidney transplantation outcomes: a systematic review of 18 observational studies: the impact of HCV on renal transplantation. Hepat Mon. 2011;11(4):247–54.
27. Cruzado JM, Bestard O, Grinyo JM. Impact of extrahepatic complications (diabetes and glomerulonephritis) associated with hepatitis C virus infection after renal transplantation. Contrib Nephrol. 2012;176:108–16. doi:10.1159/000332389.
28. Corell A, Morales JM, Mandrono A, et al. Immunosuppression induced by hepatitis C virus infection reduces acute renal-transplant rejection. Lancet. 1995;346(8988):1497–8. S0140-6736(95)92520-1 [pii].

29. Wolfe RA, Ashby VB, Milford EL, et al. Comparison of mortality in all patients on dialysis, patients on dialysis awaiting transplantation, and recipients of a first cadaveric transplant. N Engl J Med. 1999;341(23):1725–30. doi:10.1056/NEJM199912023412303.
30. Tang IY, Walzer N, Aggarwal N, Tzvetanov I, Cotler S, Benedetti E. Management of the kidney transplant patient with chronic hepatitis C infection. Int J Nephrol. 2011;2011:245823. doi:10.4061/2011/245823.
31. Fabrizi F, Martin P, Dixit V, Bunnapradist S, Kanwal F, Dulai G. Post-transplant diabetes mellitus and HCV seropositive status after renal transplantation: Meta-analysis of clinical studies. Am J Transplant. 2005;5(10):2433–40. AJT1040 [pii].
32. Campbell MS, Constantinescu S, Furth EE, Reddy KR, Bloom RD. Effects of hepatitis C-induced liver fibrosis on survival in kidney transplant candidates. Dig Dis Sci. 2007;52(10):2501–7. doi:10.1007/s10620-006-9716-x.
33. Mathurin P, Mouquet C, Poynard T, et al. Impact of hepatitis B and C virus on kidney transplantation outcome. Hepatology. 1999;29(1):257–63. S0270913999000348 [pii].
34. Morales JM, Bloom R, Roth D. Kidney transplantation in the patient with hepatitis C virus infection. Contrib Nephrol. 2012;176:77–86. doi:10.1159/000332385.
35. Morales JM, Aguado JM. Hepatitis C and renal transplantation. Curr Opin Organ Transplant. 2012;17(6):609–15. doi:10.1097/MOT.0b013e32835a2bac.
36. Bloom RD, Sayer G, Fa K, Constantinescu S, Abt P, Reddy KR. Outcome of hepatitis C virus-infected kidney transplant candidates who remain on the waiting list. Am J Transplant. 2005;5(1):139–44. AJT652 [pii].
37. Pereira BJ, Natov SN, Bouthot BA, et al. Effects of hepatitis C infection and renal transplantation on survival in end-stage renal disease. The New England Organ Bank Hepatitis C Study Group. Kidney Int. 1998;53(5):1374–81. doi:10.1046/j.1523-1755.1998.00883.x.
38. Espinosa M, Martin-Malo A, Alvarez de Lara MA, Aljama P. Risk of death and liver cirrhosis in anti-HCV-positive long-term haemodialysis patients. Nephrol Dial Transplant. 2001;16(8):1669–74.
39. Roth D, Gaynor JJ, Reddy KR, et al. Effect of kidney transplantation on outcomes among patients with hepatitis C. J Am Soc Nephrol. 2011;22(6):1152–60. doi:10.1681/ASN.2010060668.
40. Paramesh AS, Davis JY, Mallikarjun C, et al. Kidney transplantation alone in ESRD patients with hepatitis C cirrhosis. Transplantation. 2012;94(3):250–4. doi:10.1097/TP.0b013e318255f890.
41. Garcia-Tsao G, Parikh CR, Viola A. Acute kidney injury in cirrhosis. Hepatology. 2008;48(6):2064–77. doi:10.1002/hep.22605.
42. Angeli P, Sanyal A, Moller S, et al. Current limits and future challenges in the management of renal dysfunction in patients with cirrhosis: report from the International Club of Ascites. Liver Int. 2013;33(1):16–23. doi:10.1111/j.1478-3231.2012.02807.x.
43. Eason JD, Gonwa TA, Davis CL, Sung RS, Gerber D, Bloom RD. Proceedings of consensus conference on simultaneous liver kidney transplantation (SLK). Am J Transplant. 2008;8(11):2243–51. doi:10.1111/j.1600-6143.2008.02416.x.
44. Lawitz E, Sulkowski MS, Ghalib R, et al. Simeprevir plus sofosbuvir, with or without ribavirin, to treat chronic infection with hepatitis C virus genotype 1 in non-responders o pegylated interferon and ribavirin and treatment-naive patients: The COSMOS randomised study. Lancet. 2014;384(9956):1756–65. doi:10.1016/S0140-6736(14)61036-9.
45. Sorbera MA, Friedman ML, Cope R. New and emerging evidence on the use of second-generation direct acting antivirals for the treatment of hepatitis C virus in renal impairment. J Pharm Pract. 2016. pii: 0897190016632128. [Epub ahead of print].
46. Saxena V, Koraishy FM, Sise ME, et al. Safety and efficacy of sofosbuvir-containing regimens in hepatitis C infected patients with impaired renal function. Liver Int. 2016; doi:10.1111/liv.13102.
47. Saxena V, Terrault NA. Treatment of hepatitis C infection in renal transplant recipients: the long wait is over. Am J Transplant. 2015; doi:10.1111/ajt.13697.

48. Sawinski D, Kaur N, Ajeti A, et al. Successful treatment of hepatitis C in renal transplant recipients with direct-acting antiviral agents. Am J Transplant. 2015; doi:10.1111/ajt.13620.
49. Hussein NR, Sidiq Z, Saleem M. Successful treatment of hepatitis C virus genotype 4 in renal transplant recipients with direct-acting antiviral agents. Am J Transplant. 2016; doi:10.1111/ajt.13767.

# Chapter 18
# Gynecological Procedures and Pregnancy in Women with Liver Cirrhosis

Uma Perni, Haider Mahdi, and Tommaso Falcone

## Introduction

Women with liver cirrhosis are more likely to have menstrual problems and vaginal bleeding than healthy women. This is likely related to altered homeostasis, clotting factor deficiency, and high concentration of estrogen [1, 2]. The incidence of hysterectomy has been reported to be higher in women with liver cirrhosis due to higher rate of vaginal bleeding [3]. Postoperative mortality and morbidity are significantly higher in women with liver cirrhosis. The overall risk of postoperative complications and/or mortality is related to several factors including severity of liver disease quantified by Model of End-stage Liver Disease (MELD score), comorbid conditions, age, ASA class, type of surgery, and surgical expertise [4]. Cardiac surgery has the highest risk, while extra-thoracic/extra-abdominal procedures have the lowest risk [5]. The mortality for abdominal surgery fluctuates between 11 and 76% [5]. In one report in women with liver cirrhosis undergoing hysterectomy, the risk of death within 30 days after discharge was 11-fold higher compared to women with no liver cirrhosis [6].

U. Perni, MD, MPH
Section of Maternal-Fetal Medicine, Cleveland Clinic Lerner College of Medicine, Cleveland, OH, USA
e-mail: perniu@ccf.org

H. Mahdi, MD, MPH
Section of Gynecologic Oncology, Cleveland Clinic Lerner College of Medicine, Cleveland, OH, USA
e-mail: madhih@ccf.org

T. Falcone, MD, FRCSC, FACOG (✉)
Cleveland Clinic Lerner College of Medicine and Chair Obstetrics, Gynecology and Women's Health Institute, 9500 Euclid Avenue – A81, Cleveland, OH, USA
e-mail: falcont@ccf.org

© Springer International Publishing AG 2017
B. Eghtesad, J. Fung (eds.), *Surgical Procedures on the Cirrhotic Patient*,
DOI 10.1007/978-3-319-52396-5_18

## Menstrual Abnormalities and Liver Cirrhosis

Heavy menstrual bleeding and amenorrhea are common in women with chronic liver disease and liver cirrhosis. High estrogen concentration associated with chronic liver disease often results in unopposed stimulation and proliferation of the endometrial linings which consequently lead to heavy menstrual or anovulatory cycle. In a study of postmenopausal women with chronic liver disease, free estrogen concentrations and free estrogen to androgen ratio were found to be higher than in age-matched controls [3]. In women undergoing liver transplant for liver disease, 28% had irregular and unpredictable bleeding and 30% had amenorrhea [7]. After transplant, 26% had irregular bleeding and 26% had amenorrhea. A total of 95% of women under the age of 46 had return of menstrual bleeding within the first year after transplantation. Liver function did not correlate with menstrual pattern [7]. After liver transplant, the majority of the patients are expected to resume their sexual activity and can get pregnant [7]. The average time for recovery of menstrual function is about 3 months [8]. In one report and among the 24 patients under 45 year old, six women conceived seven pregnancies [7].

## Tumor Markers in Liver Cirrhosis

CA-125 level is a marker often used in patients with adnexal masses or suspected ovarian/tubal or primary peritoneal malignancies. CA-125 is often elevated in patients with liver cirrhosis especially in those with ascites. The average CA-125 levels in patients with liver cirrhosis with ascites is about 275–321 U/ml vs. 13–72 U/ml in those with no ascites [9, 10]. The average CA-125 level in patients with liver cirrhosis and ascites is not different from those with malignant ascites. The level does correlate with presence and amount of ascites and degree of liver insufficiency but not to the etiology of ascites or liver cirrhosis [9–11]. Therefore, it is important to take this into consideration in evaluating ascites and adnexal masses among patients with liver cirrhosis and elevated CA-125 to avoid unnecessary surgery especially given the high rate of postoperative morbidity and mortality.

## Risk Factors and Timing of Surgery

Abdominal surgery is associated with significant morbidity and mortality risks in patients with liver cirrhosis. The perioperative morality from nonhepatic abdominal surgery range from 16 to 75%. Reported risk factors include low hemoglobin, low albumin levels, being on dialysis, high ASA class, respiratory failure, gastrointestinal (GI) bleeding, active infection, and emergency surgery. In one study of 772 patients with liver cirrhosis undergoing major surgery, patients with liver cirrhosis were at increased risk of mortality up to 90 days after surgery. In multivariate analysis, Model of End-Stage Liver Disease (MELD) score, ASA class, and age were the only risk factors that predicted mortality within 30 days, 90 days, 1 year, and long term regardless of type of surgery [4].

MELD score is a continuous score based on only laboratory data, which include serum bilirubin, serum creatinine and International Normalized Ratio (INR) levels. It has been created and validated to predict short-term outcome in patients with liver disease. Child–Turcotte–Pugh score is based on both objective laboratory data and assessment of ascites and encephalopathy. Compared to MELD's score, Child's score places patients in categories and it is not a continuous score. The two scoring system has been shown to predict perioperative outcome including morbidity and mortality. The 30-day mortality range from 5.7% in patients with MELD score of <8 and can be as high as >50% in those with MELD score of >20 [4]. In patients undergoing elective colorectal surgery, the 30-day mortality, major complications, and respiratory complications were significantly correlated with MELD score. The 30-day mortality was 0.69% for patients with MELD score of 6, 1.6% for those with score of 7–11, 4.5% for those with score of 11–15, and 5% for those with score of >15 [12]. In general surgery literature, for every 1-point increase greater than the mean MELD score, there was a 7.8–11.6% increase in any postoperative complication [13]. In the study of 30-day postoperative outcome after hysterectomy in patients with liver cirrhosis, Nielsen et al. reported 30-day mortality of 7.6% in patients with liver cirrhosis compared to 0.6% in patients without liver cirrhosis [6]. Postoperative mortality after major abdominal surgery in patients with MELD score of 9 or more has been reported to be 29% in one report while the mortality in patients with Child's score of A, B, and C are 10%, 30–31%, and 76–82%, respectively [14]. Teh et al. in the study of operative mortality following surgery reported that patients with a MELD score of 7 or less had a mortality rate of 5.7%; patients with a MELD score of 8–11 had a mortality rate of 10.3%; and patients with a MELD score of 12–15 had a mortality rate of 25.4% [4]. In this study, age and ASA class were also a predictor of mortality beside MELD score. ASA class of IV was equivalent to MELD score of 5.5 and ASA class of V was associated with 100% mortality. Age greater 70 years was equivalent to MELD score of 3 [4].

## Preoperative Work Up and Operative Planning

Preoperative management of patients with liver cirrhosis relies on optimal medical management of expected conditions associated with liver cirrhosis including management of ascites, coagulopathy, prevention of encephalopathy and treatment of postoperative complications like acaluculus acute cholecystitis [15]. Patients with liver cirrhosis tend to have reduced hepatic blood flow related to decreased portal blood flow. Further, anesthetic agents can lead to decrease in hepatic blood flow by 40–50%. Therefore, agents that have less effect on hepatic arterial blood flow are preferred [14, 16].

Risk factors for acute intraoperative hypoxemia include ascites, hepatic hydrothorax, hepatopulmonary syndrome, and portopulmonary hypertension.

Patients with ascites or hepatic hydrothorax should be managed and optimized before surgery. On the other hand, elective major surgery should be avoided if possible and replaced with alternative nonsurgical options for patients with hepatopulmonary syndrome or portopulmonary hypertension [14, 17].

Patients with liver cirrhosis might need larger doses of muscle relaxant due to the increased volume of distribution in these patients. Sedative, narcotics, and intravenous induction agents are safe in patients with compensated liver disease but should be used with caution in patients with hepatic dysfunction as they may lead to hepatic encephalopathy and prolonged time of depressed consciousness [14].

Patients with known liver disease need extensive preoperative work up and should be optimized for an elective surgery. Minimally invasive surgery using either robotic or traditional laparoscopic platforms has been found to be associated with faster recovery time, favorable perioperative outcome, and shorter hospital stay compared to open laparotomy [18–21]. Therefore, all efforts should be directed to utilize the minimally invasive approach in those patients. Further, these surgeries need to be done by an expert surgeon and in a tertiary center with expertise in taking care of those patients.

Contraindications to elective surgery in patients with liver disease include acute liver or renal failures, acute viral hepatitis, alcoholic hepatitis, cardiomyopathy, severe coagulopathy, and hypoxemia [14].

## Postoperative Management

After surgery, patients with liver cirrhosis should be monitored for signs of hepatic decompensation like coagulopathy, renal dysfunction, and encephalopathy. Prothrombin time and serum bilirubin levels can be helpful. Renal function and serum glucose level should be monitored too. Maintenance of intravascular volume is very important to avoid risk of underperfusion or fluid overload [14].

## Alternative Nonsurgical Options for Abnormal Uterine Bleeding

Given the significant morbidity and mortality associated with surgery in patients with liver cirrhosis, it is important to consider other conservative nonsurgical options. These options include oral combined contraceptive pills, antifibrinolytic agents like tranexamic acid, and progesterone therapy. Progesterone can be oral, injectable, or intrauterine. Minor procedures might be considered for acute bleeding like dilation/curettage or endometrial ablation.

# Pregnancy and Cirrhosis

Pregnancy in women with liver cirrhosis is an uncommon clinical situation estimated to occur in 1 in 5,950 pregnancies [22]. The rarity of this occurrence can be attributed to the decreased fertility associated with cirrhosis as well as the low incidence of cirrhosis in women in their reproductive years. Cirrhosis is typically associated with anovulation and amenorrhea secondary to the metabolic and hormonal derangements associated with chronic liver disease. In addition, it is estimated that only 45 cases of cirrhosis occur in every 100,000 women of reproductive age [23]. However, with advances in treatment of liver disease and the increased incidence of conditions leading to cirrhosis, more women with cirrhotic liver disease are becoming pregnant [24].

The existing literature on cirrhosis and pregnancy outcomes consists mainly of small case series, case reports and retrospective reviews [22, 25–30]. Many of these are from decades ago and thus do not reflect important advances in medical care such as routine administration of antenatal steroids prior to preterm delivery and neonatal intensive care. More recent literature suggests decreased maternal mortality and pregnancy complications compared to reports from prior decades. This likely reflects advances in treatment of liver disease and its complications as well as contemporary standards in maternal and neonatal care [24, 31, 32]. Maternal and neonatal morbidity and mortality, however, are still significantly higher than the general population. Therefore, comprehensive, multidisciplinary prenatal care with specialists in maternal–fetal medicine, gastroenterology, anesthesiology, surgery, and neonatology in a tertiary care center is critical for successful outcomes in these pregnancies.

## *Preconception Evaluation*

Although the majority of pregnancies are unplanned, preconception evaluation and counseling with individualized evaluation of risk can be extremely valuable in women with cirrhosis who may be considering pregnancy. Furthermore, the decreased fertility associated with cirrhosis may lead women to seek assisted reproductive technologies posing a complex clinical situation requiring expert consultation. As with pregnancy in the setting of any preexisting medical condition, risks can be considered in two major categories: (1) what is the effect of the disease and its treatment on the pregnancy and fetus and (2) how will the pregnancy affect the natural course of the disease. Many diseases impact maternal physiology in ways that can adversely affect placental and fetal development. In addition, medications used to treat conditions must be evaluated for teratogenicity and other effects on the fetus. Dosage adjustments secondary to the increased volume of distribution during pregnancy must also be considered. Pregnancy itself can also impact the natural course of a disease secondary to the increased physiologic demands and hormonal changes. In the event of an unplanned pregnancy, termination of pregnancy may be a consideration depending on the severity of maternal disease and risk for major morbidity and mortality.

Although pregnancy outcomes with cirrhosis are typically related to the severity of disease and not necessarily the etiology, it is still important to consider the pregnancy implications of the etiology of the cirrhosis. Infectious causes such as viral hepatitis may be transmittable to the fetus and therefore necessary precautions and interventions should be considered. Genetic causes such as hemochromatosis and alpha-1 antitrypsin deficiency also pose a risk of transmission and genetic counseling and prenatal diagnosis should be offered. Fetal alcohol syndrome should be discussed in cases of alcohol related liver injury if alcohol is still being used. Fetal-alcohol syndrome, characterized by fetal growth restriction, dysmorphic facial features, and cognitive and behavioral impairments, is common when alcohol use does not cease during pregnancy [33]. Many etiologies of cirrhosis such as autoimmune hepatitis (AIH) will typically require medical treatment throughout pregnancy typically with prednisone and azathioprine [34].

The Model for End-Stage Liver Disease (MELD) score was initially developed to predict mortality after transjugular intrahepatic portosystemic shunt (TIPS) insertion but is now widely used in clinical practice to predict prognosis in patients with cirrhosis and to prioritize for liver transplantation. The MELD score has been evaluated as a tool for prediction of maternal and neonatal outcomes in pregnancies complicated by cirrhosis. In 62 pregnancies occurring in 29 women with cirrhosis, higher MELD scores at the time of conception were associated with preterm delivery (<37 weeks), Neonatal Intensive Care Unit (NICU) admission, and significant maternal complications including variceal bleeding and hepatic decompensation. In this cohort, the median MELD score at conception was 7 and a 58% live birth rate was reported of which 64% were premature births. The rate of serious maternal morbidity was 10%. A MELD score of 10 or above prior to conception had an 83% sensitivity and specificity for predicting a major maternal complication while a MELD score of 6 or less was not associated with significant morbidity. Based on these results the MELD score can useful in preconception counseling [35].

Preconception evaluation allows the opportunity for evaluation of the severity of disease, review and tailoring of maternal medication regimens and discussion of the risks and benefits of these medications during pregnancy and breastfeeding. It also allows for the identification of women at high risk for significant maternal complications in whom pregnancy may be contraindicated. A frank discussion of neonatal outcomes and prematurity should similarly be included.

## Pregnancy Complications

Maternal mortality has been reported to range from 10 to 18% in older studies however more recent reports suggest a significantly lower rate of approximately 1.6% and decompensation rates of 10% [31]. Variceal bleeding, hepatic decompensation, splenic artery aneurysm rupture, and postpartum hemorrhage are among the major maternal complications associated with cirrhosis. Fetal/neonatal complications include spontaneous abortion, stillbirth, and preterm delivery with its associated neonatal morbidity and mortality.

## Esophageal Varices

Bleeding from esophageal varices is the most common cause of death during pregnancy in the setting of cirrhotic liver disease [22]. Esophageal variceal bleeding has been reported in 18–32% of pregnant women with cirrhosis, 50% of those with cirrhosis and known portal hypertension, and up to 78% with known esophageal varices [36, 37]. The physiologic changes of pregnancy such as increased plasma volume and the compression of the inferior vena cava by the gravid uterus worsen portal hypertension and esophageal varices [23]. Bleeding is most likely to occur in the second and third trimesters when these changes are the greatest.

In the 1980s, endoscopic sclerotherapy was generally accepted as the first-line treatment procedure for bleeding esophageal varices and most reports of variceal bleeding during pregnancy were treated this way [38–41]. There are no studies regarding the safety of the conventionally used sclerosing agents on the fetus and the potential for adverse effects remains unknown. Vasoactive drugs used to achieve hemostasis such as vasopressin are contraindicated during pregnancy as they decrease placental perfusion and may lead to an increased risk of placental abruption [37].

Currently, endoscopic band ligation is the preferred method of treatment and for acute hemorrhage from esophageal varices in both pregnant and nonpregnant patients. Band ligation appears to have a greater efficacy and fewer complications compared to sclerotherapy [23, 31, 42–44]. In addition, band ligation avoids any potential fetal risk from chemical instillation of sclerosing agents. In 1998, Starkel et al. reported the first case of successful band ligation in a pregnant patient with acute bleeding from esophageal varices in a pregnant patient [42]. Transjugular intrahepatic portosystemic shunt or TIPS procedure has been successfully reported during pregnancy complicated by refractory variceal hemorrhage [45, 46].

Ideally screening endoscopy should be performed prior to pregnancy for evaluation and treatment for esophageal varices. If identified prior to conception, prophylactic endoscopic band ligation or initiation of beta-blocker treatment is thought to decrease risk of variceal bleeding during pregnancy [31]. Beta-blockers reduce pulse pressure in the varices and are widely used in the nonpregnant population for primary prophylaxis. Beta-blockers are used extensively in pregnancy to treat various conditions including hypertension, arrhythmias, and migraines. Their use has not been linked to an increase in fetal malformations and they are generally considered to be safe in pregnancy. Some studies have reported an increase in fetal growth restriction and neonatal hypoglycemia and monitoring for these conditions is suggested [47].

If not performed prior to pregnancy, some experts recommend screening endoscopy for esophageal varices in the second trimester [31]. Upper gastrointestinal endoscopy has been extensively reported during pregnancy and is considered to be a safe procedure. Careful monitoring for maternal hypoxia and avoidance of supine position should eliminate risk of fetal hypoxia [48].

The mode of delivery in women with esophageal varices is controversial. Valsalva maneuvers can increase portal hypertension and the risk of variceal bleeding. Most authors therefore recommend an elective caesarean delivery or an assisted second stage with vacuum or forceps [49]. Complications from caesarean delivery include bleeding from abdominal wall varices, increased blood loss from coagulopathy, poor wound healing, and infection.

## Splenic Artery Rupture

Rupture of splenic artery aneurysm is a rare but often fatal complication of pregnancy with portal hypertension occurring in 2.6% of cases typically in the third trimester [37]. Although the exact etiology is not clear, both pregnancy and portal hypertension are believed to be risk factors. A maternal mortality rate of 75% and fetal mortality rate of 90% have been reported [50]. The usual clinical presentation is sudden hemorrhagic shock sometimes preceded by nausea, vomiting, and sharp abdominal pain either in the epigastrium or localized in the left side. Abdominal tenderness and signs of shock are the most common objective findings [51]. It is critical to have a high index of suspicion for this diagnosis in order to initiate treatment as rapidly as possible. If an asymptomatic splenic artery aneurysm is identified prior to or during pregnancy, prophylactic treatment may be indicated secondary to the increased risk of rupture during pregnancy and high associated maternal and fetal mortality rates [52].

## Hepatic Decompensation

In the past, hepatic decompensation was reported to occur in up to 24% of pregnancies complicated by cirrhosis however more recent estimates are approximately 10% [35]. This can occur at any gestational age and often is reported after episodes of significant variceal bleeding [23]. Hepatic encephalopathy with coma, cerebral edema, hypoglycemia, and coagulopathy are the hallmarks of hepatic decompensation. Treatment of pregnant patients with hepatic failure is similar to nonpregnant patients. They should be carefully monitored in an intensive care setting and treated with blood products as needed to correct coagulopathy and mannitol diuresis with intubation and hyperventilation for cerebral edema [37]. In cases of fulminant hepatic failure, liver transplantation may be the only treatment.

In cases of acute liver failure at previable gestational ages when neonatal survival is not possible with delivery and termination of pregnancy is not desired by the patient, liver transplantation during pregnancy may be an option. Although successful pregnancy outcomes have been reported, almost half of reported cases have ended in spontaneous or induced abortion, fetal death or neonatal death. In addition, almost all live births have occurred prematurely for various indications [53]. When liver transplantation is being considered, careful preoperative counseling and consideration of risks of prematurity is of the utmost importance. Important considerations include radiation exposure to the fetus from preoperative imaging, hemodynamic compromise during the transplantation from blood loss, and the effects of immunosuppressive as well as other medications on the fetus. It is also important to consider pregnancy complications after liver transplantation including an increased risk for preeclampsia, fetal growth restriction, and preterm delivery [54]. The impact of the continuing pregnancy on health of the immediate posttransplant woman should also be taken into account. One noteworthy aspect of many of these case reports is that they involved women who were previously healthy without preexisting liver disease and this may have contributed to the favorable maternal outcomes [23]. Immunosuppression should be continued throughout pregnancy after transplantation. Commonly used medications include azathioprine, tacrolimus, cyclosporine, and steroids. These agents are generally safe and any small risk to the fetus from the medication is much outweighed by the risk of rejection and graft failure by discontinuation. Mycophenolate is teratogenic and is associated with a specific pattern of malformations including external ear and other facial malformations such as cleft lip and palate and should be avoided during pregnancy [55].

## Postpartum Hemorrhage

Postpartum uterine hemorrhage is another significant cause of maternal morbidity and mortality in patients with cirrhosis, occurring in 7–26% of pregnancies [23, 37]. This is most likely related to the higher incidence of coagulopathy and thrombocytopenia in these women. Management is similar to that in patients without cirrhosis consisting of transfusion of blood and coagulation factors, administration of uterotonic agents, and balloon tamponade. Surgical therapy including hysterectomy may be indicated when these measures fail.

## Hepatopulmonary Syndrome

Hepatopulmonary syndrome is a rare complication of liver cirrhosis and only a few cases of pregnancy with this condition have been reported [56, 57]. This syndrome is characterized by the presence of chronic liver disease, intrapulmonary vascular dilatation, and arterial hypoxemia. Although successful pregnancy outcomes have been reported, little is known about the effects of pregnancy on hepatopulmonary syndrome and because of the theoretic risks of increased pulmonary shunting, with the development of high-output congestive heart failure, pregnancy should be managed with extreme caution.

## Fetal/Neonatal Complications

Prematurity, spontaneous abortion, and perinatal death are significantly increased in pregnancies complicated by cirrhosis. Miscarriage rates can be as high as 40%, significantly greater than the 15–20% seen in the general population. Prematurity rates of up to 25% have been reported compared to the 12.8% seen in the general population. Perinatal mortality is also much greater at 18% compared to 1% [23]. Even though significant improvements in neonatal care have increased survival and outcomes in premature infants, long-term neurologic and respiratory complications are still potential problems particularly with extreme prematurity.

## *Etiology of Cirrhosis*

The impact of the etiology of cirrhosis on pregnancy outcomes remains largely unknown. Causes of cirrhosis differ significantly in high resource countries compared to developing countries. In the western world, alcoholic liver disease is the leading cause of cirrhosis, accounting for 65% of all cases. However, alcohol related cirrhosis is less frequently associated with pregnancy and carries a significantly worse prognosis. In developing countries, infectious etiologies such as viral hepatitis and schistosomiasis account for the majority of cases [37].

In cases of chronic viral hepatitis, vertical transmission from the mother to fetus is a significant risk. Chronic hepatitis B infection develops in up to 90% of exposed neonates who do not receive appropriate immunoprophylaxis. The major prevention strategy for vertical transmission of hepatitis B consists of neonatal administration of hepatitis B vaccine and hepatitis B immunoglobulin within 12 h of birth. Treatment with tenofovir may also be indicated in the third trimester to decrease transmission risk based on viral load [58]. In contrast, vertical transmission of hepatitis C is much lower at 5%. Maternal HIV coinfection is a significant risk factor for transmission of hepatitis C and anti-HIV therapy during pregnancy can reduce the transmission rate of both viruses. Presently hepatitis C treatment is not routinely recommended during pregnancy due to lack of safety data [59]. Cesarean delivery is not indicated solely for reduction of vertical transmission with hepatitis B or C infection and breastfeeding is not contraindicated. Obstetric procedures, such as amniocentesis, chorionic villous sampling, or internal fetal monitoring, can theoretically lead to fetal exposure to contaminated maternal blood, and should be avoided if possible although the real risk of these procedures is not known [58, 59].

One of the few prospective studies on cirrhosis in pregnancy compared outcomes in women with liver cirrhosis specifically from post viral hepatitis to two control groups, one of pregnant women without cirrhosis and a nonpregnant control group with cirrhosis. In this study from Egypt, 129 women with cirrhosis from viral hepatitis types B, C or both were followed during pregnancy. Higher rates of maternal and neonatal complications were reported in this cohort compared to controls similar to other studies. Interestingly, significantly higher rates of preeclampsia and HELLP syndrome were reported unlike many other reports. Whether this is secondary to the cirrhosis itself or specifically the viral etiology is unclear and further investigation is warranted. In addition, accelerated hepatic decompensation was reported in the pregnant women with cirrhosis compared to the nonpregnant group (63.6% vs. 13.6%) suggesting that pregnancy has an adverse effect on disease progression [60].

Pregnancy in the setting of liver cirrhosis specifically from autoimmune hepatitis (AIH) has also been studied. AIH is a progressive, chronic form of hepatitis with a female predominance that often requires life-long anti-inflammatory and/or immunosuppressive therapy [34]. During pregnancy, AIH activity often improves but postpartum flares are common. Poor disease control in the year preceding pregnancy and the absence of medical therapy during pregnancy is associated with worse pregnancy outcomes. In addition, disease flares are associated with hepatic decompensation [61].

In a retrospective and self-reported study, Borssen et al. reported similar outcomes in women with AIH with and without cirrhosis [62]. Results from this study must be interpreted with caution however given that all data was self-reported. Westbrook et al., however, reported a significantly lower live birth rate and increased adverse maternal outcomes in women with AIH and cirrhosis compared to those without. Maternal complications included death, hepatic decompensation, postpartum hemorrhage, and variceal bleeding [61].

Pregnancy is rare with cirrhosis caused by other liver diseases such as primary biliary cirrhosis, Wilson's disease, and hemochromatosis and little is known about pregnancy outcomes. Critical to management of such pregnancies is the tailoring of medication regimens during pregnancy and this usually requires a multidisciplinary approach [23].

# Conclusion

Although pregnancy is not contraindicated in women with liver cirrhosis, an increase in maternal and neonatal complications can be expected. Careful multidisciplinary preconception evaluation is recommended to identify women at high risk for hepatic decompensation and other morbidities. Pregnancy outcomes are generally better when cirrhosis is well compensated. Evaluation and treatment of esophageal varices and tailoring of medication regimens are essential components of preconception assessment. During pregnancy, ongoing specialized multidisciplinary care with intensive maternal and fetal monitoring is essential.

# References

1. Violi F, Leo R, Vezza E, Basili S, et al. Bleeding time in patients with cirrhosis: relation with degree of liver failure and clotting abnormalities. Coagulation Abnormalities in Cirrhosis (CALC) Study Group. J Hepatol. 1994;20:531–6.
2. Becker U. The influence of ethanol and liver disease on sex hormones and hepatic oestrogen receptors in women. Dan Med Bull. 1993;40:447–59.
3. Stellon AJ, Williams R. Increased incidence of menstrual abnormalities and hysterectomy preceding primary biliary cirrhosis. Br Med J (Clin Res Ed). 1986;293(6542):297–8.
4. Teh SH, Nagorney DM, Stevens SR, Offord KP, et al. Risk factors for mortality after surgery in patients with cirrhosis. Gastroenterology. 2007;132(4):1261–9.
5. Concha PM, Mertz KV. Perioperative risk among patients with cirrhosis. Rev Med Chil. 2010;138(9):1165–71.
6. Nielsen IL, Thulstrup AM, Nielsen GL, Larsen H, et al. Thirty-day postoperative mortality after hysterectomy in women with liver cirrhosis: a Danish population-based cohort study. Eur J Obstet Gynecol Reprod Biol. 2002;102(2):202.
7. Mass K, Quint EH, Punch MR, Merion RM. Gynecological and reproductive function after liver transplantation. Transplantation. 1996;62(4):476–9.
8. Parolin MB, Coelho JC, Balbi E, Wiederkehr JC, et al. Normalization of menstrual cycles and pregnancy after liver transplantation. Arq Gastroenterol. 2000;37(1):3–6.
9. Zuckerman E, Lanir A, Sabo E, Rosenvald-Zuckerman T, et al. Cancer antigen 125: a sensitive marker of ascites in patients with liver cirrhosis. Am J Gastroenterol. 1999;94(6):1613–8.
10. Xiao WB, Liu YL. Elevation of serum and ascites cancer antigen 125 levels in patients with liver cirrhosis. J Gastroenterol Hepatol. 2003;18(11):1315–6.
11. Qureshi MO, Dar FS, Khokhar N. Cancer Antigen-125 as a marker of ascites in patients with liver cirrhosis. J Coll Physicians Surg Pak. 2014;24(4):232–5.
12. Lange EO, Jensen CC, Melton GB, Madoff RD, et al. Relationship between model for end-stage liver disease score and 30-day outcomes for patients undergoing elective colorectal resections: an American college of surgeons-national surgical quality improvement program study. Dis Colon Rectum. 2015;58(5):494–501.
13. Zielsdorf SM, Kubasiak JC, Janssen I, Myers JA, et al. A NSQIP analysis of MELD and perioperative outcomes in general surgery. Am Surg. 2015;81(8):755–9.
14. Friedman LS. Surgery in the patient with liver disease. Trans Am Clin Climatol Assoc. 2010;121:192–204.
15. Rizvon MK, Chou CL. Surgery in the patient with liver disease. Med Clin North Am. 2003;87(1):211–27.
16. Gelman S. General anesthesia and hepatic circulation. Can J Physiol Pharmacol. 1987;65(8):1762–79.
17. Lai HC, Lai HC, Wang KY, Lee WL, et al. Severe pulmonary hypertension complicates postoperative outcome of non-cardiac surgery. Br J Anaesth. 2007;99(2):184–90.
18. Nieboer TE, Johnson N, Lethaby A, Tavender E, et al. Surgical approach to hysterectomy for benign gynaecological disease. Cochrane Database Syst Rev. 2009;3:CD003677.
19. Palomba S, Falbo A, Mocciaro R, et al. Laparoscopic treatment for endometrial cancer: a meta-analysis of randomized controlled trials (RCTs). Gynecol Oncol. 2009;112:415–21.
20. de la Orden SG, Reza MM, Blasco JA, et al. Laparoscopic hysterectomy in the treatment of endometrial cancer: a systematic review. J Minim Invasive Gynecol. 2008;15:395–401.
21. Walker JL, Piedmonte MR, Spirtos NM, et al. Laparoscopy compared with laparotomy for comprehensive surgical staging of uterine cancer: Gynecologic Oncology Group Study LAP2. J Clin Oncol. 2009;27:5331–6.
22. Aggarwal N, Sawnhey H, Suril V, Vasishta K, Jha M, Dhiman RK. Pregnancy and cirrhosis of the liver. Aust N Z J Obstet Gynaecol. 1999;39(4):503–6.
23. Tan J, Surti B, Saab S. Pregnancy and cirrhosis. Liver Transpl. 2008;14(8):1081–91.

24. Puljic A, Salati J, Doss A, Caughey AB. Outcomes of pregnancies complicated by liver cirrhosis, portal hypertension, or esophageal varices. J Matern Fetal Neonatal Med. 2016;29(3):506–9.
25. Lee NM, Brady CW. Liver disease in pregnancy. World J Gastroenterol. 2009;15(8):897–906.
26. Cheng YS. Pregnancy in liver cirrhosis and/or portal hypertension. Am J Obstet Gynecol. 1977;128(7):812–22.
27. Schreyer P, Caspi E, El-Hindi JM, Eshchar J. Cirrhosis–pregnancy and delivery: a review. Obstet Gynecol Surv. 1982;37(5):304–12.
28. Pajor A, Lehoczky D. Pregnancy in liver cirrhosis. Assessment of maternal and fetal risks in eleven patients and review of the management. Gynecol Obstet Invest. 1994;38(1):45–50.
29. Borhanmanesh F, Haghighi P. Pregnancy in patients with cirrhosis of the liver. Obstet Gynecol. 1970 Aug;36(2):315–24.
30. Whelton MJ, Sherlock S. Pregnancy in patients with hepatic cirrhosis. Management and outcome. Lancet. 1968;2(7576):995–9.
31. Westbrook RH, Dusheiko G, Williamson C. Pregnancy and liver disease. J Hepatol. 2016;64(4):933–45.
32. Shaheen AA, Myers RP. The outcomes of pregnancy in patients with cirrhosis: a population-based study. Liver Int. 2010;30(2):275–83.
33. Roozen S, Peters GJ, Kok G, Townend D, Nijhuis J, Curfs L. Worldwide prevalence of fetal alcohol spectrum disorders: a systematic literature review including meta-analysis. Alcohol Clin Exp Res. 2016;40(1):18–32.
34. Manns MP, Lohse AW, Vergani D. Autoimmune hepatitis–update 2015. J Hepatol. 2015;62(1 Suppl):S100–11.
35. Westbrook RH, Yeoman AD, O'Grady JG, Harrison PM, Devlin J, Heneghan MA. Model for end-stage liver disease score predicts outcome in cirrhotic patients during pregnancy. Clin Gastroenterol Hepatol. 2011;9(8):694–9.
36. Britton RC. Pregnancy and esophageal varices. Am J Surg. 1982;143(4):421–5.
37. Russell MA, Craigo SD. Cirrhosis and portal hypertension in pregnancy. Semin Perinatol. 1998;22(2):156–65.
38. Augustine P, Joseph PC. Sclerotherapy for esophageal varices and pregnancy. Gastrointest Endosc. 1989;35(5):467–8.
39. Kochhar R, Goenka MK, Mehta SK. Endoscopic sclerotherapy during pregnancy. Am J Gastroenterol. 1990;85(9):1132–5.
40. Iwase H, Morise K, Kawase T, Horiuchi Y. Endoscopic injection sclerotherapy for esophageal varices during pregnancy. J Clin Gastroenterol. 1994;18(1):80–3.
41. Aggarwal N, Negi N, Aggarwal A, Bodh V, Dhiman RK. Pregnancy with portal hypertension. J Clin Exp Hepatol. 2014;4(2):163–71.
42. Starkel P, Horsmans Y, Geubel A. Endoscopic band ligation: a safe technique to control bleeding esophageal varices in pregnancy. Gastrointest Endosc. 1998;48(2):212–4.
43. Sobral M, Granja C, Sampaio M, Guerreiro F. Bleeding from oesophageal varices in pregnancy. BMJ Case Rep. 2013;2013 doi:10.1136/bcr,2013-009653.
44. Chaudhuri K, Tan EK, Biswas A. Successful pregnancy in a woman with liver cirrhosis complicated by recurrent variceal bleeding. J Obstet Gynaecol. 2012;32(5):490–1.
45. Savage C, Patel J, Lepe MR, Lazarre CH, Rees CR. Transjugular intrahepatic portosystemic shunt creation for recurrent gastrointestinal bleeding during pregnancy. J Vasc Interv Radiol. 2007;18(7):902–4.
46. Lodato F, Cappelli A, Montagnani M, Colecchia A, Festi D, Azzaroli F, et al. Transjugular intrahepatic portosystemic shunt: a case report of rescue management of unrestrainable variceal bleeding in a pregnant woman. Dig Liver Dis. 2008;40(5):387–90.
47. Davis RL, Eastman D, McPhillips H, Raebel MA, Andrade SE, Smith D, et al. Risks of congenital malformations and perinatal events among infants exposed to calcium channel and beta-blockers during pregnancy. Pharmacoepidemiol Drug Saf. 2011;20(2):138–45.

48. Cappell MS. Risks versus benefits of gastrointestinal endoscopy during pregnancy. Nat Rev Gastroenterol Hepatol. 2011;8(11):610–34.
49. Jabiry-Zieniewicz Z, Dabrowski FA, Suchonska B, Kowalczyk R, Nowacka E, Kociszewska-Najman B, et al. Pregnancy and delivery in women with esophageal varices due to hepatic vein thrombosis. J Matern Fetal Neonatal Med. 2015;28(2):177–81.
50. Sadat U, Dar O, Walsh S, Varty K. Splenic artery aneurysms in pregnancy–a systematic review. Int J Surg. 2008;6(3):261–5.
51. Khurana J, Spinello IM. Splenic artery aneurysm rupture: a rare but fatal cause for peripartum collapse. J Intensive Care Med. 2013;28(2):131–3.
52. Ha JF, Phillips M, Faulkner K. Splenic artery aneurysm rupture in pregnancy. Eur J Obstet Gynecol Reprod Biol. 2009;146(2):133–7.
53. Eguchi S, Yanaga K, Fujita F, Okudaira S, Furui J, Miyamoto M, et al. Living-related right lobe liver transplantation for a patient with fulminant hepatic failure during the second trimester of pregnancy: Report of a case. Transplantation. 2002;73(12):1970–1.
54. Deshpande NA, James NT, Kucirka LM, Boyarsky BJ, Garonzik-Wang JM, Cameron AM, et al. Pregnancy outcomes of liver transplant recipients: a systematic review and meta-analysis. Liver Transpl. 2012;18(6):621–9.
55. Coscia LA, Constantinescu S, Davison JM, Moritz MJ, Armenti VT. Immunosuppressive drugs and fetal outcome. Best Pract Res Clin Obstet Gynaecol. 2014;28(8):1174–87.
56. Veitsman E, Yigla M, Thaler I, Baruch Y. Two successful pregnancies in a patient with advanced liver cirrhosis and hepatopulmonary syndrome. Gastroenterol Hepatol (N Y). 2007;3(7):546–8.
57. Sammour RN, Zuckerman E, Tov N, Gonen R. Pregnancy exacerbating hepatopulmonary syndrome. Obstet Gynecol. 2006;107(2 Pt 2):455–7.
58. Society for Maternal-Fetal Medicine (SMFM), Dionne-Odom J, Tita AT, Silverman NS. #38: Hepatitis B in pregnancy screening, treatment, and prevention of vertical transmission. Am J Obstet Gynecol. 2016;214(1):6–14.
59. Tovo PA, Calitri C, Scolfaro C, Gabiano C, Garazzino S. Vertically acquired hepatitis C virus infection: correlates of transmission and disease progression. World J Gastroenterol. 2016;22(4):1382–92.
60. Rasheed SM, Abdel Monem AM, Abd Ellah AH, Abdel Fattah MS. Prognosis and determinants of pregnancy outcome among patients with post-hepatitis liver cirrhosis. Int J Gynaecol Obstet. 2013;121(3):247–51.
61. Westbrook RH, Yeoman AD, Kriese S, Heneghan MA. Outcomes of pregnancy in women with autoimmune hepatitis. J Autoimmun. 2012;38(2–3):J239–44.
62. Danielsson Borssen A, Wallerstedt S, Nyhlin N, Bergquist A, Lindgren S, Almer S, et al. Pregnancy and childbirth in women with autoimmune hepatitis is safe, even in compensated cirrhosis. Scand J Gastroenterol. 2016;51(4):479–85.

# Chapter 19
# Cardiac Surgical Procedures in Patients with Cirrhosis

Ahmad Zeeshan and Nicholas Smedira

## Introduction

Cardiac surgery in patients with cirrhosis is fraught with high mortality and morbidity rates. Hepatic decompensation is common after cardiac surgery with cardiopulmonary bypass (CPB). The mortality rates in some studies were so high that cardiac surgery was contraindicated in patients with Child–Pugh (CP) Classes B and C cirrhosis [1–3]. A recent Cleveland Clinic study showed that the patients with liver cirrhosis had a five times higher mortality rate after cardiac surgery than the matched controls [4]. A large population-based study showed increased mortality, postoperative complications, length of stay, and hospital charges associated with coronary artery bypass grafting (CABG) in patients with cirrhosis [5]. Despite the general consensus of an associated higher risk, liver cirrhosis does not preclude cardiac surgery in carefully selected patients [4, 6].

A. Zeeshan, MD • N. Smedira, MD (✉)
Heart and Vascular Institute, Cleveland Clinic,
9500 Euclid Ave, Desk J4-1, Cleveland, OH 44195, USA

Heart and Vascular Institute, Cleveland Clinic Florida,
2950 Cleveland Clinic Blvd, Desk 23-24, Weston, FL 33331, USA
e-mail: smedirn@ccf.org

© Springer International Publishing AG 2017
B. Eghtesad, J. Fung (eds.), *Surgical Procedures on the Cirrhotic Patient*,
DOI 10.1007/978-3-319-52396-5_19

# Risk Stratification for Cardiac Surgery in Patients with Cirrhosis

## Utility of Various Scores

Various scoring systems have been employed to predict postoperative mortality and morbidity in patients with liver cirrhosis. These include CP score, Model for End-stage Liver Disease (MELD) score, Society of Thoracic Surgeons (STS) score, European System for Cardiac Operative Risk Evaluation (EuroSCORE), and Simplified Acute Physiology Score (SAPS) III. The CP Classification was initially developed empirically for patients with bleeding esophageal varices. It uses the albumin, prothrombin time, serum bilirubin, degree of ascites, and presence of encephalopathy to characterize the severity of liver cirrhosis. It has been found to be a reliable predictor of functional status of liver and overall survival [7]. It correlates strongly with postoperative mortality and morbidity in the patients who underwent cardiac surgery [2–5, 7, 8]. MELD score was developed in 2000 to stratify survival of patients after transjugular intrahepatic portosystemic shunt (TIPS) procedure. It is validated for predicting survival of patients with end-stage liver disease [4, 7, 9].

Filsoufi et al. did not find MELD scores to be significantly associated with hospital mortality [3], while the CP classification and its associated numerical score appropriately predicted mortality and morbidity [1–4, 7, 10]. Their study confirmed the predicted value of CP Classification; albeit, the sample size was small. On the other hand, Thielmann et al. found the MELD score to be the most predictive risk evaluation model with clear superiority to CP Classification and EuroSCORE. The best value for MELD score was found to be 13.5 with a sensitivity of 52% and specificity of 79%. CP Classification was found to be useful as well. The hospital and long term outcomes were better with CP Class A as compared to Classes B and C. Class C fared the worst [9].

CP Classification remains the best means for predicting mortality after cardiac surgery [3]. In the current literature, CP Classification is used most commonly. The numerical score associated with CP Classification is considered particularly helpful in stratifying the risk for cardiac surgery with CPB in patients with liver cirrhosis [4, 7].

Cirrhosis is not considered a risk factor in the STS score and EuroSCORE. EuroSCORE was not particularly useful in predicting the risk in patients with cirrhosis requiring cardiac surgery [9, 11]. However, a recent German study demonstrated a significant predictive power of EuroSCORE for 30 day mortality [12]. Simplified Acute Physiology Score (SAPS) III has been noted to have the best predictive value for long term outcomes [10].

## Beyond the Scores

If carefully examined, most of these risk scores rely on the synthetic function of the liver measured by serum bilirubin, prothrombin time, and international normalized ratio (INR); the stigmata of advanced liver disease like presence of ascites and encephalopathy; and the markers of end organ dysfunction like serum creatinine. Any patient with a high CP or MELD score reflects the advanced liver dysfunction with the derangements of coagulation, renal function, and portal hypertension associated with ascites and splenomegaly. Blood tests to estimate hepatic functional reserve, like indocyanine green clearance and asialoscintigraphy may augment the evaluation of hepatic function; but, their use as a preoperative risk evaluation tool has not been well characterized [13, 14].

Thrombocytopenia associated with splenomegaly is also considered to be a significant predictor of risk in patients with cirrhosis undergoing cardiac surgery. Filsoufi et al. reported a statistically significant in-hospital mortality associated with a low preoperative platelet count [3]. Thielmann et al. similarly noted that preoperative thrombocytopenia is adversely associated with survival after cardiac surgery in patients with cirrhosis [3, 9].

A Cleveland Clinic study by Suman et al. further delineated the correlation of a higher CP and MELD scores to hepatic decompensation after cardiac surgery with CPB. For patients with a CP score >7, there is an association of hepatic decompensation and mortality with a 86% sensitivity and 92% specificity for predicting mortality in addition to a 66% sensitivity and 97% specificity for predicting hepatic decompensation. MELD score with a value of >13 offered a 71% sensitivity and 89% specificity for mortality. Hepatic decompensation under the receiver operative curve (ROC) for mortality was similar for both scores. The best values for predicting mortality and hepatic decompensation were determined to be >7 for CP and >13 for MELD score. These findings confirm the poor prognosis noted in patients with CP Classes B and C in other studies [7]. The individual parameters of serum bilirubin, albumin, and INR were not strongly associated with mortality. This Cleveland Clinic study concluded that the risk for postoperative mortality in patients with cirrhosis considered for cardiac surgery with CPB was assessed accurately by using the numerical CP score and a score >7 was associated with higher mortality [7].

## Contemporary Outcomes

### Short-Term Outcomes

The risk of complications is high in all CP Classes; but, some studies report a comparable or acceptable risk in propensity matched population in patients with a CP score <8 [4]. Klemperer et al. noted that 100% of patients with CP Class B and 25% of those with CP Class A had major complications [1]. Arif et al. noted longer intensive care unit stay, longer duration of invasive ventilation, tracheostomy, and demand for red blood cells, plasma, and platelets in patients with cirrhosis who did not survive 30 days after cardiac surgery [12]. In this group, renal failure, neurological complications, sepsis, and gastrointestinal complications were higher. The patients with liver cirrhosis stayed twice as long in the hospital as compared to their matched controls. Prolonged hospital stay was primarily due to hepatic decompensation and renal failure rather than the need for mechanical ventilation and pressor support requiring [4]. Length of stay was substantially higher for patients with cirrhosis versus those without cirrhosis (9 vs. 6 days). Similarly, patients with cirrhosis accrued up to 34% higher hospital charges [5].

Common postoperative complications include coagulopathy and thrombocytopenia, resulting in increased postoperative bleeding. An early complication after CPB is a lack of vascular tone. It is unclear why this happens; but, most of the patients with cirrhosis show very low systemic vascular resistance (SVR) requiring high-dose vasoactive agents to maintain systemic blood pressure.

A number of studies demonstrated the high risk associated with open heart surgery in patients with liver cirrhosis [1–12]. Overall in-hospital mortality is high among patients with liver cirrhosis. Various single institution studies have reported 17–31% in-hospital mortality (Arif et al.: 30-day mortality 26% [12]; Shaheen et al.: 17.2% [5]; Filsoufi et al.: 26% [3]; Klemperer et al.: 31% [1]). Most of these studies had a small number of patients precluding definitive conclusions being drawn. Definitive conclusions could not be drawn from these studies due to small sample sizes. However, one common theme emerges that CP Classes B and C have a very high risk of mortality and morbidity. Patients with CP Class C have up to a 100% mortality associated with open heart surgery [1–12]. Mortality rates of 0–20%, 18–50%, and 67–100% have been reported in patients with CP Classes A, B, and C, respectively [1–12].

## Long-Term Outcomes

The overall 5-year survival rate is noted to be 19% for all CP Classes. Patients with CP Class C had a 0% 5-year survival, while patients with CP Class A had a 25% 5-year survival. In Arif et al.'s study, 1-year and 5-year survival rates of CP Class A patients were 70% and 26%, CP Class B patients 33% and 5%, and CP Class C patients 33% and 0%, respectively, suggesting a somewhat prohibitively high risk for elective cardiac surgery in CP Class C patients [12]. Another study shows excellent long-term survival for all CP Classes of 78.6% at 3 years and 70.2% at 5 years [8]. Their findings suggest that the survival after 3 years becomes similar to the survival in the general population undergoing cardiac surgery. In another study, long-term survival was 82.4% for CP Class A, 47.6% for CP Class B, and 33.3% for CP Class C patients [10].

## Preoperative Evaluation for Cardiac Surgery in Patients with Cirrhosis

Typical stigmata of liver cirrhosis, such as bleeding esophageal varices and ascites, may result in a complicated postoperative course due to severe hepatic decompensation. A careful diagnostic evaluation by a hepatologist should be performed before the operation [8]. Patients with a CP score of <8 may safely undergo cardiac surgery with CPB [4]. This is consistent with documented lower mortality rates for patients with CP Classes A and B. The presence of ascites or hepatic encephalopathy is associated with nearly a fivefold increase in mortality [5].

Patients with CP Class B should be thoroughly evaluated prior to any surgery. According to the current data, surgery in patients with CP Class C is contraindicated because most studies report a 100% mortality. In rare cases, an off pump coronary artery bypass grafting (OPCAB) may be possible. In high-risk patients, a combined OLT and cardiac surgery are performed with success [8].

One may wonder if a TIPS is feasible and useful in patients with cirrhosis who are to undergo elective cardiac surgery and result in a decrease in the incidence of postoperative complications [15].

Patients with CP Class C have a prohibitively high risk of mortality and morbidity. Elective cardiac surgery should be avoided in these patients, if possible. Urgent operations, like aortic valve and mitral valve replacement for endocarditis, should be carefully considered. For patients requiring emergency operations, the risk of mortality may be the same regardless of having surgery or not. Emergency procedures, such as an open repair of ruptured type A or B aortic dissection, CABG for unstable angina with multivessel coronary artery disease, and placement of left ventricular assist devices for low cardiac output state, are contraindicated due to a 100% mortality. In CP Class C patients, OPCAB, TAVR, transcatheter mitral valve repair, transcatheter endovascular aortic repair (TEVAR), and high-risk percutaneous coronary interventions (PCI) should be considered favorably to open heart surgery with CPB [3, 16, 17]. The use of a transesophageal echocardiography probe may cause injury to preexisting esophageal varices. Thus, a preoperative esophagogastroscopy may be particularly necessary in case a TAVR is planned [18].

## Intraoperative Considerations while Performing Cardiac Surgery in Patients with Cirrhosis

Longer mean operative time is associated with higher mortality [12]. An off pump approach for a CABG is associated with a lower risk of complications [3]. A longer cross clamp time is associated with adverse outcomes [9].

If CPB is used, a high pump flow specifically more than 2.4 L/min/m$^2$ with associated moderate hypothermia down to 28 °C is associated with less hepatic dysfunction. There are numerous factors that adversely affect the liver function during CPB including hypoxia, hemodilution with anemia, hypotension, and hypothermia. Additionally, hypercarbia and metabolic acidosis result in sympathetically mediated hepatic artery vasoconstriction with decreased blood flow in both hepatic artery and portal vein [19].

In a canine study, the total hepatic blood flow decreased by 50% during pulsatile flow at a perfusion pressure of 60 mmHg. Pulsatile blood flow is considered superior to nonpulsatile normothermic perfusion. A pump flow of 2.4 L/min/m$^2$ does not significantly impact hepatic blood flow (approximately a 20% decrease). This is consistent with the clinical observation of relatively lower complication rate with hypothermic, high flow CPB for routine cardiac surgery. The bottom line is hepatic blood flow is better maintained during CPB with high flows and hypothermic CPB [19].

It is important to realize that there is an increased in hepatic decompensation with the use of CPB. Probably, this occurs as a result of the inflammatory mediators released during CPB in combination with the compromised coagulation profile and related hepatic dysfunctions. This results in severe acidosis, loss of vasomotor tone, and coagulopathy. It is not the cardiac procedure itself; but, the presence or absence of the CPB that has a deleterious effect on the postoperative mortality and morbidity in patients with cirrhosis [3]. This is reflected in the outcomes associated with on pump CABG and AVR [3, 6, 9, 16].

## Postoperative Considerations after Cardiac Surgery in Patients with Cirrhosis

Careful hemodynamic management is critical in the early postoperative phase. Prompt correction of metabolic acidosis, coagulopathy, and fluid balance are essential for a good outcome. Better long-term outcomes are associated with lower arterial lactate and good urine output in the first 24 hours [10].

### Bleeding and Coagulopathy

High postoperative chest tube output due to bleeding is a common complication. The coagulation tests are abnormal and thrombocytopenia is universally present. Most patients require blood transfusions with red blood cells, fresh frozen plasma, platelets, and cryoprecipitate [5, 8, 11, 20]. Factor VII has been used in selected settings. In a center where cardiac surgery is performed on patients with liver cirrhosis, robust blood bank support should be available and utilized. It is important that the blood products are available on a short notice to prevent catastrophic complications. Long-term bleeding complications usually do not occur even under continuous therapy with platelet inhibitors [8].

### Worsening of Hepatic Function after CPB

Incidence of significant hepatic dysfunction after CPB is about 3% in the general population [21]. Risk factors associated are New York Heart Association functional class, sex, type of operation performed, operative time, low cardiac output state, cardiac arrest, and blood transfusions. Patients with cirrhosis are particularly vulnerable to hepatic decompensation because of their limited hepatocyte reserve. The above mentioned risk factors can be mitigated to a certain degree by vigilant postoperative management. It is hard to completely eliminate all the risk factors but an attempt can be made for a positive outcome in patients with CP Class A [21].

## *Gastrointestinal Bleeding*

Although not very common, gastrointestinal bleeding can be worrisome and some-times even fatal in patients with cirrhosis undergoing cardiac surgery. The exact incidence of gastrointestinal bleeding after cardiac surgery is unknown. Yet, the preoperative presence of esophageal varices and portal hypertension with advanced cirrhosis may herald the gastrointestinal bleeding. In select patients, TIPS place-ment could decrease the incidence of postoperative gastrointestinal bleeding [15]; however, it is associated with shunt thrombosis, encephalopathy, and hemodynamic changes likely to increase cardiac output and systemic vascular resistance.

## Coronary Artery Bypass Grafting (CABG)

Cirrhosis has a significant effect on mortality and morbidity in patients undergoing CABG. Gopaldas et al. reported increased mortality (adjusted odds ratio [AOR] 6.9, 95% confidence interval [CI]: 2.8–17), morbidity (AOR: 1.6, 95% CI: 1.3–2.0), length of stay (+1.2 days; $p < 0.001$), and hospital expenses (+$22,491; $p < 0.001$). In patients, who underwent OPCAB, mortality was only effected by severe liver dysfunction (mortality: AOR: 5.1, 95% CI 3.7–6.9; morbidity: AOR 2.1, 95% CI: 1.6–2.4). On pump patients had a higher mortality (4.6 fold) and morbidity regard-less of the severity of cirrhosis. Authors concluded that a CABG should only be performed in carefully selected patients and preferably without the use of CPB [6]. Marui et al. from Japan reported a lower adjusted in-hospital mortality after OPCAB as compared with on pump CABG. Although the same study reported an adjusted overall mortality to be similar between the two groups of patients with hepatic cir-rhosis. In this study, no optimal revascularization strategies for patients with liver cirrhosis were suggested and a need for a randomized controlled trial was empha-sized [16]. Filsoufi et al. and Hayashida et al. reported a 0% mortality in patients with CP Class B who underwent OPCAB. This contrasts with the high mortality rate for on pump CABG for this same patient group. These studies suggest that OPCAB should be attempted in patients with CP Class B, when feasible [2, 3].

Whereas, in a large population based study, Shaheen et al. reported that OPCAB was not associated with decreased mortality. This is in contrast with the above conclu-sions. In this study, patients older than 60 years, presence of congestive heart failure, and being female were associated with increased in-hospital mortality after CABG in patients with liver cirrhosis. The presence of ascites and hepatic encephalopathy was associated with three times increase in mortality [5]. Ben Ari et al. reported a single case of a 60-year-old male with CP Class C, who survived an OPCAB [17]. The above mentioned studies point towards the utility of OPCAB in select patients with CP Classes B and C. Careful consideration of the overall clinical picture should be made by a hepatologist and a cardiac surgeon. Referral to a tertiary care center for a combined CABG and OLT should be considered for patients with CP Class C.

## Aortic Valve Surgery

Surgical aortic valve replacement (SAVR) is uncommon in patients with cirrhosis due to high risk. Petress et al. reported seven patients with CP Class B and a median MELD score of 14 who underwent AVR using minimized extracorporeal perfusion circuits (MECC). Perioperative management included digestive decontamination, antioxidant supplements, and adjusted antibiotics. There was no mortality at 30, 60, and 90 days postoperatively with a median intensive care unit length of stay of 3 days. Only one patient required re-exploration for bleeding and another one suffered from temporary seizures. Authors concluded that the SAVR with vigilant postoperative management is feasible [22]. Nemati et al. reported a patient with CP score of 10 (Class B) who underwent a successful SAVR with a mechanical valve and then a subsequent liver transplant 2 months after the SAVR [23].

Due to the invasive nature of traditional cardiac surgery and the association of adverse outcomes with CPB in patients with liver cirrhosis, TAVR is an appealing alternative. Shah et al. reported a study of TAVR being performed in 17 patients with chronic liver disease (11 CP Class A and 6 CP Class B). TAVR was performed successfully in these patients with in-hospital mortality of 5.88% and a 90 day mortality of 17.65%. The authors concluded that TAVR is a feasible method for treating aortic stenosis in patients with chronic liver disease. The procedure associated risk is low in patients with CP Classes A and B. Patients in CP Class C warrant further study to assess the feasibility of TAVR [18].

Greason et al. reported a complication rate of 33% after TAVR as compared to 67% with SAVR. No mortality was noted in the TAVR group, while 17% of patient died in SAVR group. The authors concluded that in patients with liver cirrhosis TAVR may be a viable alternative to SAVR [24].

## *Simultaneous Liver Transplant and Elective Cardiac Surgery*

Due to the high mortality associated with CP Classes B and C, most cardiac surgeons are reluctant to offer elective procedures to these patients. A viable option is to perform these procedures in tandem with OLT. In a Cleveland Clinic study, Lima et al. reported the outcomes of 10 patients with preserved left ventricular function (7 in CP Class B and 3 in CP Class C) who underwent elective cardiac procedures in combination with OLT. In-hospital mortality was 20% and actuarial survival was

70% at 3 years. Mean postoperative length of stay was 23 ± 8 days. Both in-hospital deaths had a CP Class C and underwent SAVR. The addition of a cardiac surgical procedure to OLT did not have a long-term effect on survival (70% actuarial survival at 3 years). The authors concluded that the elimination of hepatic dysfunction as a postoperative issue improves outcomes, especially in patients with CP Class B. Patients with CP Class C did not receive any additional survival benefit from a cardiac procedure in conjunction with an OLT [25].

## Conclusion

Liver cirrhosis poses a challenging problem in patients requiring cardiac surgery. Patients with CP Class A have acceptable outcomes after open heart surgery regardless of the usage of CPB. Advanced cirrhosis with CP Classes B and C and higher MELD scores are associated with higher mortality and morbidity. Techniques that obviate the need for CPB, such as OPCAB and TAVR, may provide favorable outcomes in this high-risk patient population. Further, combined cardiac procedures and OLT may be the optimal treatment for patients with advanced cirrhosis.

## Bibliography

1. Klemperer JD, Ko W, Krieger KH, Connolly M, Rosengart TK, et al. Cardiac operations in patients with cirrhosis. Ann Thorac Surg. 1998;65(1):85–7. PubMed PMID: 9456100.
2. Hayashida N, Aoyagi S. Cardiac operations in cirrhotic patients. Ann Thorac Cardiovasc Surg. 2004;10(3):140–7. PubMed PMID: 15312008.
3. Filsoufi F, Salzberg SP, Rahmanian PB, Schiano TD, Elsiesy H, et al. Early and late outcome of cardiac surgery in patients with liver cirrhosis. Liver Transpl. 2007;13(7):990–5. PubMed PMID: 17427174.
4. Macaron C, Hanouneh IA, Suman A, Lopez R, Johnston D, et al. Safety of cardiac surgery for patients with cirrhosis and Child-Pugh scores less than 8. Clin Gastroenterol Hepatol. 2012;10(5):535–9. PubMed PMID: 22210437.
5. Shaheen AA, Kaplan GG, Hubbard JN, Myers RP. Morbidity and mortality following coronary artery bypass graft surgery in patients with cirrhosis: a population-based study. Liver Int. 2009;29(8):1141–51. PubMed PMID: 19515218.
6. Gopaldas RR, Chu D, Cornwell LD, Dao TK, Lemaire SA, et al. Cirrhosis as a moderator of outcomes in coronary artery bypass grafting and off-pump coronary artery bypass operations: a 12-year population-based study. Ann Thorac Surg. 2013;96(4):1310–5. PubMed PMID: 23891409.
7. Suman A, Barnes DS, Zein NN, Levinthal GN, Connor JT, et al. Predicting outcome after cardiac surgery in patients with cirrhosis: a comparison of Child-Pugh and MELD scores. Clin Gastroenterol Hepatol. 2004;2(8):719–23. PubMed PMID: 15290666.
8. Gundling F, Seidl H, Gansera L, Schuster T, Hoffmann E, et al. Early and late outcomes of cardiac operations in patients with cirrhosis: a retrospective survival-rate analysis of 47 patients over 8 years. Eur J Gastroenterol Hepatol. 2010;22(12):1466–73. PubMed PMID: 21346421.
9. Thielmann M, Mechmet A, Neuhäuser M, Wendt D, Tossios P, et al. Risk prediction and outcomes in patients with liver cirrhosis undergoing open-heart surgery. Eur J Cardiothorac Surg. 2010;38(5):592–9. PubMed PMID: 20413316.

10. Lopez-Delgado JC, Esteve F, Javierre C, Torrado H, Carrio ML, et al. Predictors of long term mortality in patients with cirrhosis undergoing cardiac surgery. J Cardiovasc Surg (Torino). 2015;56(4):647–54. PubMed PMID: 24670881.
11. Vanhuyse F, Maureira P, Portocarrero E, Laurent N, Lekehal M, et al. Cardiac surgery in cirrhotic patients: results and evaluation of risk factors. Eur J Cardiothorac Surg. 2012;42(2):293–9. PubMed PMID: 22290926.
12. Arif R, Seppelt P, Schwill S, Kojic D, Ghodsizad A, et al. Predictive risk factors for patients with cirrhosis undergoing heart surgery. Ann Thorac Surg. 2012;94(6):1947–52. PubMed PMID: 22921237.
13. Sheng QS, Lang R, He Q, Yang YJ, Zhao DF, et al. Indocyanine green clearance test and model for end-stage liver disease score of patients with liver cirrhosis. Hepatobiliary Pancreat Dis Int. 2009;8(1):46–9. PubMed PMID: 19208514.
14. Takami Y, Masumoto H. Preoperative evaluation using asialoscintigraphy in patients undergoing cardiac surgery with noncardiac liver cirrhosis. Jpn J Thorac Cardiovasc Surg. 2006;54(11):463–8. PubMed PMID: 17144594.
15. Bizouarn P, Ausseur A, Desseigne P, Le Teurnier Y, Nougarede B, et al. Early and late outcome after elective cardiac surgery in patients with cirrhosis. Ann Thorac Surg. 1999;67(5):1334–8. PubMed PMID: 10355407.
16. Marui A, Kimura T, Tanaka S, Miwa S, Yamazaki K, et al. Coronary revascularization in patients with liver cirrhosis. Ann Thorac Surg. 2011;91(5):1393–9. PubMed PMID: 21396626.
17. Ben Ari A, Elinav E, Elami A, Matot I. Off-pump coronary artery bypass grafting in a patient with Child Class C liver cirrhosis awaiting liver transplantation. Br J Anaesth. 2006;97(4):468–72. PubMed PMID: 16873385.
18. Shah AM, Ogbara J, Herrmann HC, Fox Z, Kadakia M, et al. Outcomes of transcatheter aortic valve replacement in patients with chronic liver disease. Catheter Cardiovasc Interv. 2015;86(5):888–94. PubMed PMID: 25963625.
19. Mathie RT. Hepatic blood flow during cardiopulmonary bypass. Crit Care Med. 1993;21(2 Suppl):S72–6. PubMed PMID: 8428501.
20. An Y, Xiao YB, Zhong QJ. Open-heart surgery in patients with liver cirrhosis: indications, risk factors, and clinical outcomes. Eur Surg Res. 2007;39(2):67–74. PubMed PMID: 17283429.
21. Michalopoulos A, Alivizatos P, Geroulanos S. Hepatic dysfunction following cardiac surgery: determinants and consequences. Hepatogastroenterology. 1997;44(15):779–83. PubMed PMID: 9222689.
22. Peterss S, Beckmann E, Bhandari R, Hadem J, Hagl C, et al. Aortic valve replacement in patients with end-stage liver disease: a modified perfusion concept in high-risk patients. J Heart Valve Dis. 2015;24(3):302–9. PubMed PMID: 26901900.
23. Nemati MH, Astaneh B, Zamirian M. Aortic valve replacement in a patient with liver cirrhosis and coagulopathy. Gen Thorac Cardiovasc Surg. 2008;56(8):430–3. PubMed PMID: 18696213.
24. Greason KL, Mathew V, Wiesner RH, Suri RM, Rihal CS. Transcatheter aortic valve replacement in patients with cirrhosis. J Card Surg. 2013;28(5):492–5. PubMed PMID: 23899420.
25. Lima B, Nowicki ER, Miller CM, Hashimoto K, Smedira NG, et al. Outcomes of simultaneous liver transplantation and elective cardiac surgical procedures. Ann Thorac Surg. 2011;92(5):1580–4. PubMed PMID: 21944439.

# Chapter 20
# Thoracic and Esophageal Procedures, Lung Transplant in Cirrhotic Patients: Safety and Limiting Factors

Toshihiro Okamoto, Haytham Elgharably, Basem Soliman, Matthew Blum, and Kenneth R. McCurry

## Introduction

Performing a surgical procedure on cirrhotic patients carries higher risks of morbidity and mortality compared to noncirrhotic patients [1–3]. For instance, the perioperative mortality associated with cholecystectomy is increased in patients with liver disease versus patients without liver disease (odd ratio 8.47, 95% confidence interval 6.34–11.33) [1]. In an earlier study, the mortality for cholecystectomy in cirrhotic patients was 11–25% compared to 1.1% in noncirrhotic patients [4]. In a Danish cohort study of outcomes after colorectal cancer surgery, the 30-day mortality in patients without liver disease was 8.7% compared to 24.1% in cirrhotic patients [5]. Regarding cardiovascular procedures, a large retrospective analysis showed that cirrhotic patients undergoing coronary artery bypass grafting had an increased risk of morbidity and mortality compared to noncirrhotic patients (43% vs. 28% and 17% vs. 3%, respectively) [6]. In a nationwide study exploring mortality in four elective surgical procedures (cholecystectomy, colectomy, coronary artery bypass graphing, or abdominal aortic aneurysm repair), mortality rates were significantly higher for cirrhotic patients, even in those without portal hypertension [7].

The poor outcomes of cirrhotic patients after surgical procedures can be attributed to several factors. Coagulopathy, thrombocytopenia, and varices increase the risk of surgical and/or upper gastrointestinal tract bleeding. Notably, intraoperative transfusion is an independent predictor of mortality [8]. The tendency for volume overload despite intravascular depletion renders perioperative fluid management

T. Okamoto • H. Elgharably • K.R. McCurry, MD (✉)
Cleveland Clinic Department of Thoracic and Cardiovascular Surgery,
Cleveland, OH, USA
e-mail: mccurrk@ccf.org

B. Soliman, MD, PhD • M. Blum
Cleveland Clinic Department of General Surgery,
Cleveland, OH, USA

© Springer International Publishing AG 2017
B. Eghtesad, J. Fung (eds.), *Surgical Procedures on the Cirrhotic Patient*,
DOI 10.1007/978-3-319-52396-5_20

challenging and increases the risk of hypoxemia and hypotension under anesthesia. Impaired nutrition and metabolic status contribute to increased susceptibility to infection and poor wound healing. Lastly, acute liver failure may develop under surgical stress leading to hepatic encephalopathy, jaundice, and ascites [3, 9].

## Thoracic and Esophageal Procedures in Cirrhotic Patients

### Lung Cancer

Lung cancer is a global epidemic. It is the second most common malignancy after prostate cancer in men and breast cancer in women [10]. For resectable non-small-cell lung cancer, surgery is the standard of care and offers a potential cure [11, 12] but with the high number of patients with lung cancer, comorbid diseases in this population are common. A recent national study indicates that there are more than 600,000 adults with liver cirrhosis in the United States, and this number is rising [13]. With both diseases being quite common, the likelihood of a cirrhotic patient presenting for surgical resection of lung lesion is increasing. Nevertheless, only a few reports explore the safety and outcomes of pulmonary resection in cirrhotic patients, especially when compared to abdominal surgery in cirrhotic patients Table 20.1 [9, 14, 15, 16, 17]. These series have shown that the prognostic factors for outcomes following pulmonary resection in cirrhotic patients can be attributed to liver cirrhosis status and/or lung cancer stage. Cirrhosis factors include Child's classification, nutritional status, platelet count, and preoperative liver function (as assessed by bilirubin level, for example). Factors related to lung cancer include pathological stage, local invasion, and surgical approach [9] [14–16]. A recent multivariate analysis of the largest published series identified age and lung cancer stage as independent prognostic factors [17].

Cirrhotic patients undergoing pulmonary resection experience perioperative complications between 5 and 45% of the time (Table 20.1). The most common complication is postoperative bleeding, either surgical site or less commonly gastrointestinal bleeding. This results in an increased requirement for perioperative blood transfusion [9, 15, 16]. Other complications include acute liver failure (5–18%) and sepsis (5.4%) transfusion [9, 15, 16]. Operative mortality related to liver cirrhosis ranges between 5 and 8% transfusion [9, 15–17].

Iwata et al. reported that 5-year survival was 37.6% in 33 cirrhotic patients who underwent lung cancer surgery [15]. Further analysis has shown that the 5-year survival from lung cancer-related death was lower than 5-year survival from liver disease-related death (59.7% vs. 62.9%, Table 20.1). The authors observed that the most common cause of death in the first three postoperative years was lung cancer, while in the subsequent 3 years, liver disease was the most common cause of death [18]. Iwasaki et al. reported long-term outcomes of lung cancer surgery in 17 patients with liver cirrhosis [14]. The 5-year overall survival was 45.6%. Liver

**Table 20.1** Pulmonary resection in patients with liver cirrhosis

| Study | n | Child–Pugh Class | MELD score | Pulmonary resection | Morbidity | Mortality (operative) | Late outcome |
|---|---|---|---|---|---|---|---|
| Iwasaki et al. [14] | 17 | Class A: 4 Class B: 13 | N/A | Lobectomies = 11 Pneumnectomies = 3 Wedge = 3 | Rate = 29.5% Respiratory complications: $n = 5$ (45.5%) | $n = 1$ (5.9%), class B | Survival: 87.8, 57, 45.6% at 1, 3, 5 year Hepatic failure related mortality: $n = 4$ Class B: 30.8% morbidity and 7.6% mortality |
| Iwata et al. [9] | 37 | Class A: 28 Class B: 9 | N/A | Lobectomies = 32 Wedge = 5 | Cirrhosis-related: $n = 7$ (18.9%) Transient liver failure: $n = 2$ (5.4%) Surgical bleeding: $n = 4$ (10.8%) | $n = 2$ (5.4%), due to sepsis | HCC death: $n = 1$ (2.7%) at 6.5 months Cirrhotic death: $n = 1$ (2.7%) at 11.3 months Lung cancer death: $n = 1$ (2.7%) at 8.1 months |
| Iwata et al. [15] | 33 | Class A: 24 Class B: 9 | N/A | ≥ Lobectomies = 29 Wedge = 4 | Transient liver failure: $n = 2$ (6.5%) Surgical bleeding: $n = 3$ (9.7%) | $n = 2$ (6.5%) | Lung cancer survival: 84, 65.1, 59.7% at 1, 3, 5 year Cirrhotic survival: 92.1, 92.1, 62.9% at 1, 3, 5 year Overall survival: 77.3, 59.9, 37.6% at 1, 3, 5 year |
| Iwata et al. [16] | 11 | Class A: 10 Class B: 1 | N/A | Lobectomies = 8 Wedge = 3 | Liver failure $n = 2$ (18.2%) Surgical bleeding $n = 2$ (18.2%) | n=0 | Lung cancer survival: 88.9, 74.1, 74.1%, at 1, 3, 5 year Cirrhotic survival: 79.5, 79.5, 39.8%, at 1, 3, 5 year Overall survival: 70.7, 58.9, 29.5%, at 1, 3, 5 year |

(continued)

**Table 20.1** (continued)

| Study | n | Child–Pugh Class | MELD score | Pulmonary resection | Morbidity | Mortality (operative) | Late outcome |
|-------|---|------------------|------------|---------------------|-----------|----------------------|--------------|
| Rivera et al. [17] | 49 | N/A | N/A | Lobectomies = 33 Pneumnectomies = 10 Wedge = 5 Explorative thoracotomy = 1 | n = 20 40.8% Hepatic vs. 24.8% nonhepatic disease (p = 0.11) | n = 4 8.2% Hepatic vs. 4.2% nonhepatic disease (p = 0.32) | 5-year survival: 35.3% Hepatic vs. 43.8% nonhepatic disease (p = 0.0021) |

cirrhosis–related mortality was 7.6%, with all mortalities occurring in Child–Pugh class B patients while none was noted among Child–Pugh class A patients. Recently, Rivera et al. reported that the 5-year survival was significantly lower among cirrhotic patients who underwent lung cancer surgery compared to those without liver disease (35.3% vs. 43.8%, $p = 0.0021$) [17].

Chronic liver dysfunction is associated with impaired clearance of systemic vasodilators leading to a prolonged effect on various tissue beds. In the lung, it causes increased pulmonary vasculature vasodilatation and/or formation of arteriovenous shunting in the tissue bed. Subsequently, mild hypoxemia, hyperventilation, hypocapnia, and decreased diffusion capacity occur [18, 19]. Collectively, hepatic dysfunction, hypoxemia, and intrapulmonary vasodilatation are known as hepatopulmonary syndrome [20]. Portoplumonary hypertension is another unique entity in which liver cirrhosis and portal hypertension lead to pulmonary hypertension, which complicates any pulmonary resection procedure [21]. Cirrhosis contributes to pulmonary dysfunction in other ways too, including atelectasis and poor respiratory mechanics secondary to ascites, and hepatic hydrothorax.

Liver fibrosis is associated with portal venous congestion and splenomegaly, resulting in chronic anemia and thrombocytopenia [18, 19]. Impairment of liver synthetic function results in coagulopathy, which along with thrombocytopenia increases the risk of surgical bleeding. Moreover, cirrhotic patients are at risk of gastrointestinal bleeding (from esophageal or gastric varices or congested gastric mucosa) in the setting of surgical stress. The congestion of Intestinal mucosa interrupts nutrient absorption and, along with impaired albumin synthesis, causes malnutrition and increased susceptibility to infection. Impaired bile acid synthesis affects fat and fat-soluble vitamin absorption, including vitamin K. All of these pathophysiological changes increase the risk of perioperative complications in cirrhotic patients [18, 19].

## Gastrointestinal Reflux Disease and Achalasia

The incidence of gastrointestinal reflux disease (GERD) in cirrhotic patients is higher than the general population with a reported incidence of 25–55% [22, 23] and as high as 64% in patients with esophageal varices [24]. If medical treatment fails to control symptoms in these patients, surgery can be considered based with the patient's Child classification used to predict risk/benefit ratio of Nissen fundoplication (either open or laparoscopic) [25].

Achalasia is uncommon esophageal motility disorder characterized by loss of peristalsis and insufficient lower esophageal sphincter relaxation. Surgical management of this condition is considered if nitrates and calcium channel blockers fail to control symptoms. Coexistence of achalasia and cirrhosis is seldom reported and complicates potential surgical therapy especially if the patient has portal hypertension and esophageal varices [26]. Management of these patients depends first on presence of portal hypertension and esophageal varices and then on their Child's classification to predict operative risk. If the cirrhotic patient has no signs of portal hypertension or esophageal varices, pneumatic dilation or surgical myotomy may be considered based on Child classification. If the cirrhotic patient has esophageal varices, most authors suggest minimal intervention with botulinum toxin injection [26] or, recently, endoscopic ultrasound-guided botulinum injection to avoid inadvertent laceration of the varices [27].

## Esophageal Cancer

Surgery remains the mainstay treatment for early and locally advanced esophageal adenocarcinoma in conjunction with adjuvant or neoadjuvant chemotherapy or chemoradiation [28]. Moreover, salvage esophagectomy is the only curative option if chemo/radiotherapy or chemoradiation fails to control the disease [28]. The incidence of liver cirrhosis in esophageal cancer patients is about 7% [29], with overall morbidity after esophageal surgery in these patients twice that observed in noncirrhotic patients (17–21% vs. 3–8%) [30, 31]. Therefore, with reported unsatisfying results of esophagectomy in these patients, a comprehensive preoperative evaluation including liver function assessment is mandatory along with selection of appropriate procedure and preoperative phase management according to patient evaluation and nutritional status [32].

The incidence of perioperative complications in cirrhotic patents following esophagectomy ranges between 31 and 89% in the published series (Table 20.2). The most common reported complication was ascitic effusion, which is the cause of death in one-third of patients [30, 33, 34], and pneumonia in other series [34]. Other reported complications includes, respiratory failure [35], anastomotic leak, hepatorenal syndrome, portal thrombosis [33], and sepsis [30]. Reported operative blood loss during esophagectomy in cirrhotic patients has been variable. Fekete et al. reported that no massive intraoperative blood loss occurred and attributed that to cautious dissection and hemostasis during surgery [33].

Reported perioperative mortality rates are still high in the published series, ranging from 10 to 26%, which is comparable to the mortality rate associated with other gastrointestinal surgeries in cirrhotic patients [36]. It is much higher, however, in Child's B and C patients, 50%, and 100%, respectively, as reported in one series [37]. Tachibana et al. reported 1- and 3-year survival of 50% and 21%, respectively,

**Table 20.2** Published series for esophagectomy in cirrhotic patients

| Study | Country | Number of patients | Child classification | | | Thoracotomy | Postoperative morbidity | Perioperative mortality | Survival |
|---|---|---|---|---|---|---|---|---|---|
| | | | A | B | C | | | | |
| Fekete et al. [33] | France | 23 | 21 | 2 | 0 | In 20 patients | 83% Ascites, 65% Respiratory failure, 17% Anastomotic leak, 13% Hepato-renal syndrome, 13% | 26% | N/A |
| Belghiti et al. [30] | France | 30 | 30 | 0 | 0 | In all patients | 89% Ascites in 68% Sepsis 21% | 21% | N/A |
| Belghiti [65] | France | 53 | N/A | N/A | N/A | All patients | 72% Ascites 26% Pleural effusion 26% Anastomotic leak 24% Infection 22% | 26% | N/A |
| Tachibana et al. [31] | Japan | 18 | 11 | 7 | 0 | In all patients with three fields LND | 83.3% | 16.7% | 1 year, 50%, 3 years, 21% |
| Lu et al. [34] | Taiwan | 16 | 10 | 4 | 2 | In all patients | 31.75% Pneumonia, 18.75% Respiratory failure, 12.5% | 25%, 10%, 50%, and 100% in Child A, B, and C, respectively | N/A |

in a series of 18 patients [31]. Preoperative predictors of mortality include (1) hepatic functional reserve reflected by Child's score (Fekete et al. reported an acceptable postoperative mortality rate in patients with Child's A or selected Child B cases [31] and an unacceptable rate in Child's B patients with disturbed liver functions and low prothrombin value [33] and in Child's C patients), (2) presence of acute viral hepatitis [30, 33], and (3) prothrombin time above 160% of normal.

The impact of surgical approach on mortality rate in these patients has been addressed in several publications. Fekete et al. reported no difference in mortality rates between patients who underwent abdominal, thoracic, or a combined approach [33]. Similarly, Ueda et al. suggested that thoracotomy does not add more risk to cirrhotic patients even in advanced disease provided skilled postoperative management is applied [38]. However, Baker et al. reported 2 deaths out of 23 patients with cirrhosis who underwent transhiatal esophagectomy [39].

## Thoracic Procedures in Cirrhotic Patients: When to Operate and When Not to Operate?

A number of conditions are associated with unacceptably high risk for elective or semiurgent thoracic procedures including acute or fulminant hepatitis, acute viral hepatitis, acute alcoholic hepatitis, and American Society of Anesthesiologists Physical Status class V [19]. Existing data suggest that elective procedures should not be performed in Child–Pugh class C patients or those with a MELD score >15 [3, 19]. Emergency surgery in patients with cirrhosis carries high risk and poor outcomes compared to elective surgery [19].

The general consensus is that surgery is tolerated in Child–Pugh class A patients or those with a MELD score <10, while it is accepted in Child–Pugh class B or MELD score 10–15 after adequate preoperative optimization [3, 19]. With regard to lung cancer surgery, Iwata suggested that pulmonary resection can be carried out if life expectancy is expected to be more than 3 years based on liver condition [18].

## Lung Transplantation in Cirrhotic Patients

### Pulmonary Complications in Liver Transplantation Candidates

In liver transplant candidates with cirrhosis, the following pulmonary complications might be encountered: hepatopulmonary syndrome, portopulmonary hypertension, hepatic hydrothorax, advanced chronic obstructive pulmonary disease (COPD), pulmonary nodules, and interstitial lung disease.

Hepatopulmonary syndrome (HPS) is characterized by liver disease, poor oxygenation, and intrapulmonary vascular dilatations. Reduced metabolism of vasodilators in the liver causes pulmonary shunting, resulting in severe hypoxemia

(PaO$_2$ < 60 mmHg). Usually, hypoxemia resolves following liver transplantation. Although preoperative hypoxemia is associated with increased mortality [40], HPS is not a contraindication for liver transplantation if other morbidities are not identified [41]. Recently, Iyer et al. reported good outcomes for these patients: 76% 5-year survival of HPS patients with preoperative PaO$_2$ < 50 mmHg [42]. The Model for End-stage Liver Disease (MELD) score for patients with PaO$_2$ < 60 mmHg is upgraded by 10% every 3 months.

Portopulmonary hypertension is defined by the following criteria in patients with portal hypertension: (1) mean pulmonary artery pressure >25 mmHg; (2) pulmonary vascular resistance >240 dyne·s/cm$^5$; or (3) pulmonary capillary wedge pressure <15 mmHg. Although most portopulmonary hypertension patients have cirrhosis, the cause of portopulmonary hypertension remains unclear. The following pathogeneses are hypothesized: humoral substance, including serotonin and interleukin-1, genetic predisposition, and thromboembolism. Proliferative pulmonary angiopathy, including intimal and medial thickening, is the typical pathological finding. Patients with mild to moderate portopulmonary hypertension have good liver transplantation outcomes [43], whereas increased postoperative risk and poor clinical outcomes are associated with severe portopulmonary hypertension (systolic pulmonary artery pressure >60 mmHg) [44]. Portopulmonary hypertension is one of chronic liver diseases, which are not accounted for in the MELD scoring system. A MELD exception is applied if the following improvement is achieved: mean pulmonary artery pressure <35 mmHg and pulmonary vascular resistance <400 dyne·s/cm$^5$. Therefore, in the patients with severe portopulmonary hypertension, combined liver–lung transplantation or liver–heart–lung transplant should be considered.

Xiol et al. reported improvement of hepatic hydrothorax following liver transplantation. Of 29 patients with hepatic hydrothorax, 36% had hydrothorax at 1 month but all had resolved within 3 months. Therefore, hepatic hydrothorax is not a contraindication of liver transplantation [45].

In an analysis of COPD patients ($n = 67$, 18% of total population) receiving liver transplant, COPD severity was not associated with the risk of death [46]. However, severe COPD might be a contraindication for liver transplant, and such a patient could be a candidate of combined liver–lung transplantation, if the criteria for lung transplant are met.

Although interstitial lung disease may be rare in liver transplant candidates, deciding to perform a liver transplant for these patients requires careful consideration. This is because interstitial lung disease is rapidly progressive, resulting in 20–40% 5-year survival [47]. Liver transplant is contraindicated for patients with severe interstitial lung disease, though combined liver–lung transplantation might be considered.

## Combined Liver–Lung Transplantation

Because combined liver–lung transplantation (CLLT) is performed in a limited number of programs for a small population of candidates, there is limited information regarding patient demographics and outcomes. The clinical case series of CLLT are listed in Table

20.3 [48–54]. Originally, the Cambridge group reported heart–lung–liver transplantation [49]. In the United States, Barshes et al. reported 11 cases from the United Network for Organ Sharing (UNOS) database between 1984 and 2004 [50]. Arnon et al. reported 15 cystic fibrosis patients from UNOS database between 1987 and 2008 [52]. Recently, the Leuven group published 10 cases performed between 2000 and 2015 [54].

A CLLT candidate must to be sick enough to meet criteria for both liver and lung transplantation. CLLT is the only option to save patients with end-stage lung disease and end-stage liver disease. Performing either of the two transplants alone is insufficient to save the patients for whom CLLT is necessary. According to 2014 International Society for Heart and Lung Transplantation (ISHLT) consensus document for the selection lung transplant candidates, cirrhosis should be proven by biopsy and a portal gradient should be more than 10 mmHg. CLLT should not be considered in patients with a serum albumin less than 2.0 g/dl, an international normalized ratio higher than 1.8, or the presence of severe ascites or encephalopathy. However, a patient with milder liver or lung disease might be a candidate for CLLT if postoperative complications, such as bleeding or pulmonary failure, are expected when the patient receive a single organ transplantation. Lung allocation score (LAS) might be an important factor to predict postoperative complications. In an eight-patient series from the University of Kentucky during 2009 to 2012, Yi et al. reported that patients with high LAS (>50) might be poor candidates for CLLT, since two patients with LAS > 50 died within 90 days, while all patients with a median LAS of 39.5 had survived at 1 year [53].

Patients receiving CLLT fit either of the following scenarios: (1) a single systemic disease affects both organs—such as cystic fibrosis and alpha-1 antitrypsin deficiency, (2) a primary single organ disease caused the failure of the other organ, like hepatic cirrhosis leading to portopulmonary hypertension or HPS, or (3) a primary independent disease of both organs occurred (e.g., COPD and end-stage alcoholic cirrhosis). The majority of previously CLLT was performed for patients with cystic fibrosis.

**Table 20.3** Published case series of combined liver–lung transplantation

| Study | Institute | Term | Patient | CF | Procedures | 1-year survival (%) | 5-year survival (%) |
|---|---|---|---|---|---|---|---|
| Praseedom et al. [49] | Cambridge | 1986–1999 | 9 | 7 | LHL, 9 | 56 | 44 |
| Couetil et al. [48] | Paris | 1990–1995 | 10 | 10 | LHL, 5; LL, 5 | 70 | – |
| Grannas et al. [51] | Hannover | 1999–2003 | 13 | 5 | LHL, 1; LL, 12 | 69 | 49 |
| Barshes et al. [50] | Houston, UNOS | 1984–2004 | 11 | 11 | LL, 11 | 79 | 63 |
| Arnon [52] | UNOS | 1987–2008 | 15 | 15 | LL, 15 | 80 | 80 |
| Yi et al. [53] | Kentucky | 2009–2012 | 8 | 3 | LHL, 1; LL, 7 | 71 | – |
| Ceulemans et al. [54] | Leuven | 2000–2015 | 11 | 5 | LHL, 1; LL, 10 | 90 | – |

*CF* cystic fibrosis, *LHL* liver–heart–lung transplantation, *LL* liver–lung transplantation

Cystic fibrosis is an autosomal recessive disorder, characterized by epithelial electrolyte transport abnormalities and elevated sweat chloride concentration. It affects multiple organs including the lungs, pancreas, and liver. Chronic respiratory failure is the most frequent manifestation (45%). Hepatic manifestations include biliary cirrhosis, portal hypertension, cholelithiasis, and sclerosing cholangitis with the incidence of 4–10% of all cystic fibrosis patients. In this disease, liver failure accounts for 20% of deaths and respiratory failure for 33% [55]. Therefore, CLLT is indicated in a certain limited population of cystic fibrosis patients.

Historically, an en bloc double-lung–heart–liver graft was transplanted with cardiopulmonary bypass [49]. Following the evolution of lung transplant, the Paris group initiated sequential double lung transplant, followed by the discontinuation of cardiopulmonary bypass and laparotomy for liver transplant. Chest incision is a clamshell (anterolateral thoracotomies with transverse sternotomy), sternotomy, or bilateral thoracotomy. Given that the acceptable cold ischemic time is shorter in lungs than in liver, lung transplantation is typically performed before liver transplantation [48, 50, 51]. The Kentucky group advocated that performing abdominal dissection before initiating cardiopulmonary bypass might reduce bleeding and blood transfusions [53]. Conversely, a patient's abnormal coagulation status led the Leuven group to perform the liver transplantation first to ensure improvement in coagulation status prior to lung transplantation. In this case, ex vivo lung perfusion machine was utilized to maintain donor lungs during the liver procedures [56]. In one of three cases, severe hypoxia and hypercarbia was reported during the liver transplantation procedure.

A high postoperative infection rate has been reported in CLLT. In a series of nine cases, the Cambridge group reported four deaths (44%) sepsis during the early postoperative period (cystic fibrosis, $n = 7$; primary biliary cirrhosis, $n = 1$; alpha-1 antitrypsin deficiency, $n = 1$). The Kentucky group also reported that three of eight patients (37%) died of sepsis (series included three cystic fibrosis patients). In a series of 13 cases (cystic fibrosis, $n = 5$), Grannas et al. reported that only two of five patients were free of severe infections, while the remaining cases died from infection. Patients with cystic fibrosis tend to experience complications of infection and malnutrition in liver disease might contribute to this group's susceptibility to infection. To minimize this risk factor, the Hannover group established a body mass index threshold of >18 kg/m² for CLLT [51].

Relatively lower rates of rejection were observed in a CLLT case series. Bhama et al. reported that the incidence of acute cellular rejection in the first year following lung transplantation was significantly lower in CLLT group than in the control group [57]. Faro et al. demonstrated that pediatric CLLT recipients with cystic fibrosis had a lower incidence of bronchiolitis obliterans than the control [58]. Similar results have been reported in other multiorgan transplants [59, 60]. Several possible mechanisms have been postulated to explain the potential protective effect of transplanting the liver in conjunction with other solid organs [57, 61, 62].

The 1-year survival in a relatively large case series ($n \geq 8$) of CLLT was 56–90% and the 5-year survival was 44–90%. This is comparable to that of isolated bilateral lung transplant (80% at 1 year, and 54% at 5 years) [63]. Given that CLLT is the only option to save patients with end-stage lung disease and end-stage liver disease and provides similar outcomes to lung transplantation in experienced hands, the use of more than one organ for a single recipient in CLLT can be ethically justified.

## Conclusions

Although existing surgical risk models can be applied to cirrhotic patients in the setting of thoracic surgeries, they were not developed for this purpose, and current recommendations using these models are based on retrospective data. As of now, there are no standardized evidence-based guidelines developed to predict surgical outcomes of patients with cirrhosis. The care of cirrhotic patients should be individualized based on the indication for the procedure and the liver condition. Further research is warranted to develop a reliable scoring model that specifically can estimate the risk for surgical procedures in patients with cirrhosis.

## References

1. Patel T. Surgery in the patient with liver disease. Mayo Clin Proc. 1999;74(6):593–9.
2. O'Leary JG, Yachimski PS, Friedman LS. Surgery in the patient with liver disease. Clin Liver Dis. 2009;13(2):211–31.
3. Nicoll A. Surgical risk in patients with cirrhosis. J Gastroenterol Hepatol. 2012;27(10):1569–75.
4. Aranha GV, Sontag SJ, Greenlee HB. Cholecystectomy in cirrhotic patients: a formidable operation. Am J Surg. 1982;143(1):55–60.
5. Montomoli J, Erichsen R, Christiansen CF, Ulrichsen SP, Pedersen L, Nilsson T, et al. Liver disease and 30-day mortality after colorectal cancer surgery: a Danish population-based cohort study. BMC Gastroenterol. 2013;13:66.
6. Shaheen AA, Kaplan GG, Hubbard JN, Myers RP. Morbidity and mortality following coronary artery bypass graft surgery in patients with cirrhosis: a population-based study. Liver Int. 2009;29(8):1141–51.
7. Csikesz NG, Nguyen LN, Tseng JF, Shah SA. Nationwide volume and mortality after elective surgery in cirrhotic patients. J Am Coll Surg. 2009;208(1):96–103.
8. Neeff H, Mariaskin D, Spangenberg HC, Hopt UT, Makowiec F. Perioperative mortality after non-hepatic general surgery in patients with liver cirrhosis: an analysis of 138 operations in the 2000s using Child and MELD scores. J Gastrointest Surg. 2011;15(1):1–11.
9. Iwata T, Inoue K, Nishiyama N, Nagano K, Izumi N, Tsukioka T, et al. Factors predicting early postoperative liver cirrhosis-related complications after lung cancer surgery in patients with liver cirrhosis. Interact Cardiovasc Thorac Surg. 2007;6(6):720–30.
10. Siegel RL, Miller KD, Jemal A. Cancer statistics, 2016. CA Cancer J Clin. 2016;66(1):7–30.
11. Van Schil PE, Balduyck B, De Waele M, Hendriks JM, Hertoghs M, Lauwers P. Surgical treatment of early-stage non-small-cell lung cancer. EJC Suppl. 2013;11(2):110–22.
12. Deslauriers J, Gregoire J. Surgical therapy of early non-small cell lung cancer. Chest. 2000;117(4 Suppl 1):104S–9S.
13. Scaglione S, Kliethermes S, Cao G, Shoham D, Durazo R, Luke A, et al. The epidemiology of cirrhosis in the United States: a population-based study. J Clin Gastroenterol. 2015;49(8):690–6.

14. Iwasaki A, Shirakusa T, Okabayashi K, Inutsuka K, Yoneda S, Yamamoto S, et al. Lung cancer surgery in patients with liver cirrhosis. Ann Thorac Surg. 2006;82(3):1027–32.
15. Iwata T, Inoue K, Nishiyama N, Nagano K, Izumi N, Mizuguchi S, et al. Long-term outcome of surgical treatment for non-small cell lung cancer with comorbid liver cirrhosis. Ann Thorac Surg. 2007;84(6):1810–7.
16. Iwata T, Nishiyama N, Nagano K, Izumi N, Mizuguchi S, Morita R, et al. Pulmonary resection for non-small cell lung cancer in patients with hepatocellular carcinoma. World J Surg. 2008;32(10):2204–12.
17. Rivera C, Chevalier B, Fabre E, Pricopi C, Badia A, Arame A, et al. Lung cancer surgery and cirrhosis. Rev Pneumol Clin. 2015;71(1):12–9.
18. Chen KC, Lin JW, Tseng YT, Kuo SW, Huang PM, Hsu HH, et al. Thoracic empyema in patients with liver cirrhosis: clinical characteristics and outcome analysis of thoracoscopic management. J Thorac Cardiovasc Surg. 2012;143(5):1144–51.
19. Im GY, Lubezky N, Facciuto ME, Schiano TD. Surgery in patients with portal hypertension: a preoperative checklist and strategies for attenuating risk. Clin Liver Dis. 2014;18(2):477–505.
20. Huffmyer JL, Nemergut EC. Respiratory dysfunction and pulmonary disease in cirrhosis and other hepatic disorders. Respir Care. 2007;52(8):1030–6.
21. Lai HC, Lai HC, Wang KY, Lee WL, Ting CT, Liu TJ. Severe pulmonary hypertension complicates postoperative outcome of non-cardiac surgery. Br J Anaesth. 2007;99(2):184–90.
22. Arsene D, Bruley des Varannes S, Galmiche JP, Denis P, Chayvialle JA, Hellot MF, et al. Gastro-oesophageal reflux and alcoholic cirrhosis. A reappraisal. J Hepatol. 1987;4(2):250–8.
23. Zhang J, Cui PL, Lv D, Yao SW, Xu YQ, Yang ZX. Gastroesophageal reflux in cirrhotic patients without esophageal varices. World J Gastroenterol (WJG). 2011;17(13):1753–8.
24. Ahmed AM, al Karawi MA, Shariq S, Mohamed AE. Frequency of gastroesophageal reflux in patients with liver cirrhosis. Hepatogastroenterology. 1993;40(5):478–80.
25. Cobb W, Heniford B, Burns J, Carbonell A, Matthews B, Kercher K. Cirrhosis is not a contraindication to laparoscopic surgery. Surg Endosc Other Interventional Techniques. 2005;19(3):418–23.
26. Pinillos H, Legnani P, Schiano T. Achalasia in a patient with gastroesophageal varices: problematic treatment decisions. Dig Dis Sci. 2006;51(1):31–3.
27. Lakhtakia S, Monga A, Gupta R, Kalpala R, Pratap N, Wee E, et al. Achalasia cardia with esophageal varix managed with endoscopic ultrasound-guided botulinum toxin injection. Indian J Gastroenterol (Official Journal of the Indian Society of Gastroenterology). 2011;30(6):277–9.
28. Ajani JA, D'Amico TA, Almhanna K, Bentrem DJ, Besh S, Chao J, et al. Esophageal and esophagogastric junction cancers, version 1.2015. J Natl Compr Canc Netw (JNCCN). 2015;13(2):194–227.
29. Pessaux P, Msika S, Atalla D, Hay JM, Flamant Y. Risk factors for postoperative infectious complications in noncolorectal abdominal surgery: a multivariate analysis based on a prospective multicenter study of 4718 patients. Arch Surg. 2003;138(3):314–24.
30. Belghiti J, Cherqui D, Langonnet F, Fekete F. Esophagogastrectomy for carcinoma in cirrhotic patients. Hepatogastroenterology. 1990;37(4):388–91.
31. Tachibana M, Kotoh T, Kinugasa S, Dhar DK, Shibakita M, Ohno S, et al. Esophageal cancer with cirrhosis of the liver: results of esophagectomy in 18 consecutive patients. Ann Surg Oncol. 2000;7(10):758–63.
32. Shimakawa T, Naritaka Y, Asaka S, Isohata N, Murayama M, Konno S, et al. Surgical treatment for superficial esophageal cancer with liver cirrhosis and esophageal varices: report of a case. Anticancer Res. 2007;27(5B):3507–11.
33. Fekete F, Belghiti J, Cherqui D, Langonnet F, Gayet B. Results of esophagogastrectomy for carcinoma in cirrhotic patients. A series of 23 consecutive patients. Ann Surg. 1987;206(1):74.
34. Lu M-S, Liu Y-H, Wu Y-C, Kao C-L, Liu H-P, Hsieh M-J. Is it safe to perform esophagectomy in esophageal cancer patients combined with liver cirrhosis? Interact Cardiovasc Thorac Surg. 2005;4(5):423–5.

35. Masoomi H, Nguyen B, Smith BR, Stamos MJ, Nguyen NT. Predictive factors of acute respiratory failure in esophagectomy for esophageal malignancy. Am Surg. 2012;78(10):1024–8.
36. Mansour A, Watson W, Shayani V, Pickleman J. Abdominal operations in patients with cirrhosis: still a major surgical challenge. Surgery. 1997;122(4):730–6.
37. Li B, Zhang B, Ma JW, Li P, Li L, Song YM, et al. High prevalence of reflux esophagitis among upper endoscopies in Chinese patients with chronic liver diseases. BMC Gastroenterol. 2010;10:54.
38. Ueda H, Iwasaki A, Kusano T, Shirakusa T. Thoracotomy in patients with liver cirrhosis. Scand J Thorac Cardiovasc Surg. 1994;28(1):37–41.
39. Baker Jr JW, Schechter GL. Management of panesophageal cancer by blunt resection without thoracotomy and reconstruction with stomach. Ann Surg. 1986;203(5):491–9.
40. Krowka MJ, Mandell MS, Ramsay MA, Kawut SM, Fallon MB, Manzarbeitia C, et al. Hepatopulmonary syndrome and portopulmonary hypertension: a report of the multicenter liver transplant database. Liver Transpl (Official Publication of the American Association for the Study of Liver Diseases and the International Liver Transplantation Society). 2004;10(2):174–82.
41. Krowka MJ, Wiesner RH, Heimbach JK. Pulmonary contraindications, indications and MELD exceptions for liver transplantation: a contemporary view and look forward. J Hepatol. 2013;59(2):367–74.
42. Iyer VN, Swanson KL, Cartin-Ceba R, Dierkhising RA, Rosen CB, Heimbach JK, et al. Hepatopulmonary syndrome: favorable outcomes in the MELD exception era. Hepatology. 2013;57(6):2427–35.
43. Taura P, Garcia-Valdecasas JC, Beltran J, Izquierdo E, Navasa M, Sala-Blanch J, et al. Moderate primary pulmonary hypertension in patients undergoing liver transplantation. Anesth Analg. 1996;83(4):675–80.
44. Ramsay MA, Simpson BR, Nguyen AT, Ramsay KJ, East C, Klintmalm GB. Severe pulmonary hypertension in liver transplant candidates. Liver Transpl Surg. 1997;3(5):494–500.
45. Xiol X, Tremosa G, Castellote J, Gornals J, Lama C, Lopez C, et al. Liver transplantation in patients with hepatic hydrothorax. Transpl Int (Official Journal of the European Society for Organ Transplantation). 2005;18(6):672–5.
46. Rybak D, Fallon MB, Krowka MJ, Brown Jr RS, Reinen J, Stadheim L, et al. Risk factors and impact of chronic obstructive pulmonary disease in candidates for liver transplantation. Liver Transpl (Official Publication of the American Association for the Study of Liver Diseases and the International Liver Transplantation Society). 2008;14(9):1357–65.
47. Olson AL, Swigris JJ, Lezotte DC, Norris JM, Wilson CG, Brown KK. Mortality from pulmonary fibrosis increased in the United States from 1992 to 2003. Am J Respir Crit Care Med. 2007;176(3):277–84.
48. Couetil JP, Soubrane O, Houssin DP, Dousset BE, Chevalier PG, Guinvarch A, et al. Combined heart-lung-liver, double lung-liver, and isolated liver transplantation for cystic fibrosis in children. Transpl Int (Official Journal of the European Society for Organ Transplantation). 1997;10(1):33–9.
49. Praseedom RK, McNeil KD, Watson CJ, Alexander GJ, Calne RY, Wallwork J, et al. Combined transplantation of the heart, lung, and liver. Lancet. 2001;358(9284):812–3.
50. Barshes NR, DiBardino DJ, McKenzie ED, Lee TC, Stayer SA, Mallory GB, et al. Combined lung and liver transplantation: the United States experience. Transplantation. 2005;80(9):1161–7.
51. Grannas G, Neipp M, Hoeper MM, Gottlieb J, Luck R, Becker T, et al. Indications for and outcomes after combined lung and liver transplantation: a single-center experience on 13 consecutive cases. Transplantation. 2008;85(4):524–31.
52. Arnon R, Annunziato RA, Miloh T, Padilla M, Sogawa H, Batemarco L, et al. Liver and combined lung and liver transplantation for cystic fibrosis: analysis of the UNOS database. Pediatr Transplant. 2011;15(3):254–64.
53. Yi SG, Burroughs SG, Loebe M, Scheinin S, Seethamraju H, Jyothula S, et al. Combined lung and liver transplantation: analysis of a single-center experience. Liver Transpl (Official

Publication of the American Association for the Study of Liver Diseases and the International Liver Transplantation Society). 2014;20(1):46–53.

54. Ceulemans LJ, Strypstein S, Neyrinck A, Verleden S, Ruttens D, Monbaliu D, et al. Combined liver-thoracic transplantation: Single-center experience with introduction of the 'liver-first' principle. Transpl Int (Official Journal of the European Society for Organ Transplantation). 2016;29(6):715–26.

55. Feigelson J, Anagnostopoulos C, Poquet M, Pecau Y, Munck A, Navarro J. Liver cirrhosis in cystic fibrosis–therapeutic implications and long term follow up. Arch Dis Child. 1993;68(5):653–7.

56. Ceulemans LJ, Monbaliu D, Verslype C, van der Merwe S, Laleman W, Vos R, et al. Combined liver and lung transplantation with extended normothermic lung preservation in a patient with end-stage emphysema complicated by drug-induced acute liver failure. Am J Transpl (Official Journal of the American Society of Transplantation and the American Society of Transplant Surgeons). 2014;14(10):2412–6.

57. Bhama JK, Pilewski JM, Zaldonis D, Fontes PA, DeVera ME, Shullo MA, et al. Does simultaneous lung-liver transplantation provide an immunologic advantage compared with isolated lung transplantation? J Thorac Cardiovasc Surg. 2011;141(5):e36–8.

58. Faro A, Shepherd R, Huddleston CB, Lowell J, Gandhi S, Nadler M, et al. Lower incidence of bronchiolitis obliterans in pediatric liver-lung transplant recipients with cystic fibrosis. Transplantation. 2007;83(11):1435–9.

59. Rana A, Robles S, Russo MJ, Halazun KJ, Woodland DC, Witkowski P, et al. The combined organ effect: protection against rejection? Ann Surg. 2008;248(5):871–9.

60. Pinderski LJ, Kirklin JK, McGiffin D, Brown R, Naftel DC, Young Jr KR, et al. Multi-organ transplantation: is there a protective effect against acute and chronic rejection? J Heart Lung Transplant (The Official Publication of the International Society for Heart Transplantation). 2005;24(11):1828–33.

61. Gugenheim J, Amorosa L, Gigou M, Fabiani B, Rouger P, Gane P, et al. Specific absorption of lymphocytotoxic alloantibodies by the liver in inbred rats. Transplantation. 1990;50(2):309–13.

62. Narula J, Bennett LE, DiSalvo T, Hosenpud JD, Semigran MJ, Dec GW. Outcomes in recipients of combined heart-kidney transplantation: multiorgan, same-donor transplant study of the International Society of Heart and Lung Transplantation/United Network for Organ Sharing Scientific Registry. Transplantation. 1997;63(6):861–7.

63. Yusen RD, Edwards LB, Kucheryavaya AY, Benden C, Dipchand AI, Goldfarb SB, et al. The registry of the International Society for Heart and Lung Transplantation: thirty-second Official Adult Lung and Heart-Lung Transplantation Report–2015; Focus Theme: Early Graft Failure. J Heart Lung Transplant (The Official Publication of the International Society for Heart Transplantation). 2015;34(10):1264–77.

64. Belghiti J. Chirurgie oesophagienne chez le cirrhotique. La chirurgie digestive chez le cirrhotique Paris: Monographies de l'AFC. 1993:61–72.

Chapter 21

# Neurosurgical Procedures in Patients with Cirrhosis and Acute Liver Failure: Indications, Safety, and Feasibility of Intracranial Pressure Monitor Devices

Jeffrey P. Mullin, Connor Wathen, Alvin Chan, and Edward C. Benzel

## Encephalopathy Derived from Acute Liver Failure and Cirrhosis

### *Introduction*

Hepatic encephalopathy (HE) is a well-known complication of liver failure. The exact pathophysiology of HE is not entirely understood, although hyperammonemia, among other neurotoxins, plays a central role. One of the most feared complications of HE is intracranial hypertension. Clinically, HE can present across a broad spectrum from mild cognitive impairment to coma. A very high percentage of patients with severe HE suffer from elevated intracranial pressure (ICP). The most accurate way to measure ICP is via invasive monitoring, although this has risks. In this chapter, we review the current indications and outcomes for invasive monitoring.

J.P. Mullin, MD, MBA • E.C. Benzel, MD (✉)
Department of Neurosurgery, Cleveland Clinic, Neurological Institute,
9500 Euclid Avenue, Cleveland, OH 44195, USA
e-mail: benzele@ccf.org

C. Wathen, BS
Cleveland Clinic Lerner College of Medicine, Cleveland, OH, USA

A. Chan, BS
Medical College of Wisconsin, Milwaukee, WI, USA

© Springer International Publishing AG 2017
B. Eghtesad, J. Fung (eds.), *Surgical Procedures on the Cirrhotic Patient*,
DOI 10.1007/978-3-319-52396-5_21

## *Pathophysiology*

The pathophysiology of hepatic encephalopathy (HE) is complex and not completely understood. Several factors play a role in the pathogenesis of HE, including toxins, alterations in neurotransmission, inflammatory mediators, and structural damage. Furthermore, there are differences in terms of pathophysiology and clinical progression between patients experiencing HE with acute liver failure and those with chronic liver disease.

Hyperammonemia is central to the pathophysiology of HE [1]. The net result of dysfunctional ammonia metabolism by the gut, liver, kidney, and muscle in liver disease is increased ammonia delivery to the brain. Astrocytes are the primary cells in the brain that contain glutamine synthetase, responsible for the detoxification of ammonia, and consequently they are the cells primarily affected by hyperammonemia [2, 3]. The astrocyte takes up ammonia, which is converted to glutamine via cytosolic glutamine synthetase. Because glutamine is osmotically active, states of hyperammonemia overwhelm the astrocytic capacity for osmoregulation via myo-inositol degradation. The ultimate result is cellular swelling and cytotoxic edema (Fig. 21.1) [4]. In addition, glutamine is transported into astrocytic mitochondria where it is hydrolyzed by phosphate activated glutaminase to form ammonia. Accumulation of ammonia within the mitochondria results in increased reactive

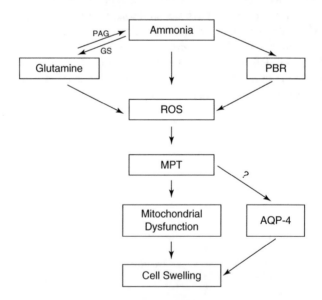

**Fig. 21.1** Hypothetical scheme of ammonia-HE-induced astrocyte swelling. Note the interconversion between ammonia and glutamine and that both result in the formation of ROS. While the role of aquaporin-4 (AQP-4) in this scheme is uncertain, inhibition of the MPT was able to block the upregulation of AQP-4 by ammonia. (*GS* glutamine synthetase, *MPT* mitochondrial permeability transition, *PAG* phosphate-activated glutaminase, *PBR* peripheral benzodiazepine receptor, *ROS* reactive oxygen species.)

oxygen species, leading to mitochondrial dysfunction, induction of inflammatory signaling cascades, and further exacerbation of cellular swelling [5].

Through undefined mechanisms, neurotoxins, especially ammonia, induce changes in neurotransmission. The peripheral-type benzodiazepine receptor (PTBR) in particular is thought to contribute to HE pathogenesis [6]. Increased PTBR signaling leads to increased cholesterol uptake and neurosteroid synthesis. Neurosteroids such as allopregnanolone act as positive allosteric modulators of the $GABA_A$ receptor [7]. The net result is a significant increase in GABA-ergic tone [8].

In addition to altered inhibitory neurotransmission, alterations in excitatory neurotransmission are seen in experimental models and patients with HE as well. Interestingly, despite a total decrease in total brain glutamate, extracellular glutamate is increased in animal models of HE [9–11]. The increase in extracellular glutamate is thought to be caused by astrocytic dysfunction leading to decreased glutamate reuptake or excessive neuronal release of glutamate due to depolarization via ammonia [12, 13]. Increased NMDA signaling has also been implicated in the pathogenesis of HE by increasing sodium influx and subsequent cellular swelling [14].

Systemic inflammation and neuroinflammation also play critical roles in the pathogenesis of HE [15]. The development of systemic inflammatory response syndrome (SIRS) is a potent predictor of developing HE. Circulating tumor necrosis factor alpha (TNF-α) levels are also correlated with the severity of HE and known polymorphisms of TNF are known to influence prognosis [16, 17]. Studies have also shown that microglia are activated in HE, providing direct evidence of neuroinflammation [18]. Once activated, microglia produce inflammatory cytokines, especially TNF-α, interleukin (IL)-1β, and IL-6. Deletion of either the gene encoding TNF or IL-1β resulted in a delay in the onset of HE and attenuated cerebral edema [19]. There remains debate over how the integrity of the BBB changes in response to this proinflammatory setting and the associated effects on HE and cerebral edema [20].

## Intracranial Hypertension

HE associated with acute liver failure and cirrhosis can result in intracranial hypertension. Intracranial hypertension is defined as intracranial pressure (ICP) exceeding 20 mmHg. ICP is determined by the brain, blood, and cerebrospinal fluid (CSF). Brain parenchyma composes 80% of the contents of the skull while blood and cerebrospinal fluid account for approximately 10% each [21]. ICP increases with an increase in the volume of the brain parenchyma, which can occur with an expanding mass or an increase in cerebral water content, an increase in blood volume, which may occur when cerebral autoregulation is impaired, or an increase in CSF volume either due to increased production or impaired resorption [22]. The driving force for blood flow within the brain is the cerebral perfusion pressure (CPP). Cerebral perfusion pressure (CPP) is dependent upon the mean arterial pressure (MAP) and ICP. More specifically, CPP is equal to the ICP subtracted from the MAP (i.e., CPP = MAP – ICP). Thus if the MAP is held constant, as ICP increases, cerebral perfusion pressure (and consequently blood flow) decreases, increasing the risk for ischemia. ICP elevation can also result in various herniation syndromes that are frequently fatal.

In HE, ammonia is converted to glutamine within astrocytes, as discussed previously. As glutamine is osmotically active, this results in astrocytic swelling and is a primary contributor to cerebral edema in HE [23]. Proinflammatory signaling molecules may also contribute to astrocyte swelling and increased ICP [24]. A number of other factors are thought to mediate the effects of ammonia and inflammatory signals, including reactive oxygen species (ROS), nuclear factor kappa B (NF-κB) signaling, mitogen activated protein kinase (MAPK) signaling, mitochondrial permeability transition, and various ion transporters and aquaporins [25, 26]. Consequently, great care must be taken to manage cerebral perfusion pressure, cerebral blood volume, and cerebral blood flow to reduce the risk of herniation or ischemia [27].

## Clinical Manifestations

Hepatic encephalopathy presents clinically as a wide spectrum of cognitive and neuromuscular dysfunction. HE is classified by the underlying etiology, clinical signs and symptoms, the time course, and precipitating factors [28]. Type A HE occurs in the setting of acute liver failure, type B HE occurs in the setting of porto-systemic bypass with no intrinsic hepatic disease, and type C HE occurs in the setting of cirrhosis. The time course is classified as episodic, recurrent, or persistent. In patients with acute liver failure (i.e., type A HE), the onset of symptoms is typically sudden and patients rapidly progress through the grades of HE. Type A HE is associated with elevated ICP and frequently results in death within hours to days of symptom onset [29]. HE in the setting of chronic liver disease (i.e., type C HE) is typically more insidious and often occurs episodically.

The most common grading system to classify the clinical manifestations of HE is the West Haven Criteria (WHC) [28]. Patients with minimal hepatic encephalopathy (MHE), sometimes referred to as Grade 0 HE, demonstrate limited clinically recognizable signs and may often only be identified following abnormal neuropsychological testing [30]. Sleep disturbances, both insomnia and hypersomnia, are frequently an initial manifestation of HE [31]. Furthermore, the absence of excessive daytime sleepiness has a strong negative predictive value for the development of HE in patients with cirrhosis [32].

Patients with grade I HE typically present with impaired attention and increased difficulty with basic arithmetic and other similar cognitive skills. Neuromuscular findings in these patients include mild tremor, slurred speech, and impaired handwriting [33]. Asterixis may also become evident in patients with grade I HE. Grade I HE is associated with behavioral changes including irritability, depression, or euphoria [34].

Grade II HE results in further cognitive impairment, including amnesia and gross deficits in basic computation. Behaviorally, patients may exhibit disorientation or inappropriate behavior in addition to marked lethargy. Grade II HE is also characterized by more prominent asterixis, hypoactive reflexes, and muscular rigidity [35].

Patients with grade III HE demonstrate somnolence and significant confusion, typically disorientation to time and place. Neuromuscular dysfunction is especially pronounced and may result in incontinence, incoherent speech, hyperreflexia, clonus, and a positive Babinski's sign [34].

In grade IV HE, patients are comatose and may or may not respond to noxious stimuli. Decerebrate posturing is also seen in these patients. Although infrequent, focal neurologic deficits may also be seen in patients with HE, most commonly hemiplegia [36].

## Diagnosis

The diagnosis of HE starts with a thorough history and physical examination to identify (1) the characteristic signs and symptoms of HE, (2) the evaluation of other possible causes of altered mental status, (3) the evaluation of possible precipitating factors, and (4) response to empiric therapy. Several diagnostic tools have been developed to aid in the process of identifying patients with HE. Among these tools are the hepatic encephalopathy scoring algorithm (HESA), clinical hepatic encephalopathy staging scale (CHESS), and modified-orientation log (MO-log) [37–39]. While these various tools provide an objective measure of severity and can increase the precision with which HE is diagnosed and classified, which is particularly useful in therapeutic trials, their clinical use is often limited due to concerns about the length of time it takes to administer these tests.

There is limited utility in additional laboratory testing or imaging in the evaluation of HE. The levels of ammonia, which play in important role in HE pathogenesis, are consistently elevated in patients with HE [40]. The correlation between the degree of hepatic encephalopathy and arterial ammonia levels only holds true for ammonia concentrations up to two times the upper limit of normal [41]. A potential alternative laboratory biomarker for MHE is 3-nitrotyrosine, a product of protein nitrosylation via peroxynitrite, a derivative of nitric oxide, which is elevated in MHE. 3-Nitrotyrosine was shown to have a sensitivity of 93% and a specificity of 89% in the diagnosis of MHE in patients with cirrhosis [5, 42].

## Pharmacologic Treatment-Encephalopathy

The treatment of overt HE consists of managing precipitating factors, ammonia reducing therapies, reduction of elevated ICP, and prevention of recurrent bouts of HE. Correction or treatment of the precipitating cause of HE is typically associated with improvement or resolution of HE [43]. Common precipitating causes that should be investigated and treated include gastrointestinal (GI) bleeding, infection, metabolic alkalosis, hypovolemia, hypoglycemia, and renal failure. The mainstay of HE therapy is the reduction of ammonia. Lactulose and lactitol, both nonabsorbable disaccharides, are first-line therapies [44].

Antibiotics also play an important role in the treatment of overt HE. Antibiotics improve HE through the elimination of ammonia producing bacteria that reside in the GI tract. The current antibiotic of choice is rifaximin [45]. In patients with overt HE, rifaximin has been shown to be more efficacious than lactulose therapy in both treating HE and improving patient reported quality of life [46]. Furthermore, randomized, placebo-controlled studies of rifaximin in patients already receiving lactulose showed that rifaximin therapy was more effective than placebo as a secondary prevention measure to reduce recurrent bouts of HE [47].

Nutritional support is also essential in the management of HE. In the past, patients with HE were placed on protein restricted diets under the assumption that it would reduce the total amount of ammonia absorbed through the gut and improve HE [48]. However, in patients with chronic liver disease and HE, protein restriction exacerbates malnutrition and increases mortality compared to patients with a diet containing protein [49]. Current recommendations are for a diet that provides 35–40 kcal/kg/day, including 1.2–1.5 g/kg/day of protein [50]. In addition, corrections of zinc deficiency and supplementation with l-ornithine-l-aspartate, both necessary components of the urea cycle, have shown benefits in treating HE and reducing circulating ammonia [51, 52]. Branched-chain amino acids have also shown a therapeutic benefit in HE, but the data do not show any survival advantage [53, 54].

## Feasibility of Invasive Intracranial Monitoring

An estimated 86–95% of patients with grade III–IV encephalopathy have intracranial hypertension [61]. Moreover, complications from intracranial hypertension account for a large portion of death in patients with acute liver failure, as an estimate is likely around 20–35% [62]. There is some debate in terms of whether implanting an invasive intracranial pressure (ICP) device is necessary, where some centers suggest that patients are managed optimally without it while others find that invasive ICP monitoring can be beneficial [63, 64].

The frequency of invasive ICP monitoring varies widely among different institutions. For example, Vaquero et al. found that 28% of the studied cohort among 24 different centers used ICP monitoring [65]. However, the variability is high among different centers globally, possibly due to the perceived high potential of serious complications [66]. Indeed, frequency of ICP monitoring can range from 0 to 85% in the USA, depending on institution [65].

Screening patients for the risk of intracranial hypertension is complex and involves a number of factors. Those with cerebral edema will likely also suffer from intracranial hypertension. Risk factors for cerebral edema include (1) a high-grade hepatic encephalopathy (e.g., grade III or IV), (2) elevated serum ammonia levels (i.e., higher than 100 μmol/L), (3) a rapidly progressive deterioration of hepatic function (i.e., progression from jaundice to encephalopathy in less than 1 week), (4) the presence of a systemic inflammatory response syndrome (SIRS), and (5) a requirement for vasopressors or renal replacement therapy [67, 68]. Intracranial hypertension should be suspected in AFL patients who experience newly onset hypertension, worsening encephalopathy, or deterioration in their neurological examination [62]. Furthermore, risk of edema increases to 25–35% with progression to grade III and 65–75% or higher in patients reaching grade IV encephalopathy [69].

Imaging is usually inadequate in diagnosing intracranial hypertension or cerebral edema. For example, computed tomography (CT) imaging of the brain is usually not sensitive enough to determine intracranial hypertension or rule out cerebral edema [62]. There are specific markers in CT findings that are suggestive of cerebral edema (e.g., sulci effacement, compression of basal cisterns, midline shifts), but the absence of these does not exclude the possibility of cerebral edema [70, 71]. Rather, CT imaging in ALF patients is used to rule out pathology other than intracranial hypertension or cerebral edema (e.g., intracranial hemorrhage, hydrocephalus) [72]. Magnetic resonance imaging (MRI) has not been shown to properly assess cerebral edema in ALF patients most likely because of the prolonged time required for obtaining images [62].

## Advantages of Invasive Intracranial Monitoring

The benefits of invasive ICP monitoring are the following: (1) ICP can be monitored accurately and precisely, allowing for quick detection of elevated ICP, (2) it can allow for an immediate evaluation of ICP response to therapy, (3) it provides knowledge of intracranial perfusion pressure, (4) it provides information that allows for accurate patient prognosis, and (5) anesthetic management during liver transplant is improved with ICP monitoring because ICP surges intraoperatively are common [73]. Ultimately, these benefits may allow for longer patient survival prior to transplant, which would increase the chance allocating a graft [73].

The main goal of monitoring ICP is to maintain appropriate cerebral profusion. Ideally, this means keeping ICP below 20 mmHg and CPP above 70 mmHg [62]. When patients are monitored, they may be more likely to receive appropriate treatment in a timely manner (e.g., mannitol, barbituates, vasopressors) [65]. Recommendations of the US Acute Liver Failure Study Group for the intensive care of patients with ALF state that ICP monitoring should be considered in all patients listed for liver transplantation with grade III/IV hepatic encephalopathy, and in patients with advanced hepatic encephalopathy who are not transplant candidates but have reasonable chances of recovery (e.g., patients with acetaminophen toxicity ALF) [74].

While there are no published reports listing cut-off criteria with regards to ICP and liver transplant Vaquero et al. found that patients who have invasive monitors are more likely to receive vasopressors and ICP-related medications [65]. However, they also found no difference in 30-day survival between liver transplant patients who undergo invasive monitoring and those that do not. They theorize that the real benefit of ICP monitoring is not in the 30-day survival but possibly in the impact on long-term neurological recovery following liver transplant [65].

## Safety of Intracranial Monitoring

The main risk associated with invasive ICP monitoring is bleeding because of the coagulopathy associated with liver failure. Arguably, intracranial hemorrhage though is the main complication that prevents invasive ICP monitoring from being used widely in the care of ALF patients [62]. A study showed that bleeding occurred in 20% of patients, where 5% of patients had a fatal hemorrhage; moreover, invasively monitored patients did not experience improved outcomes when compared to the control [75]. However, these percentages are inconsistent. Another study showed that out of 92 patients who were invasively monitored, the rate of hemorrhages for roughly 10% (half of them found incidentally via imaging) with only two deaths [65]. Further, another study of 101 patients showed there was no significant difference in mortality between ALF patients who were invasively monitored and those who were not [76]. Although hemorrhage is a serious risk of invasive ICP monitoring, its likelihood is probably determined by protocol and management.

## Why Is Invasive Intracranial Monitoring Not Associated with Better Outcomes?

There is little evidence associating invasive ICP monitoring with better outcomes. There could be a number of hypotheses to explain why, as described by Bernuau and Durand [66]. First, the risks associated with implanting the device may offset the potential benefits that are conferred by ICP monitoring. Second, there is no established standardized algorithm for determining which patients require invasive ICP monitoring, thus there likely has not been accurate investigation of the cohort whom ICP monitoring could actually help. Third, invasive monitoring itself is not therapeutic and thus not directly beneficial, which means that the benefits exacted are likely to be more mild and modest in comparison to a direct therapy.

As previously mentioned, supportive evidence for the use of invasive ICP monitoring may be lacking because patient selection is likely crucial. For example, a retrospective study investigating ICP monitoring in ALF patients with high-grade encephalopathy found that in patients with ALF due to acetaminophen toxicity, ICP monitoring did not impact 21-day mortality, while ICP monitoring was associated with high 21-day mortality in patients with ALF not associated with acetaminophen toxicity [77]. Conversely, another study showed that ICP monitoring resulted in higher survival rates in pediatric patients in comparison to those who were not monitored while maintaining low complication rates [78]. Therefore, ICP monitoring is likely beneficial in a specific patient population while detrimental in another and the specific characteristics of either has yet to be fully elucidated.

## Indications for Invasive ICP Monitoring

There are a number of factors that are incorporated into the algorithm for deciding who should undergo invasive ICP monitoring. Gasco et al. state that based on their review of the literature, invasive monitoring is based on level 2 evidence, at best [79]. Generally, patients who have liver failure and known elevated ICP, as graded by an ammonia levels >200 μmol/L, grade III or IV encephalopathy, acute renal failure, or a need for vasopressor support [80]. CT scans likely do not provide reliable evidence that demonstrates cerebral edema, especially during the early grades [70]. Further, the American Association for the Study of Liver Diseases established a recommendation that invasive ICP monitoring should be considered in patients with high-grade hepatic encephalopathy (e.g., grade III or IV) if their care center has experience with ICP monitoring or patients who are awaiting or undergoing liver transplantation [81]. After transplantation, intracranial hypertension could be more likely to develop because rapid shifts in electrolytes and hemodynamic changes associated with surgery may cause large ICP fluctuations [80].

## Types of Invasive Intracranial Monitoring

Different methods are typically dependent on the anatomic location of the reading, which include intraventricular, intraparenchymal, epidural, subdural, and subarachnoid. External ventricular drainage (EVD), where a catheter is placed into a ventricle, is considered to be the most accurate method [82]. EVD placement is not considered to be a major procedure, but it does carry the highest risk of hemorrhage or infection [83]. Although some believe EVD to be the most beneficial monitor because they allow the potential therapeutic option of CSF drainage [85]. ICP microtransducers are widely used and can be divided into multiple categories (e.g., fiber optic devices, strain gauge, pneumatic sensors) [83]. Using microtransducers to measure intraparenchymally or intraventricularly is most common, as epidural and subdural measurements are typically not as accurate. For example, a study showed that epidural measurements consistently overestimated ICP [84]. However, intraparenchymal or intraventricular measurements are not always possible, thus the most accurate method that does not jeopardize patient safety should be utilized. A sterilized environment should always be used to minimize the risk of infection. Prophylactic antibiotics may be considered, though there is the concern of infection from drug-resistant organisms.

## Liver Failure ICP Monitoring Protocol

In collaboration with the Department of Neurosurgery, the Cleveland Clinic has developed the following algorithm for invasive ICP monitoring of liver failure patients (Fig. 21.2). Patients must be under consideration for liver transplantation and be in grade III or IV coma secondary to liver failure. First, invasive procedures (e.g., central lines, implantation of an ICP monitoring device) should be scheduled and performed as close together temporally as possible. Second, critical care and hepatology should do a preliminary discussion with the patient's family regarding the rationale behind implanting the ICP monitoring device, but formal consent should be obtained by neurosurgery. Critical care must be consulted to determine the optimal efficacy of implantation and subsequent management of the ICP monitor. Third, the implantation should be done at the bedside regardless of INR. Fourth, if the platelet count is under 80,000 platelets/μL, platelets should be administered. Fifth, one unit of FFP should be administered for at least 10 min in preparation for the procedure and another unit should be administered for 20 min simultaneously with the procedure. One unit of FPP should be administered at least 20 min after the procedure. Sixth, if a hematoma develops after implantation of the monitor, surgical evacuation should not be offered if the INR is greater than 1.3 or the platelet count is fewer than 100,000 platelets/μL.

The use of FFP may need to be adjusted depending on the patient. Study of the USALF showed that FFP was most common in 91% of patients and FPP was used

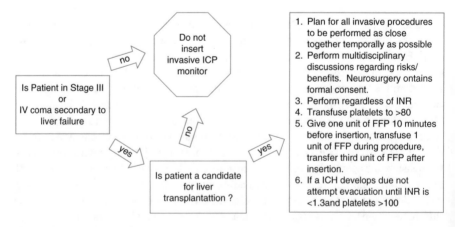

**Fig. 21.2** Cleveland Clinic Algorithm for ICP monitor insertion in liver failure

in conjunction with another treatment in 59% of patients; others (e.g., platelets, cryoprecipitate, and factor VIIa) were used 18–31% of the time [65].

Traditionally, coagulopathy was managed by infusion of FFP, platelets, and vitamin K, but more recent evidence has suggested that administering recombinant factor VIIa may help optimally minimize the risk of bleeding [86, 87]. Le et al. reported a case series of 11 patients who received recombinant factor VIIa prior to ICP monitor implantation and they reported that there were no complications associated with invasive monitoring [87]. However, they had a small sample size and did not repeat laboratory findings after factor VIIa was administered [87]. It is possible that because factor VIIa has a relatively short half-life (2–5 h), it is the first factor to become deficient in liver failure patients, and thus replenishing it likely helps to play a role in preventing bleeding complications [86]. Another study compared eight liver failure patients who received only FFP and seven who received FFP and recombinant factor VIIa and found that only 38% of the patients who received FFP had acceptable laboratory values that allowed for ICP monitoring while all of the patients who received FFP and recombinant factor VIIa had acceptable laboratory values for ICP monitoring [88]. The study also found that those who received the recombinant factor VIIa were also less likely to develop anasarca in comparison with those who did not; the authors hypothesized that this was due to better fluid management secondary to data provided by ICP monitoring and less high volume FFP required to reverse coagulopathy [88].

## Managing Invasive ICP Monitoring

The cerebral perfusion pressure (CPP) is the intracranial pressure (ICP) subtracted from the mean arterial pressure (MAP) (i.e., CPP = MAP – ICP); therefore to maintain adequate CPP, clinicians can either increase MAP or decrease ICP. Practically, CPP can be maintained by (1) optimizing the patient's position and (2) appropriate pharmacologic management. Optimizing the patient's position means that the head of the bed should be elevated over 30° (i.e., putting the bed in a sitting position) with nothing compressing the neck and protecting the blood flow through the jugular veins. Hyperventilation for short periods can also help by causing vasoconstriction.

In terms of pharmacologic agents, indomethacin can cause vasoconstriction that may reduce ICP while maintaining adequate perfusion and causing no significant changes in cerebral microdialysis [89]. There are potential risks though, such as nephrotoxicity, platelet dysfunction, or GI bleeding/ischemia [89]. Additionally, osmotic diuretics can help decrease ICP pressure by increasing blood osmolality, which draws fluid out of the cerebral tissue and into the intravascular space (i.e., decreasing volume of fluid in the brain). For example, administrating mannitol has been shown to reduce ICP and increase survival among grade IV encephalopathic ALF patients [90]. Further, hypertonic saline solutions and propofol may also help lower ICP in patients with IV encephalopathic ALF patients [91, 92]. Pentobarbital is typically not used in ALF patients due to prolonged clearance [62].

Induced hypothermia has been shown in limited settings to also reduce ICP in ALF patients, though further research is still required to determine efficacy and safety. Optimal therapeutic temperature has yet to be elucidated, as 32 and 35 °C have been shown to be effective [93, 94]. Induced hypothermia is most likely not a first-line therapy, but it may have usefulness in specific situations.

## Noninvasive Methods of Monitoring Intracranial Pressure

There are a number of noninvasive methods for monitoring intracranial pressure. First, transcranial Doppler (TCD) ultrasound recording is a noninvasive technique that measures cerebral vascular flow velocity [95]. Research has shown that the pulsatility index (PI) derived from TCD is strongly correlated with ICP [33], thus TCD may be a viable alternative to monitoring ICP in patients who are unable to undergo implantation of an invasive ICP monitor. Second, a few studies have investigated whether the optic nerve, as it is part of the central nervous system (CNS) and surrounded by dura, can be used to estimate ICP, but the results are currently unreliable and further investigation is required prior to routine clinical application. Ultimately, there are no noninvasive methods that can measure ICP as accurately as invasive methods, which remain the "gold standard."

## Elective and Emergent Surgery in Patients with Cirrhosis

As in other fields, cirrhosis significantly increases the risk of neurosurgical complications, especially hemorrhage. Although there is sparse literature directly reporting on these complications in elective neurological surgery, one large study showed that as Child classification progressed from A to C, the overall complication rate rose from 38.7 to 84.2% and hemorrhage increased from 29.3 to 63.2% in patients undergoing cranial operations [55]. Similar results are seen in patients undergoing spine surgery where patients with cirrhosis had significantly elevated blood loss and increased length of stay [56]. If the decision to undergo an elective procedure is made, however, clotting parameters should be normalized prior to surgery and for 1 week after. Common indications for emergent surgery in patients with cirrhosis are subdural hematoma (SDH), spontaneous intracerebral hemorrhage (SICH), and epidural hematoma (EDH). In these cases clotting function and urgency of surgery must be balanced.

Intraoperatively, several tools can be utilized to minimize blood loss in cirrhotic patients. Surgicel and other absorbable hemostatic agents have been widely used in neurosurgical procedures for control of capillary, venous, and small arterial hemorrhage [57]. Thrombin, often used in conjunction with other hemostatic agents such as Floseal (gelatin-thrombin matrix sealant) or Gelfoam, can provide additional hemostatic control [58]. One study has also shown benefit in using thrombin containing irrigation solution over saline in the prevention of rebleeding following SDH evacuation [59]. The use of thrombin, however, may also result in the production of thrombin associated factor V antibodies that may increase the risk for subsequent hemorrhage.

The Aquamantys bipolar system has also been used successfully in neurological surgery [60]. The Aquamantys system allows for effective hemostasis while minimizing thermal damage to underlying nervous tissue. The use of the above tools is essential is maintaining adequate hemostasis in cirrhotic patients at high risk of complications from excessive blood loss.

## Conclusions

Hepatic encephalopathy (HE) is associated with intracranial hypertension; therefore, there may be benefit to monitoring ICP in patients with liver failure. The most accurate way of measuring ICP is invasively, but there are associated risks involved. Moreover, the benefits of ICP monitoring have yet to truly be examined. It has been shown that ICP monitoring can be done with minimal complications; therefore, the likelihood of the risks associated with ICP monitoring is likely contingent on proper protocol and management. Regardless, invasive ICP monitoring is currently the most accurate way of measuring ICP and should be considered in the management of patients with liver failure.

## References

1. Tapper EB, Jiang ZG, Patwardhan VR. Refining the ammonia hypothesis. Mayo Clin Proc. 2015;90:646–58.
2. Norenberg MD, Rao KVR, Jayakumar AR. Mechanisms of ammonia-induced astrocyte swelling. Metab Brain Dis. 2005;20:303–18.
3. Rose C. Effect of ammonia on astrocytic glutamate uptake/release mechanisms. J Neurochem. 2006;97(Suppl 1):11–5.
4. Laubenberger J, et al. Proton magnetic resonance spectroscopy of the brain in symptomatic and asymptomatic patients with liver cirrhosis. Gastroenterology. 1997;112:1610–6.
5. Skowrońska M, Albrecht J. Oxidative and nitrosative stress in ammonia neurotoxicity. Neurochem Int. 2013;62:731–7.
6. Panickar KS, Jayakumar AR, Rama Rao KV, Norenberg MD. Downregulation of the 18-kDa translocator protein: effects on the ammonia-induced mitochondrial permeability transition and cell swelling in cultured astrocytes. Glia. 2007;55:1720–7.
7. Butterworth RF. The astrocytic ('peripheral-type') benzodiazepine receptor: role in the pathogenesis of portal-systemic encephalopathy. Neurochem Int. 2000;36:411–6.
8. Ahboucha S, et al. Reduced brain levels of DHEAS in hepatic coma patients: significance for increased GABAergic tone in hepatic encephalopathy. Neurochem Int. 2012;61:48–53.
9. Norenberg MD. Astrocytic-ammonia interactions in hepatic encephalopathy. Semin Liver Dis. 1996;16:245–53.
10. Moroni F, Lombardi G, Moneti G, Cortesini C. The release and neosynthesis of glutamic acid are increased in experimental models of hepatic encephalopathy. J Neurochem. 1983;40:850–4.

11. de Knegt RJ, et al. Extracellular brain glutamate during acute liver failure and during acute hyperammonemia simulating acute liver failure: an experimental study based on in vivo brain dialysis. J Hepatol. 1994;20:19–26.
12. Michalak A, Rose C, Butterworth J, Butterworth RF. Neuroactive amino acids and glutamate (NMDA) receptors in frontal cortex of rats with experimental acute liver failure. Hepatology (Baltimore, MD). 1996;24:908–13.
13. Oppong KN, Bartlett K, Record CO, al Mardini H. Synaptosomal glutamate transport in thioacetamide-induced hepatic encephalopathy in the rat. Hepatology (Baltimore, MD). 1995;22:553–8.
14. Llansola M, et al. NMDA receptors in hyperammonemia and hepatic encephalopathy. Metab Brain Dis. 2007;22:321–35.
15. Butterworth RF. The liver-brain axis in liver failure: neuroinflammation and encephalopathy. Nat Rev Gastroenterol Hepatol. 2013;10:522–8.
16. Odeh M, Sabo E, Srugo I, Oliven A. Relationship between tumor necrosis factor-alpha and ammonia in patients with hepatic encephalopathy due to chronic liver failure. Ann Med. 2005;37:603–12.
17. Bernal W, Donaldson P, Underhill J, Wendon J, Williams R. Tumor necrosis factor genomic polymorphism and outcome of acetaminophen (paracetamol)-induced acute liver failure. J Hepatol. 1998;29:53–9.
18. Dennis CV, et al. Microglial proliferation in the brain of chronic alcoholics with hepatic encephalopathy. Metab Brain Dis. 2014;29:1027–39.
19. Bémeur C, Qu H, Desjardins P, Butterworth RF. IL-1 or TNF receptor gene deletion delays onset of encephalopathy and attenuates brain edema in experimental acute liver failure. Neurochem Int. 2010;56:213–5.
20. Skowrońska M, Albrecht J. Alterations of blood brain barrier function in hyperammonemia: an overview. Neurotox Res. 2011;21:236–44.
21. Kofke WA. In Textbook of critical care. Philadelphia, PA: Saunders/Elsevier. 2011. p. 134–45.
22. Rangel-Castillo L, Gopinath S, Robertson CS. Management of intracranial hypertension. Neurol Clin. 2008;26:521–41.
23. Scott TR, Kronsten VT, Hughes RD, Shawcross DL. Pathophysiology of cerebral oedema in acute liver failure. World J Gastroenterol (WJG). 2013;19:9240–55.
24. Rama Rao KV, Jayakumar AR, Tong X, Alvarez VM, Norenberg MD. Marked potentiation of cell swelling by cytokines in ammonia-sensitized cultured astrocytes. J Neuroinflammation. 2010;7:66.
25. Rama Rao KV, Jayakumar AR, Tong X, Curtis KM, Norenberg MD. Brain aquaporin-4 in experimental acute liver failure. J Neuropathol Exp Neurol. 2010;69:869–79.
26. Rama Rao KV, Jayakumar AR, Norenberg MD. Brain edema in acute liver failure: mechanisms and concepts. Metab Brain Dis. 2014;29:927–36.
27. Larsen FS, Wendon J. Prevention and management of brain edema in patients with acute liver failure. Liver Transplant Off Publ Am Assoc Study Liver Dis Int Liver Transplant Soc. 2008;14(Suppl 2):S90–6.
28. Dharel N, Bajaj JS. Definition and nomenclature of hepatic encephalopathy. J Clin Exp Hepatol. 2015;5(Supplement 1):S37–41.
29. Shawcross DL, Wendon JA. The neurological manifestations of acute liver failure. Neurochem Int. 2012;60:662–71.
30. Wang J-Y, et al. Prevalence of minimal hepatic encephalopathy and quality of life evaluations in hospitalized cirrhotic patients in China. World J Gastroenterol. 2013;19:4984–91.
31. Samanta J, et al. Correlation between degree and quality of sleep disturbance and the level of neuropsychiatric impairment in patients with liver cirrhosis. Metab Brain Dis. 2013;28:249–59.
32. Rui MD, et al. Excessive daytime sleepiness and hepatic encephalopathy: it is worth asking. Metab Brain Dis. 2012;28:245–8.
33. Gill RQ, Sterling RK. Acute liver failure. J Clin Gastroenterol. 2001;33:191–8.

34. Jones EA, Weissenborn K. Neurology and the liver. J Neurol Neurosurg Psychiatry. 1997;63:279–93.
35. Martinez-Camacho A, Fortune BE, Everson G. In Textbook of critical care. Philadelphia, PA: Saunders/Elsevier. 2011. p. 760–70.
36. Cadranel JF, et al. Focal neurological signs in hepatic encephalopathy in cirrhotic patients: an underestimated entity? Am J Gastroenterol. 2001;96:515–8.
37. Hassanein TI, Hilsabeck RC, Perry W. Introduction to the Hepatic Encephalopathy Scoring Algorithm (HESA). Dig Dis Sci. 2008;53:529–38.
38. Ortiz M, et al. Development of a clinical hepatic encephalopathy staging scale. Aliment Pharmacol Ther. 2007;26:859–67.
39. Salam M, et al. Modified-orientation log to assess hepatic encephalopathy. Aliment Pharmacol Ther. 2012;35:913–20.
40. Ong JP, et al. Correlation between ammonia levels and the severity of hepatic encephalopathy. Am J Med. 2003;114:188–93.
41. Kramer L, et al. Partial pressure of ammonia versus ammonia in hepatic encephalopathy. Hepatology (Baltimore, MD). 2000;31:30–4.
42. Montoliu C, et al. 3-nitro-tyrosine as a peripheral biomarker of minimal hepatic encephalopathy in patients with liver cirrhosis. Am J Gastroenterol. 2011;106:1629–37.
43. Waghray A, Waghray N, Kanna S, Mullen K. Optimal treatment of hepatic encephalopathy. Minerva Gastroenterol Dietol. 2014;60:55–70.
44. Patidar KR, Bajaj JS. Covert and overt hepatic encephalopathy: diagnosis and management. Clin Gastroenterol Hepatol Off Clin Pract J Am Gastroenterol Assoc. 2015;13:2048–61.
45. Kimer N, Krag A, Møller S, Bendtsen F, Gluud LL. Systematic review with meta-analysis: the effects of rifaximin in hepatic encephalopathy. Aliment Pharmacol Ther. 2014;40:123–32.
46. Iadevaia MD, et al. Rifaximin in the treatment of hepatic encephalopathy. Hepatic Med Evid Res. 2011;3:109–17.
47. Sharma BC, et al. A randomized, double-blind, controlled trial comparing rifaximin plus lactulose with lactulose alone in treatment of overt hepatic encephalopathy. Am J Gastroenterol. 2013;108:1458–63.
48. Cabral CM, Burns DL. Low-protein diets for hepatic encephalopathy debunked: let them eat steak. Nutr Clin Pract Off Publ Am Soc Parenter Enter Nutr. 2011;26:155–9.
49. Eghtesad S, Poustchi H, Malekzadeh R. Malnutrition in Liver Cirrhosis:The Influence of Protein and Sodium. Middle East J Dig Dis. 2013;5:65–75.
50. Rahimi RS, Rockey DC. Hepatic encephalopathy: how to test and treat. Curr Opin Gastroenterol. 2014;30:265–71.
51. Chavez-Tapia NC, et al. A systematic review and meta-analysis of the use of oral zinc in the treatment of hepatic encephalopathy. Nutr J. 2013;12:74.
52. Bai M, Yang Z, Qi X, Fan D, Han G. l-ornithine-l-aspartate for hepatic encephalopathy in patients with cirrhosis: a meta-analysis of randomized controlled trials. J Gastroenterol Hepatol. 2013;28:783–92.
53. Dam G, Ott P, Aagaard NK, Vilstrup H. Branched-chain amino acids and muscle ammonia detoxification in cirrhosis. Metab Brain Dis. 2013;28:217–20.
54. Gluud LL, et al. Branched-chain amino acids for people with hepatic encephalopathy. Cochrane Database Syst Rev. 2015;2:CD001939.
55. Chen C-C, et al. Brain surgery in patients with liver cirrhosis. J Neurosurg. 2012;117:348–53.
56. Liao J-C, et al. Complications associated with instrumented lumbar surgery in patients with liver cirrhosis: a matched cohort analysis. Spine J Off J North Am Spine Soc. 2013;13:908–13.
57. Keshavarzi S, MacDougall M, Lulic D, Kasasbeh A, Levy M. Clinical experience with the surgicel family of absorbable hemostats (oxidized regenerated cellulose) in neurosurgical applications: a review. Wounds Compend Clin Res Pract. 2013;25:160–7.
58. Yao HHI, Hong MKH, Drummond KJ. Haemostasis in neurosurgery: what is the evidence for gelatin-thrombin matrix sealant? J Clin Neurosci. 2013;20:349–56.

59. Shimamura N, Ogasawara Y, Naraoka M, Ohnkuma H. Irrigation with thrombin solution reduces recurrence of chronic subdural hematoma in high-risk patients: preliminary report. J Neurotrauma. 2009;26:1929–33.
60. Grasso G, Giambartino F, Iacopino DG. Hemostasis in brain tumor surgery using the Aquamantys system. Med Sci Monit Int Med J Exp Clin Res. 2014;20:538–43.
61. Sasbón JS, Centeno M, Ciocca M, et al. Fulminant hepatic failure. Results with liver transplantation. World Federation J Crit Care Med. 2004;1:17–22.
62. Mohsenin V. Assessment and management of cerebral edema and intracranial hypertension in acute liver failure. J Crit Care. 2013;28:783–91.
63. Bernuau J, Durand F. Intracranial pressure monitoring in patients with acute liver failure: a questionable invasive surveillance. Hepatology. 2006;44(2):502–4. PubMed PMID: 16871566.
64. Wendon JA, Larsen FS. Intracranial pressure monitoring in acute liver failure. A procedure with clear indications. Hepatology. 2006;44(2):504–6. PubMed PMID: 16871578.
65. Vaquero J, Fontana RJ, Larson AM, Bass NM, Davern TJ, Shakil AO, Han S, Harrison ME, Stravitz TR, Muñoz S, Brown R, Lee WM, Blei AT. Complications and use of intracranial pressure monitoring in patients with acute liver failure and severe encephalopathy. Liver Transpl. 2005;11(12):1581–9. PubMed PMID:16315300.
66. Bernuau J, Durand F. Intracranial pressure monitoring in patients with acute liver failure: a questionable invasive surveillance. Hepatology. 2006;44(2):502–4. PubMed PMID: 16871566.
67. Tofteng F, Hauerberg J, Hansen BA, et al. Persistent arterial hyperammonemia increases the concentration of glutamine and alanine in the brain and correlates with intracranial pressure in patients with fulminant hepatic failure. J Cereb Blood Flow Metab. 2006;26:21–7.
68. Bernal W, Hall C, Karvellas CJ, et al. Arterial ammonia and clinical risk factors for encephalopathy and intracranial hypertension in acute liver failure. Hepatology. 2007;46:1844–52.
69. Munoz SJ. Difficult management problems in fulminant hepatic failure. Semin Liver Dis. 1993;13:395–413.
70. Munoz SJ, Robinson M, Northrup B, et al. Elevated intracranial pressure and computed tomography of the brain in fulminanthepatocellular failure. Hepatology. 1991;13:209–12.
71. Wijdicks EF, Plevak DJ, Rakela J, et al. Clinical and radiologic features of cerebral edema in fulminant hepatic failure. Mayo Clin Proc. 1995;70:119–24.
72. Rabinstein AA. Treatment of brain edema in acute liver failure. Curr Treat Options Neurol. 2010;12:129–41.
73. Fortea JI, Bañares R, Vaquero J. Intracranial pressure in acute liver failure: to bolt or not to bolt-that is the question. Crit Care Med. 2014;42(5):1304–5. doi:10.1097/CCM.0000000000000242. PubMed PMID: 24736348.
74. Stravitz RT, Kramer AH, Davern T, Shaikh AO, Caldwell SH, Mehta RL, Blei AT, Fontana RJ, BM MG, Rossaro L, Smith AD, Lee WM, Acute Liver Failure Study Group. Intensive care of patients with acute liver failure: recommendations of the U.S. Acute Liver Failure Study Group. Crit Care Med. 2007;35(11):2498–508. PubMed PMID: 17901832.110.
75. Blei AT, Olafsson S, Webster S, et al. Complications of intracranial pressure monitoring in fulminant hepatic failure. Lancet. 1993;341:157–8.
76. Schmidt L, Larsen FS. Prognostic implications of hyperlactatemia, multiple organ failure, and systemic inflammatory response syndrome in patients with acetaminophen-induced acute liver failure. Crit Care Med. 2006;34:337–43.
77. Karvellas CJ, Fix OK, Battenhouse H, Durkalski V, Sanders C, Lee WM. Outcomes and complications of intracranial pressure monitoring in acute liver failure: a retrospective cohort study. Crit Care Med. 2014;42:1157–67.
78. Kamat P, Kunde S, Vos M, Vats A, Heffron T, Romero R, Fortenberry JD. Invasive intracranial pressure monitoring is a useful adjunct in the management of severe hepatic encephalopathy associated with pediatric acute liver failure. Pediatr Crit Care Med. 2012;13:e33–8.
79. Gasco J, Rangel-Castilla L, Franklin B, Thomas PG, Patterson JT. State-of-the-art management and monitoring of brain edema and intracranial hypertension in fulminant hepatic failure. A proposed algorithm. Acta Neurochir Suppl. 2010;106:311–4. doi:10.1007/978-3-211-98811-4_58. PubMed PMID: 19812970.

80. Datar S, Wijdicks EF. Neurologic manifestations of acute liver failure. Handb Clin Neurol. 2014;120:645–59. doi:10.1016/B978-0-7020-4087-0.00044-9. Review. PubMed PMID: 24365344.
81. Krisl JC, Meadows HE, Greenberg CS, Mazur JE. Clinical usefulness of recombinant activated factor VII in patients with liver failure undergoing invasive procedures. Ann Pharmacother. 2011;45:1433–8.
82. Le TV, Rumbak MJ, Liu SS, et al. Insertion of intracranial pressure monitors in fulminant hepatic failure patients: early experience using recombinant factor VII. Neurosurgery. 2010;66:455–8. [discussion 458].
83. Shami VM, Caldwell SH, Hespenheide EE, et al. Recombinant activated factor VII for coagulopathy in fulminate hepatic failure compared with conventional therapy. Liver Transpl. 2003;9:138–43. doi:10.1053/jlts.2003.50017.
84. Tofteng F, Larsen FS. The effect of indomethacin on intracranial pressure, cerebral perfusion and extracellular lactate and glutamate concentrations in patients with fulminant hepatic failure. J Cereb Blood Flow Metab. 2004;24:798–804.
85. Canalese J, Gimson AE, Davis C, et al. Controlled trial of dexamethasone and mannitol for the cerebral oedema of fulminant hepatic failure. Gut. 1982;23:625–9.
86. Wijdicks EFM, Nyberg SL. Propofol to control intracranial pressure in fulminant hepatic failure. Transplant Proc. 2002;34:1220–2.
87. Murphy N, Auzinger G, Bernel W, et al. The effect of hypertonic sodium chloride on intracranial pressure in patients with acute liver failure. Hepatology. 2004;39:464–70.
88. Jalan R, Damink O, Steven SW, Deutz NE, et al. Moderate hypothermia for uncontrolled intracranial hypertension in acute liver failure. Lancet. 1999;354:1164–8.
89. Stravitz RT, Larsen FS. Therapeutic hypothermia for acute liver failure. Crit Care Med. 2009;37(7 Suppl):S258–64. doi:10.1097/CCM.0b013e3181aa5fb8. Review. PubMed PMID: 19535956.
90. Aaslid R, Markwalder TM, Nomes H. Noninvasive transcranial Doppler ultrasound recording of flow velocity in basal cerebral arteries. J Neurosurg. 1982;57:769–74.
91. Bellner J, Romner B, Reinstrup P, Kristiansson K-A, Ryding E, Brandt L. Transcranial Doppler sonography pulsatility index (PI) reflects intracranial pressure (ICP). Surg Neurol. 2004;62:45–51.
92. Geeraerts T, Launey Y, Martin L, et al. Ultrasonography of the optic nerve sheath may be useful for detecting raised intracranial pressure after severe brain injury. Intensive Care Med. 2007;33:1704–11.
93. Kimberly HH, Shah S, Marill K, Noble V. Correlation of optic nerve sheath diameter with direct measurement of intracranial pressure. Acad Emerg Med. 2008;15:201–4.
94. Soldatos T, Karakitsos D, Chatzimichail K, Papathana M, Gouliamos A, Karabinis A. Optic nerve sonography in the diagnostic evaluation of adult brain injury. Crit Care. 2008;12:R67.
95. Weissenborn K, Heidenreich S, Giewekemeyer K, Rückert N, Hecker H. Memory function in early hepatic encephalopathy. J Hepatol. 2003;39:320–5.

# Chapter 22
# Endocrine Surgery in Cirrhotic Patients

Nisar Zaidi and Eren Berber

## Management of Thyroid Disease and Thyroid Nodules

### Thyroid Dysfunction

Thyroid hormone and hepatocytes share a reciprocal relationship. Thyroid hormone is necessary for the growth and function of hepatocytes. In turn, the liver is the primary site of metabolism of thyroxine (T4) to its active form, triiodothyronine (T3) [1]. Thus thyroid dysfunction is a frequent finding in patients with advanced liver disease, seen in up to 25% of patients with nonalcoholic fatty liver disease, 13% in primary biliary cirrhosis, and 11% in primary sclerosing cholangitis [2]. Similarly, in patients with alcohol-related liver disease, the severity of liver dysfunction was noted to correlate with a decrease in circulating free T3 [3].

### Thyroid Nodules

Thyroid nodules appear to have a similar prevalence between cirrhotic and non-cirrhotic patients, occurring in approximately 5% of all women and 1% of all men in iodine-replete environments [5]. Papillary thyroid cancer, however, has been demonstrated to occur more frequently in HCV-infected patients [4]. Management of nodules is according to published evidence-based American

N. Zaidi, MD (✉)
EssentiaHealth/Duluth Clinic, 300 East 3rd St, Duluth, MN 55805, USA
e-mail: nisar.zaidi@essentiahealth.org

E. Berber, MD
Cleveland Clinic, 9500 Euclid Ave F-20, Cleveland, OH 44195, USA
e-mail: berbere@ccf.org

© Springer International Publishing AG 2017
B. Eghtesad, J. Fung (eds.), *Surgical Procedures on the Cirrhotic Patient*,
DOI 10.1007/978-3-319-52396-5_22

Thyroid Association guidelines [5]. Initial work-up of any clinically palpable or suspected nodule begins with an assessment of thyroid function by means of serum thyrotropin (TSH) and neck ultrasound. Nodules greater than 1 cm should lend consideration for fine needle cytologic evaluation to exclude thyroid malignancy, which occurs in 7–15% of cases. The most recent ATA guidelines published in 2015 recommended a risk stratification of nodules based on ultrasound characteristics, allowing for nodules with less suspicious features a larger size threshold for fine needle aspiration (FNA). Such characteristics are summarized in Table 22.1. TSH levels below the reference range should prompt radionucleotide iodine scanning to assess for autonomous, or "hot" thyroid nodule. In these instances, fine needle biopsy may be deferred, as the risk of malignancy is approximately 1%.

FNA cytologic diagnosis of nodules is graded according to a standardized reporting of thyroid cytology known as the Bethesda score [6]. Nodules are graded into one of six diagnostic categories: Bethesda I, nondiagnostic; Bethesda II, benign; Bethesda III, atypia/follicular lesion of undetermined significance; Bethesda IV, follicular neoplasm or suspicion for follicular neoplasm; Bethesda V, suspicion for malignancy; and Bethesda VI, malignant. Each diagnostic category corresponds to an associated risk of malignancy with recommended management summarized in Table 22.2.

**Table 22.1** Ultrasound risk stratification for thyroid nodules

| Sonographic risk | Sonographic features | Risk of malignancy (%) | Size threshold for FNA |
|---|---|---|---|
| High | Hypoechoic solid or solid component with one or more of following findings: infiltrative margins, microlobular margins, MC, rim calcification, taller than wide shape, evidence of ETE | Up to 70–90 | 1 cm |
| Intermediate | Hypoechoic solid or solid component with smooth margins without MC, ETE, or taller than wide shape | 10–20 | 1 cm |
| Low | Isoechoic or hyperechoic solid nodule or partially cystic nodule without MC, irregular margins, ETE, or taller than wide shape | 5–10 | 1.5 cm |
| Very low | Spongiform or partially cystic nodule without features described above | <3 | 2 cm |
| Benign | Purely cystic | <1 | No FNA recommended |

Adapted from 2015 American Thyroid Association Management Guidelines for Adult Patients with Thyroid Nodules and Differentiated Thyroid Cancer. *MC* microcalcifications, *ETE* extrathyroidal extension

**Table 22.2** Bethesda system for reporting thyroid cytology

| Bethesda class | Cytologic diagnosis | Risk of malignancy (%) | Treatment recommendation |
|---|---|---|---|
| I | Nondiagnostic | 1–4 | Repeat FNA |
| II | Benign | 0–3 | Clinical surveillance |
| III | Atypia of undetermined significance or follicular lesion of undetermined significance | 5–15 | Repeat FNA, consider gene expression analysis |
| IV | Follicular neoplasm or suspicion for follicular neoplasm | 15–30 | Thyroid lobectomy |
| V | Suspicious for malignancy | 60–75 | Total thyroidectomy or lobectomy |
| VI | Malignant | 97–99 | Total thyroidectomy |

Adapted from Cibas and Ali [8]

## Thyroidectomy in Cirrhotic Patients

The decision to proceed with thyroidectomy in patients with advanced liver dysfunction should be made only after thorough examination of its indications and assessment of perioperative risk. Along with nodules in which malignancy cannot be excluded, benign diagnoses for which thyroidectomy may be necessary include multinodular and/or substernal goiter with symptoms of compression, and thyrotoxicosis—due to autonomous nodule, toxic nodular goiter, or Graves' disease.

## Preoperative Risk Assessment and Patient Selection

Several retrospective studies have shown the increased risk of complications in cirrhotic patients undergoing a variety of surgical procedures [7–9]. Estimated 30-day mortalities have ranged from 9.8 to 28% in patients who underwent nonhepatic surgical procedures. The majority of these studies evaluated intraabdominal procedures. Outcomes data looking specifically at thyroidectomy in cirrhotic patients are extremely limited, though most authors agree that any thyroidectomy is considered at the least moderate risk based on the amount of tissue dissection and manipulation necessary for the procedure [10].

Historically, the Childs–Turcotte–Pugh (CTP) score and associated Childs–Pugh class have been utilized to gauge the severity of a patient's underlying liver dysfunction. High Childs–Pugh class has been shown to be independently associated with perioperative complications and mortality in multivariate analysis [8]. More recently, due to subjective nature of estimating encephalopathy and degree of ascites in the Childs–Pugh system, other more objective means of estimating liver dysfunction have been derived. The model for end-stage liver disease (MELD) score, initially utilized to assess prognosis in liver failure patients undergoing transjugular portosystemic shunt (TIPS) procedure [11], has been accepted as a useful risk strati-fication method in patients undergoing nontransplant surgery. Northup et al. have suggested estimating 1% increase in mortality for every MELD point below 20 and 2% increase in mortality for every MELD point beyond 20 [12].

Certainly any decision to consider thyroidectomy in a cirrhotic patient needs to account for factors other than the severity of liver disease. A patient's functional status, cardiovascular risk factors, social factors, and expected benefit from surgery need to be carefully considered. In our experience, cirrhotic patients with well-compensated liver disease—generally Childs–Pugh class A or B or MELD score less than 15 with clear indications for thyroidectomy may proceed to surgery after thorough optimization of their liver disease and other comorbidities. We addition-ally ensure patients have platelet counts above 60,000 to limit the risk of postopera-tive hematoma.

## Operative Technique

Once the decision is made to proceed with surgery, thyroidectomy is performed via the standard cervical incision with the patient in semifowler position and the neck in extension. A thorough preoperative ultrasound is necessary to exclude central or lateral neck metastasis in the case of suspicion for or known malignancy [5]. Cervical incision is placed at the level of the thyroid isthmus with elevation of sub-platysmal flaps. The strap muscles are then separated at the midline raphe and retracted laterally. The thyroid isthmus is next identified, followed by mobilization of the inferior and superior pole vessels. The parathyroid glands are preserved in situ, taking care not to disturb their vascular pedicles. The thyroid lobe is then rotated medially and the recurrent laryngeal nerve (RLN) is identified along the tracheoesophageal groove. The nerve is traced cephalad to its insertion into the larynx typically at the lower border of the inferior constrictor muscle. The thyroid lobe is delivered after dissection off of the trachea and division of Berry's ligament.

Although a variety of vessel sealers have been introduced that may safely reduce operating time by obfuscating the need for knot tying [13–15], we have recently employed a hybrid approach to vessel ligation in patients at particular risk for hem-orrhage such as cirrhotics. Here, conventional 3–0 ties are utilized on larger vessels along the upper and lower pole and the inferior thyroid artery and vessel sealers such as harmonic scalpel are utilized to seal and divide the vessel on the distal (specimen) side. In instances where the RLN is at risk of thermal injury, only ties are employed for vessel ligation. Following thyroidectomy, the strap muscles and platysma are reapproximated with absorbable sutures. Skin is then reapproximated with 4–0 absorbable monofilament suture. Drains are not routinely placed except in instances of very large goiters in which a sizeable dead space is left after thyroidec-tomy. Patients are monitored overnight and discharged to home on the first postop-erative day on levothyroxine replacement and calcium supplementation.

**Case Presentation**
A 75-year-old male patient with alcoholic cirrhosis status post-transplant 2 years ago and an incidental 1 cm hepatocellular cancer in explanted liver was found to have a 7 mm thyroid nodule on his follow-up CT scans (Fig. 22.1a). On surgeon-performed ultrasound, this corresponded to a 0.88 × 0.75 × 1.02 cm isoechoic nodule with irregular borders (Fig. 22.1b, c). Fine-needle aspiration biopsy showed benign findings. This nodule was then followed up with an initial ultrasound at 6 months and then annually.

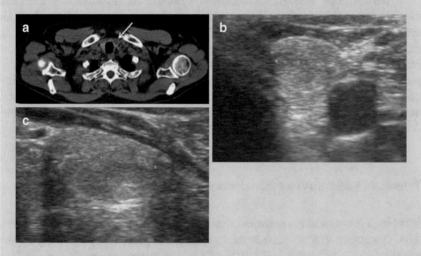

**Fig. 22.1** (a) Incidental left thyroid nodule on CT; (b, c) transverse and longitudinal ultrasound of same nodule demonstrating isoechoic nodule with border irregularity

# Parathyroid Disease and Vitamin D Deficiency

## *Hypercalcemia and Diagnosis of Primary Hyperparathyroidism*

Hypercalcemia is frequently encountered in clinical practice. Although the differential diagnosis of hypercalcemia is quite broad, primary hyperparathyroidism remains the most common cause of hypercalcemia in the nonhospitalized patient, affecting on average 25–60 individuals per 100,000 [16]. Classic signs and symptoms of severe primary hyperparathyroidism in the developed world are now mainly of historical interest. Osteitis fibrosa cystica, severe bone loss, severe peptic ulcer disease, and nephrocalcinosis are now rarely seen in patients with primary hyperparathyroidism. Rather, hypercalcemia due to primary hyperparathyroidism is typically noted incidentally with patients presenting with asymptomatically or with less dramatic versions of the classically taught "bones, moans, stones, and psychiatric overtones".

Biochemical diagnosis of primary hyperparathyroidism begins with confirmation of elevated serum calcium and measurement of serum parathyroid hormone (PTH) levels. In malnourished or in patients with advanced liver disease, albumin-corrected levels of calcium should be obtained as 40% of circulating calcium is bound to albumin and levels may be erroneously interpreted in a hypoproteinemic state. Additionally, ionized calcium levels may be tested, particularly in patients with chronic acid–base disorders. Diagnosis of primary hyperparathyroidism is confirmed with the finding or elevated serum calcium or ionized calcium with concomitant elevated or inappropriately normal PTH level.

In the cirrhotic patient, incidental or symptomatic hypercalcemia should also prompt evaluation for malignancy as both cholangiocarcinoma and hepatocellular carcinomas (HCC) have been associated with hypercalcemia [17]. In the case of hepatocellular carcinoma, paraneoplastic syndrome is not an uncommon occurrence, noted in up to 30.9% of patients [18]. Hypercalcemic paraneoplastic syndrome is seen in 4–7% of HCC and is thought to be due to secretion of parathyroid hormone-related peptide (PTH-rP). Such patients have been noted to have poorer prognosis than HCC patients without paraneoplastic syndrome [19]

## Vitamin D Metabolism in Advanced Liver Disease

Vitamin D is a steroid hormone intimately involved in calcium and bone metabolism. Deficiency in vitamin D is more prevalent in patients with primary hyperparathyroidism, occurring in 53–91% of patients compared a prevalence of 36% in the general United States population [20, 21]. In patients with chronic liver disease, vitamin D deficiency has been reported ranging between 64 and 92% [22]. The mechanism of vitamin D deficiency in chronic liver disease is likely multifactorial. Apart from decreased biosynthesis of inactive precursors in cutaneous epithelium and decreased absorption of dietary vitamin D due to malnutrition, production of the active metabolite is impaired due to the liver's inability to produce necessary binding proteins and catalyze hydroxylation [23]. With end-organ harm from primary hyperparathyroidism accelerated by vitamin D deficiency, recognition and careful correction of vitamin D is recommended to limit ongoing bone loss.

In addition to its role in calcium and bone metabolism, recent studies have demonstrated compelling anti-inflammatory, antifibrotic, and immune-modulating functions of vitamin D [24–27]. Several studies have demonstrated that low levels of vitamin D are associated with poorer response to therapy in the treatment of hepatitis C virus (HCV) [24, 25]. Other studies have suggested an association between initiation and progression of liver fibrosis in chronic HCV infection and vitamin D deficiency [26]. Severe vitamin D deficiency (<12 ng/mL) has also been implicated in organ rejection following liver transplantation [27].

## Indications for Parathyroidectomy

Though any patient with symptomatic primary hyperparathyroidism should be considered for surgery, for most patients exhibiting asymptomatic disease, the decision to proceed with surgery for primary hyperparathyroidism needs an assessment to gauge the degree of end-organ damage. Measurement of phosphate, alkaline phosphatase, blood urea nitrogen, and creatinine should be included with the measurements of calcium, PTH, and 25-hydroxyvitamin D mentioned above. In addition, 24-h urine calcium will help identify patients with hypercalciuria, an indication of surgery, and familial hypercalcemic hypocalciuria, a contraindication. Bone mineral density of the spine, hip, and distal radius is indicated to identify patients with osteoporosis and risk of fragility fracture. The 4th International Workshop for the Management of Asymptomatic Primary Hyperparathyroidism also recommends routine abdominal imaging by means of ultrasound, x-ray or computed tomography (CT) to rule out nephrocalcinosis or nephrolithiasis [28]. Recommendations for surgery by the Workshop are summarized below in Table 22.3.

## Patient Selection and Techniques of Parathyroidectomy

After establishing biochemical diagnosis of primary hyperparathyroidism, localizing studies are recommended to identify the abnormal parathyroid gland or glands. A cervical ultrasound and technetium-99 m sestamibi scanning allow for anatomic and functional imaging with sensitivities generally ranging from 70 to 90% for each modality [29, 30]. Cervical sonography provides the additional benefit of identifying concomitant thyroid pathology, present in 24–76% of patients with primary

Table 22.3 Summary guidelines of the 4th International Workshop for the Management of Asymptomatic Primary Hyperparathyroidism

| Patient factor | Recommendation for surgery |
|---|---|
| Age | <50 years |
| Measured serum calcium | >1.0 mg/dL (0.25 mmol/L) above upper limit of normal |
| Skeletal findings | A. BMD by DXA: T-score < = −2.5 at lumbar spine, total hip, femoral neck, or distal forearm [a] <br> B. Evidence of vertebral fracture by X-ray, CT, MRI, or VFA |
| Renal findings | A. Creatinine Clearance <= 60 mL/min <br> B. 24-h urine calcium >10 mmol/day (400 mg/day) <br> C. Presence of nephrolithiasis or nephrocalcinosis by X-ray, ultrasound, or CT |

*BMD* bone mineral density, *DXA* dual-energy X-ray absorptiometry, *VFA* vertebral fracture assessment

[a]In premenopausal women and men below the age of 50, Z-score equal to or less than −2.5 is utilized over the T-score

hyperparathyroidism with thyroid cancer noted in 6–17% of patients [31]. The addition of single photon emission computed tomography (SPECT) to sestamibi scanning additionally aids in identifying ectopic parathyroid glands high in the neck or in the mediastinum [32].

The decision to bring a patient with advanced liver disease for parathyroid surgery mirrors that of thyroidectomy. Patients with Childs class A or B cirrhosis, who are medically optimized and with adequate platelet counts, may proceed with parathyroidectomy. There remains considerable debate among parathyroid surgeons with regard to the extent of parathyroid exploration. Proponents of routine four-gland exploration advocate examination of all parathyroid glands by means of a bilateral neck exploration. Surgeons cite lower recurrence rate with bilateral exploration [33] as up to 15% of patients with preoperatively localized disease and appropriate drop in intraoperative parathyroid hormone (normalization of PTH level with 50% drop in value 10–15 min after excision) have an additional enlarged gland [34]. Proponents of focused parathyroidectomy, frequently called minimally invasive parathyroidectomy, argue that as 85% of primary hyperparathyroidism patients have a single adenoma, focused unilateral exploration with intraoperative parathyroid hormone measurement obviates the risk of bilateral recurrent laryngeal nerve injury and permanent hypoparathyroidism [35]. Several studies cite recurrence rates of focused parathyroidectomy between 95 and 98% [36–38]. In August of 2016, the American Association of Endocrine Surgeons published their first set of evidence-based guidelines for the definitive management of primary hyperparathyroidism [39]. In their guidelines, the authors state that both bilateral and focused parathyroidectomy are acceptable options for surgery, except in patients with known or suspected multigland disease.

## Adrenal Masses in Cirrhotic Patients

### Diagnostic Evaluation of Adrenal Mass

It is not uncommon to discover incidental adrenal masses during the work-up and surveillance of a patient with advanced liver disease. According to autopsy studies, adrenal incidentalomas occur with a prevalence of approximately 1–8.7% among the general population [40]. The prevalence appears to increase with age [41]. Patients with hepatocellular carcinoma frequently exhibit adrenal metastases, occurring in 11–20% of patients [42]. In light of these findings, proper work-up of an adrenal neoplasm is essential.

The diagnostic work-up of an adrenal neoplasm begins with biochemical evaluation to assess for hormonal excess. We recommend morning fasting adrenocorticotropic hormone and cortisol levels, serum aldosterone and plasma renin activity, and plasma fractionated metanephrines and catecholamines, and a 1-mg overnight dexamethasone suppression test. These tests will provide an effective and sensitive screen for the most common secreting adrenal tumors, namely, cortisol-secreting adenoma, aldosterone-secreting adenoma, and pheochromocytoma. Clinical suspicion for malignancy should also include testing for dihydoepiadrosterone sulfate (DHEA-S), which is frequently elevated in cases of adrenocortical carcinoma [43].

There are several caveats, diagnostic pitfalls, and occasionally necessary confirmatory testing in the biochemical diagnosis of adrenal tumors. Interfering medications, cyclic hormonal secretion, and differing methods of laboratory collection and analysis can make the proper diagnosis of such tumors a challenge [44, 45]. Thus we advocate a multi-disciplinary approach with involvement of an experienced adrenal endocrinologist.

Proper imaging of an adrenal neoplasm should include a dedicated noncontrast adrenal CT. Findings of adrenocortical adenoma, adrenocortical carcinoma, pheochromocytoma, and adrenal metastasis are summarized in Table 22.4. Benign neoplasms typically have smooth, homogeneous, well-circumscribed margins; lack internal calcifications or associated lymphadenopathy; and have noncontrast Hounsfield density <10 units. On pre- and postcontrast imaging, benign neoplasms will demonstrate >50% washout at 10 min [46].

## Indications for Adrenal Surgery in Cirrhotic Patients

In the presence of a confirmed hormonal hypersecretion, adrenalectomy is indicated regardless of the size of the neoplasm. In the case of primary hyperaldosteronism secondary to aldosterone-secreting adenoma, hypokalemia is normalized in all patients and previously refractory hypertension is markedly improved in nearly all patients with cure of hypertension in 30–60% of patients [47]. Results of adrenalectomy for cortisol-secreting adenomas are equally dramatic, with rapid resolution of the myriad symptoms and complications related to cortisol excess [48]. Similarly, patients with pheochromocytoma are at risk for early cardiac death and should undergo adrenalectomy after appropriate preoperative blockade [49]. We prefer a 3-week treatment with incremental doses of phenoxybenzamine.

In scenarios in which a hormonal hypersecretion has been ruled out, the decision for surgery hinges primarily on the suspicion for malignancy. In patients with no previous history of malignancy, incidental adrenal masses greater than 6 cm proved to be adrenocortical cancer 15–25% of the time [50]. Thus historically, 6 cm became a size threshold at which surgery was recommended. Over recent years, as minimally invasive techniques have become the gold-standard for adrenal surgery and substantial numbers of adrenocortical cancers are found to be less than 6 cm in size, the size threshold has decreased [51]. In our practice adrenalectomy is recommend on good surgical candidates with tumors >4 cm.

In patients with known cirrhosis, history of malignancy, or who are post-liver transplantation for cirrhosis or malignancy, the finding of an adrenal lesion should prompt consideration of metastatic disease. In a retrospective series of over 95 patients with metastatic disease to the adrenal of unknown primary, 8% proved to have hepatocellular cancer [52]. Various studies have shown that in highly select

**Table 22.4** Biochemical and CT-imaging phenotype of incidental adrenal masses

| Neoplasm | Hormonal workup | Size/laterality | Growth | Borders/internal features | Non-contrast CT density | Contrast washout feature |
|---|---|---|---|---|---|---|
| Benign adenoma | 80–90% non-secreting | <4 cm, unilateral | Slow over years | Homogeneous, Sharp, Well-Defined Borders | <10 HU | >50% at 10 min |
| Adrenocortical carcinoma | Increased steroid precursors (i.e. DHEA-S) | >4 cm, unilateral | Rapid over months | Irregular, Inhomogenous, Internal Calcification, Central Necrosis, Infiltrative | >20 HU | <50% at 10 min |
| Pheochromocytoma | Increased plasma metanephrines | Variable, occasionally bilateral | Variable; typically slow over years | Typically well-defined, cystic components | >20 HU | <50% at 10 min |
| Adrenal metastasis | Negative | Variable, frequently bilateral | Variable; typical growth seen over months | Irregular, Inhomogenous | >10–15 HU | <50% at 10 min |

patients with preserved liver function, either synchronous or metachronous adrenalectomy for metastatic hepatocellular carcinoma may improve survival [53, 54]. In one study, patients with metachronous adrenal metastasis from HCC who had previously undergone liver resection or transplantation were found to have 5-year survival of 20.3% and 85.7%, respectively [54].

The surgical approach to the adrenal gland has evolved over the past two decades. Whereas in the past, adrenalectomy was performed in an open transabdominal, thoracoabdominal, or retroperitoneal fashion; today, minimally invasive adrenalectomy has become the gold standard. Several studies have shown that a laparoscopic approach is feasible even for large adrenal tumors up to 10 cm [55–57]. In recent years, retroperitoneoscopic adrenalectomy has been popularized as it avoids the need for mobilization of the liver or spleen, and avoids entry into the peritoneum in those patients with significant adhesions from prior surgery [58]. In our experience, robotic adrenalectomy has been shown to reduce operating time, presumably due to the ease in dissecting in a manner that may prove difficult with conventional laparoscopic robotic instruments [59].

Careful patient selection and planning of surgical approach are necessary for adrenalectomy in the cirrhotic patient. The need to enter the peritoneal cavity and mobilize the liver or spleen risk further derangement in liver physiology and hemorrhage. In such patients, as well as patient who have undergone prior liver surgery, the retroperitoneal approach avoids many of these potential dangers and thus is the procedure of choice for tumors less than 6 cm in size. In the case of dense adhesions, however, the surgeon should be prepared to convert to a laparoscopic transabdominal or open approach. Regardless of approach, however, any cirrhotic patients undergoing adrenal surgery should have preserved liver function (Childs class A or B) with platelet counts above 70,000. In patients in whom a synchronous liver resection is planned, we recommend platelet counts above 100,000. Patients deemed unsuitable for surgery have the option of undergoing percutaneous thermal ablation with or without transarterial chemoembolization. Small

## Case Presentation
### Case 1

A 61-year-old female patient with cryptogenic cirrhosis and portal hypertension was found to have a 3.5 cm indeterminate right adrenal mass on an IV contrast CT of the liver (Fig. 22.2a). When the patient was referred, blood and urine hormonal testing were performed and found to be negative. A noncontrast CT of the adrenal glands demonstrated a 2.8 × 2.4 × 3.0 cm right adrenal mass with a Hounsfield density of 7 in the noncontrast phase (Fig. 22.2b). With the findings, this adrenal mass was characterized to be benign and a decision was made to follow this lesion up with repeat imaging in 6 months. This case emphasizes the importance of obtain a complete hormonal work-up and a noncontrast CT scan in patients with adrenal incidentalomas.

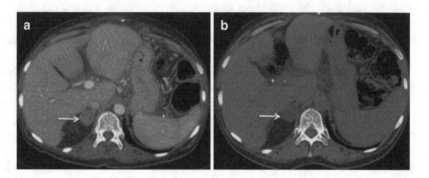

**Fig. 22.2** (**a**) CT with IV contrast demonstrating 3.5 cm indeterminate right adrenal mass; (**b**) noncontrast CT of same adrenal mass

## Case 2

A 65-year-old male patient with end-stage liver disease related to hepatitis C associated cirrhosis was found to have an enlarging right adrenal mass with irregular borders and heterogeneity (Fig. 22.3). Hormonal work up was negative. The lesion was initially approached with a right posterior retroperitoneal technique. However, due to the adhesions of this mass with the inferior vena cava and retroperitoneum, the case was converted to an open right adrenalectomy on a supine position. Pathology showed metastatic hepatocellular carcinoma with clear margins.

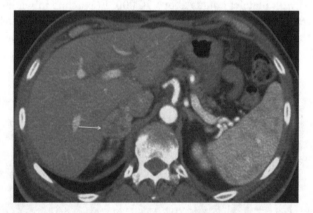

**Fig. 22.3** Contrast CT demonstrating irregular, heterogeneous right adrenal mass in patient with hepatitis C associated cirrhosis

studies have shown this to be a safe option although local recurrence rates have ranged from 18 to 25% [60].

## Conclusion

Endocrine disorders and neoplasms of endocrine organs are not uncommon finding. The finding of endocrine neoplasm requires proper assessment of endocrine function and hormonal excess. Although at risk for increased surgical complications, patients with preserved liver function, well-optimized medical comorbidities, and good functional status should be considered for necessary endocrine surgical procedures.

## References

1. Bianco AC, Larsen PR. Intracellular pathways of iodothyronine metabolism. In: Braverman LE, Utiger RD, editors. The Thyroid: Fundamental and Clinical Text. Philadelphia: Lippincott Williams and Wilkins; 2005.
2. Burra P. Liver abnormalities and endocrine diseases. Best Pract Res Clin Gastroenterol. 2013;27:553–63.
3. Burra P, Franklyn JA, Ramsden DB, Elias E, Sheppard MC. Severity of alcoholic liver disease and markers of thyroid and steroid status. Postgrad Med J. 1992;68:804–10.
4. Antonelli A, Ferri C, Fallahi P, et al. Thyroid cancer in HCV-related chronic hepatitic patients: a case-control study. Thyroid. 2007;17:447–51.
5. Haugen BR, Alexander EK, Bible KC, et al. 2015 American Thyroid Association Management Guidelines for Adult Patients with Thyroid Nodules and Differentiated Thyroid Cancer: The American Thyroid Association Guidelines Task Force on Thyroid Nodules and Differentiated Thyroid Cancer. Thyroid. 2016;26:1.
6. Cibas ES, Ali SZ. The Bethesda system for reporting thyroid cytopathology. Thyroid. 2009;19:1159.
7. Friedman LS. The risk of surgery in patients with liver disease. Hepatology. 1999;29:1617.
8. Ziser A, Plevak DJ, Wiesner RH, et al. Morbidity and mortality in cirrhotic patients undergoing anesthesia and surgery. Anesthesiology. 1999;90:42.
9. Teh SH, Nagorney DM, Stevens SR, et al. Risk factors for mortality after surgery in patients with cirrhosis. Gastroenterology. 2007;132:1261.
10. Friedman LS, Maddrey WC. Surgery in the patient with liver disease. Med Clin North Am. 1987;71:453.
11. Malinchoc M, Kamath PS, Gordon FD, et al. A model to predict poor survival in patients undergoing transjugular intrahepatic portosystemic shunts. Hepatology. 2000;31:864.
12. Northup PG, Wanamaker RC, Lee VD, Adams RB, Berg CL. Model for end-stage liver disease (MELD) predicts non-transplant surgical mortality in patients with cirrhosis. Ann Surg. 2005;242:244–51.
13. Pons Y, Gauthier J, Ukkola-Pons E, et al. Comparison of LigaSure vessel sealing system, harmonic scalpel, and conventional hemostasis in total thyroidectomy. Otolaryngol Head Neck Surg. 2009;141:496.
14. Siperstein AE, Berber E, Morkoyun E. The use of the harmonic scalpel vs. conventional knot tying for vessel ligation in thyroid surgery. Surgery. 2002;137:137–42.

15. Ecker T, Carvalho AL, Choe JH, et al. Hemostasis in thyroid surgery: harmonic scalpel versus other techniques–a meta-analysis. Otolaryngol Head Neck Surg. 2010;143:17.
16. Silverberg SJ, Bilezikian JP. Evaluation and management of primary hyperparathyroidism. J Clin Endocrinol Metab. 1996;81:2036.
17. Oldenburg WA, Van Heerden PA, Sizemore GW, Abbound CF, Sheedy PF. Hypercalcemia and primary hepatic tumors. Arch Surg. 1982;117:1363–6.
18. Luo JC, Hwang SJ, Wu JC, et al. Paraneoplastic syndromes in patients with hepatocellular carcinoma in Taiwan. Cancer. 1999;86:799–804.
19. Luo JC, Hwang SJ, Wu JC, Lai CR, Li CP, Chang FY, Chiang JH, Lui WY, Chu CW, Lee SD. Clinical characteristics and prognosis of hepatocellular carcinoma patients with paraneoplastic syndromes. Hepatogastroenterology. 2002;49:1315–9.
20. Forrest KY, Stuhldreher WL. Prevalence and correlates of vitamin D deficiency in US adults. Nutr Res. 2011;31:48.
21. Grey A, Lucas J, Horne A, et al. Vitamin D repletion in patients with primary hyperparathyroidism and coexistent vitamin D insufficiency. J Clin Endocrinol Metab. 2005;90:2122.
22. Compston JE. Hepatic osteodystrophy: vitamin D metabolism in patients with liver disease. Gut. 1986;27:1073.
23. Kumar R. Hepatic and intestinal osteodystrophy and the hepatobiliary metabolism of vitamin D. Ann Intern Med. 1983;98:662.
24. Sun J. Vitamin D and mucosal immune function. Curr Opin Gastroenterol. 2010;26:591–5.
25. Bitetto D, Fabris C, Fornasiere E, Pipan C, Fumolo E, Cussigh A, et al. Vitamin D supplementation improves response to antiviral treatment for recurrent hepatitis C. Transpl Int. 2011;24:43–50.
26. Petta S, Camma C, Scazzone C, Tripodo C, Di Marco V, Bono A, et al. Low vitamin D serum level is related to severe fibrosis and low responsiveness to interferon-based therapy in genotype 1 chronic hepatitis C. Hepatology. 2010;51:1158–67.
27. Bitetto D, Fabris C, Falleti E, Fornasiere E, Fumolo E, Fontanini E, et al. Vitamin D and the risk of acute allograft rejection following human liver transplantation. Liver Int. 2010;30:417–44.
28. Bilezikian JP, Brandi ML, Eastell R, et al. Guidelines for the management of asymptomatic primary hyperparathyroidism: summary statement from the Fourth International Workshop. J Clin Endocrinol Metab. 2014;99:3561.
29. Haber RS, Kim CK, Inabnet WB. Ultrasonography for preoperative localization of enlarged parathyroid glands in primary hyperparathyroidism: comparison with (99 m)technetium sestamibi scintigraphy. Clin Endocrinol (Oxf). 2002;57:241.
30. Eslamy HK, Ziessman HA. Parathyroid scintigraphy in patients with primary hyperparathyroidism: 99mTc sestamibi SPECT and SPECT/CT. Radiographics. 2008;28:1461.
31. Kwon JH, Kim EK, Lee HS, et al. Neck ultrasonography as preoperative localization of primary hyperparathyroidism with an additional role of detecting thyroid malignancy. Eur J Radiol. 2013;82:e17.
32. Nichols KJ, Tomas MB, Tronco GG, et al. Preoperative parathyroid scintigraphic lesion localization: accuracy of various types of readings. Radiology. 2008;248:221.
33. Norman J, Lopez J, Politz D. Abandoning unilateral parathyroidectomy: why we reversed our position after 15,000 parathyroid operations. J Am Coll Surg. 2012;214(3):260–9.
34. Siperstein A, Berber E, Mackey R, Alghoul M, Wagner K, Milas M. Prospective evaluation of sestamibi scan, ultrasonography, and rapid PTH to predict the success of limited exploration for sporadic primary hyperparathyroidism. Surgery. 2004;136(4):872–80.
35. Day KM, Elsayed M, Monchik JM. No need to abandon focused unilateral exploration for primary hyperparathyroidism with intraoperative monitoring of intact parathyroid hormone. J Am Coll Surg. 2015;221(2):518–23.

36. Norlén O, Wang KC, Tay YK, et al. No need to abandon focused parathyroidectomy: a multicenter study of long-term outcome after surgery for primary hyperparathyroidism. Ann Surg. 2015;261(5):991–6.
37. Slepavicius A, Beisa V, Janusonis V, Strupas K. Focused versus conventional parathyroidectomy for primary hyperparathyroidism: a prospective, randomized, blinded trial. Langenbecks Arch Surg. 2008;393:659.
38. Westerdahl J, Bergenfelz A. Unilateral versus bilateral neck exploration for primary hyperparathyroidism: five-year follow-up of a randomized controlled trial. Ann Surg. 2007;246:976.
39. Wilhelm SM, Wang TS, Ruan DT, et al. The American Association of Endocrine Surgeons Guidelines for Definitive Management of Primary Hyperparathyroidism. JAMA Surg (Published online August). 2016;10 doi:10.1001/jamasurg.2016.2310.
40. Bovio S, Cataldi A, Reimondo G, et al. Prevalence of adrenal incidentaloma in a contemporary computerized tomography series. J Endocrinol Invest. 2006;29:298.
41. Terzolo M, Stigliano A, Chiodini I, et al. AME position statement on adrenal incidentaloma. Eur J Endocrinol. 2011;164:851.
42. Katyal S, Oliver 3rd JH, Peterson MS, Ferris JV, Carr BS, Baron RL. Extrahepatic metastases of hepatocellular carcinoma. Radiology. 2000;216:698–703.
43. Fassnacht M, Allolio B. Clinical management of adrenocortical carcinoma. Best Pract Res Clin Endocrinol Metab. 2009;23:273.
44. Eisenhofer G, Goldstein DS, Walther MM, Friberg P, Lenders JWM, Keiser HR, Pacak K. Biochemical diagnosis of pheochromocytoma: how to distinguish true- from false-positive test results. J Clin Endocrinol Metab. 2003;88:2656–66.
45. Vilar L, Freitas Mda C, Faria M, et al. Pitfalls in the diagnosis of Cushing's syndrome. Arq Bras Endocrinol Metabol. 2007;51:1207–16.
46. Hamrahian AH, Ioachimescu AG, Remer EM, et al. Clinical utility of noncontrast computed tomography attenuation value (hounsfield units) to differentiate adrenal adenomas/hyperplasias from nonadenomas: Cleveland Clinic experience. J Clin Endocrinol Metab. 2005;90:871.
47. Rossi H, Kim A, Prinz RA. Primary hyperaldosteronism in the era of laparoscopic adrenalectomy. Am Surg. 2002;68:253.
48. Välimäki M, Pelkonen R, Porkka L, et al. Long-term results of adrenal surgery in patients with Cushing's syndrome due to adrenocortical adenoma. Clin Endocrinol (Oxf). 1984;20:229.
49. Amar L, Servais A, Gimenez-Roqueplo AP, et al. Year of diagnosis, features at presentation, and risk of recurrence in patients with pheochromocytoma or secreting paraganglioma. J Clin Endocrinol Metab. 2005;90:2110.
50. Herrera MF, Grant CS, van Heerden JA, et al. Incidentally discovered adrenal tumors: an institutional perspective. Surgery. 1991;110:1014.
51. Angeli A, Osella G, Alì A, Terzolo M. Adrenal incidentaloma: an overview of clinical and epidemiological data from the National Italian Study Group. Horm Res. 1997;47:279.
52. Lee JE, Evans DB, Hickey RC, et al. Unknown primary cancer presenting as an adrenal mass: frequency and implications for diagnostic evaluation of adrenal incidentalomas. Surgery. 1998;124(6):1115–22.
53. Hornstein I, Schwarz C, Ebbing S, Hoppe-Lotichius M, Otto G, Lang H, Musholt TJ. Surgical resection of metastases to the adrenal gland: a single center experience. Langenbecks Arch Surg. 2015;400(3):333–9. doi:10.1007/s00423-015-1293-z. Epub 2015 Mar 1. PubMed PMID: 25726026.
54. Ha TY, Hwang S, Ahn CS, Kim KH, Lee YJ, Moon DB, Song GW, Jung DH, Park GC, Lee SG. Resection of metachronous adrenal metastasis after liver resection and transplantation for hepatocellular carcinoma. Dig Surg. 2014;31(6):428–35. doi:10.1159/000370078. Epub 2015 Jan 7.
55. Lee J, El-Tamer M, Schifftner T, et al. Open and laparoscopic adrenalectomy: analysis of the National Surgical Quality Improvement Program. J Am Coll Surg. 2008;206:953.

56. Henry J, Sebag F, Iacobone M, et al. Results of laparoscopic adrenalectomy for large and potentially malignant tumors. World J Surg. 2002;26:1043.
57. Ramacciato G, Mercantini P, Torre ML, et al. Is laparoscopic adrenalectomy safe and effective for adrenal masses larger than 7 cm? Surg Endosc. 2008;22:516.
58. Walz MK, Alesina PF, Wenger FA, et al. Posterior retroperitoneoscopic adrenalectomy–results of 560 procedures in 520 patients. Surgery. 2006;140:943.
59. Taskin HE, Berber E. Robotic adrenalectomy. Cancer J. 2013;19:162.
60. Yamakado K, Anai H, Takaki H, et al. Adrenal metastasis from hepatocellular carcinoma: radiofrequency ablation combined with adrenal arterial chemoembolization in 6 patients. AJR Am J Roentgenol. 2009;192:W300–5.

# Chapter 23
# Head and Neck Issues in Cirrhotic Patients

**Robert R. Lorenz and Dennis Tang**

## Introduction

The primary head and neck issues that are prevalent in patients with liver failure can be divided into upper aerodigestive bleeding, need for tracheostomy, and head and neck cancer.

## Epistaxis

Epistaxis is a common medical problem affecting 7–14% of the general population each year. In the majority of patients, epistaxis is a self-limiting disease and many do not require medical attention. However, in patients with liver failure who have coagulopathy, these events can become difficult to manage and at times life threatening.

There have been multiple reports of severe epistaxis in patients with liver failure. Patients who present signs and symptoms of severe upper gastrointestinal hemorrhage should also be evaluated for epistaxis. Around 4.3% of patients diagnosed with upper gastrointestinal bleeding in cirrhotic patients ultimately were determined to be from epistaxis [1]. Mortality in patients with posterior epistaxis in cirrhotic patients is five times higher compared to the general population [1].

The majority of the blood supply of the nose originates from the external carotid system with the internal carotid system supplying a smaller component. The major terminal branches off the internal maxillary artery include the sphenopalatine artery, the greater palatine artery, and the pharyngeal artery. Bleeding from the nose

R.R. Lorenz, MD (✉) • D. Tang, MD
Cleveland Clinic Head and Neck Institute, Cleveland Clinic Main Campus,
9500 Euclid Avenue, Cleveland, OH 44195, USA
e-mail: lorenzr@ccf.org; tangd@ccf.org

© Springer International Publishing AG 2017
B. Eghtesad, J. Fung (eds.), *Surgical Procedures on the Cirrhotic Patient*,
DOI 10.1007/978-3-319-52396-5_23

can originate from the lateral nasal wall or the septum. Lateral nasal wall bleeding is most commonly seen from the region of the sphenopalatine artery, where it enters through the sphenopalatine foramen at the posterior end of the middle turbinate. Septal bleeding is most common from the anterior portion of the septum. This occurs at a region of anastomosis between the posterior nasal artery, greater palatine artery, anterior and posterior ethmoidal arteries, and branches of the labial artery entering from the nose. This is commonly known as Kiesselbach's plexus or Little's area and can be found about 1.5 cm posterior to the anterior mucocutaneous junction.

Treatment of epistaxis depends on the severity. Nonsurgical management should be attempted first. Initial management of epistaxis should start with nasal pressure. Compression of nasal ala against the septum is often enough to resolve anterior epistaxis. Administration of topical vasoconstrictors is a useful adjuvant when pressure alone is not sufficient. If a source of bleeding is visualized on anterior rhinoscopy, chemical cautery, or electric bipolar cautery has shown to have a high success rate. The main risk of this procedure is septal perforation and bilateral cauterization concurrently on opposing sides should be avoided.

Nasal packing is often a simple and effective mean of stopping nasal bleeding. Multiple options exist for nasal packing including layered ribbon gauze, balloon or catheter packing, or nasal tampons. The wide availability of nasal packing, ease of use by nonspecialists, and low cost make these a reasonable first line option. Application should begin with local anesthesia via cotton balls or aerosolization. Surgical lubricant should be applied to the nasal packing for ease of insertion and the packing should be placed as far posteriorly as possible. Despite their advantages, nasal packing can be uncomfortable and may be responsible for multiple complications. These include eustachian tube dysfunction, epiphora, and vasovagal reaction. Infections can also occur including vestibulitis, sinusitis, giant pyogenic granuloma, or more severe and potentially lethal systemic reactions such as toxic shock syndrome and infectious endocarditis. Concurrent use of prophylactic antibiotics should be considered in all patients with nasal packing.

Patients who fail conservative therapy or have massive hemorrhage will need more invasive intervention. Surgical interventions include anterior ethmoid artery ligation, maxillary artery ligation, or ligation of the sphenopalatine artery. Performed by experienced otolaryngologist, success rates approach 95–100% [2]. Familiarity with anatomy is critical for proper identification and avoiding complications, which include cerebrospinal fluid leak, edema, facial ecchymosis, and orbital injury. Embolization of the maxillary arteries or sphenopalatine arteries are well-described interventions. These are performed by neurointerventional radiology and are effective options for patients who are poor surgical candidates or continue to have epistaxis despite surgical intervention. Control rates range from 71% to 95% [2]. Complication rates are between 14% and 28% and range from stroke to facial numbness. Severe complications are low when performed by experienced practitioners.

## Oral Bleeding

Patients with liver failure are at high risk of oral or oropharyngeal bleeding. These commonly occur after procedures. Around 65% of patients with liver disease require dental surgical intervention for oral sanitation [3]. These include residual roots, unrestorable dental caries, periapical lesions, and advanced periodontal disease. Optimization prior to intervention includes correction of thrombocytopenia and elevated prothrombin time or partial thromboplastin time. Secondary bleeding occurs in around 15% of all procedures despite optimization [4]. Multiple local and systemic therapies have been shown to be effective in controlling oral bleeding. Local therapies include periodontal packing, oxidized cellulose, tranexamic acid, cyanoacrylate spray, aminocaproic acid, human fibrinogen concentrate, thrombin powder, fibrin glue, or suture closure. Systemic therapies include blood product infusion, tranexamic acid, and vitamin K injection.

## Tracheostomy

Acute respiratory failure with need for mechanical ventilation is a common complication in patients with liver failure who are critically ill. Prolonged translaryngeal endotracheal intubation is associated with multiple complications including increased risk of ventilator-associated pneumonia, severe laryngeal and tracheal damage, and prolonged need for sedation [5]. These complications are minimized by performing a tracheostomy. In the United States, over 100,000 tracheostomy tubes are placed annually. Indications for tracheostomy include (1) anticipated long-term intubation, (2) failure to wean from mechanical ventilation, (3) upper airway obstruction, (4) facilitation of pulmonary hygiene, and (5) airway protection [6].

Tracheostomy is historically one of the oldest known surgical intervention with descriptions dating back to 3600 BC. Despite this, optimal timing for performing a tracheostomy remains controversial. Many observational studies have documented a wide variability in tracheostomy timing. A Cochrane meta-analysis in 2015 showed no mortality difference between early vs late tracheotomy defined as before or after 10 days of intubation [7]. This is in congruence with the TracMan trial [8] performed in United Kingdom in 2013, which is a randomized controlled trial where patients expected to require prolonged mechanical ventilation were randomized to early tracheostomy (within 4 days after intubation) or late tracheostomy (after 10 days of intubation). The study showed no difference in 30-day mortality, 2-year mortality, length of intensive care unit stay, or duration of mechanical ventilation; however, while 91.9% of patients of the patient randomized to early tracheostomy underwent the procedure as planned, only 45.5% of patient in the late tracheostomy group underwent the procedure. This reflects a limited ability for clinicians to predict which patients require extended ventilator support. Based on this evidence, it is reasonable to wait at least 10 days to ensure a patient has ongoing need for mechanical ventilation prior to performing a tracheostomy.

Liver failure patients present a unique challenge when performing tracheostomy. These patients have coagulopathy and impaired tissue healing accentuating the need for reducing complications. Complications from tracheostomy can be divided into immediate, early (within 1 week), and late complications (>1 week) [9]. Complications are listed in Table 23.1. Immediate, early, and late complications rates have been shown to be 1.4%, 5.6%, and 7.1%, respectively.

Intraoperative complications are lowest when performed by an experienced surgeon. Nonotolaryngologists are 9.1 times more likely to have an intraoperative complications compared to otolaryngologist, specifically in prolonged desaturation and mortality [9]. Preoperative optimizations to reduce the rate of intraoperative complications include minimizing ventilator setting, weaning vasopressors, and correction of coagulopathy. The most common early complication is bleeding which occurs in approximately 2.6% of cases. Percutaneous tracheotomy has a significantly higher rate of postoperative bleeding compared to an open method with a rate of 6.6% compared to 1.9% [9]. The use of security sutures to anchor the tracheostomy tube has been shown to decrease rates of early complications, specifically bleeding and accidental decannulation [9]. Placement of anchoring sutures is highly encouraged. Late complications are directly related to injury during placement of the tube, abnormal healing at site of injured tracheal mucosa, or prolonged need for inflated cuff [10]. The development of high-volume low-pressure tracheostomy tube cuffs has led to a ten-fold reduction in cuff site stenosis [10]. Insertion of appropriately sized tracheostomy tube and avoidance of overinflation of the cuff can assist in avoiding tracheal mucosal injury. Given that, it is the belief of this author that tracheostomies in critical ill patients such as those with end-stage liver failure should be performed in the operating room by an experienced otolaryngologist to minimize complications.

Appropriate decannulation is critical in avoiding long-term consequences of tracheostomy. Decannulation can be considered once the indication for tracheostomy tube placement has resolved. A consensus statement was published by the American Academy of Otolaryngologist in 2012, based on the Delphi survey outlining 77 statements to reduce variations in practice in management of tracheostomy [11]. A list of prerequisites for decannulation has been provided in Table 23.2. The decannulation process should be performed in the following manner: (1) Remove the

**Table 23.1** Complication of tracheostomy

| Immediate complications | Early complications | Late complication |
|---|---|---|
| Desaturation | Bleeding | Airway stenosis |
| Stroke | Mucous plug | Granulation tissue |
| Pneumothorax | Infection/Tracheitis | Tracheoinnominate fistula |
| Severe blood loss | Accidental decannulation | Tracheoesophageal fistula |
| | | Tracheomalacia |
| | | Aspiration |

**Table 23.2** Prerequisites for decannulation in adult patients

| Answer the following to determine readiness of patient for decannulation of tracheostomy tube: |
| --- |
| Have the indications for the tracheostomy placement resolved or significantly improved? |
| Is the patient tolerating a decannulation cap on an appropriately sized uncuffed tracheostomy tube without stridor? |
| Does fiberoptic laryngoscopy confirm airway patency to the level of the glottis and immediate subglottis? |
| Does the patient have an adequate level of consciousness and laryngopharyngeal function to protect the lower airway from aspiration? |
| Does the patient have an effective cough while the tracheostomy tube is capped? |
| Have all procedures that require general endotracheal anesthesia been completed? |

tracheostomy tube; (2) Clean the site; (3) Cover the site with a dry gauze dressing; (4) Instruct the patient to apply pressure over the dressing with fingers when talking or coughing; (5) Change dressing daily and as needed if moist with secretions until the site has healed; and (6) Monitor for decannulation failure.

# Head and Neck Cancer

Head and neck cancer is a major health issue with an incidence of over 60,000 new cases in the United States each year. These include cutaneous malignancies, malignancies of the aerodigestive tract, and salivary gland cancers.

The two greatest risk factors for developing head and neck cancer include alcohol and tobacco use. Other risk factors include human papillomavirus infection, betel quid use, radiation exposure, and poor oral health. Many of these are also risk factors for developing liver cirrhosis. In patients who have undergone liver transplant, there is a 3.7 times greater overall incidence of de novo head and neck tumors compared to the general population ranging from 3% to 26% [12].

# Cutaneous Malignancies

The majority of head and neck malignancy in transplant patients are skin cancers of the head and neck. In patients who have undergone transplantation, around 80% of patient will develop a cutaneous malignancy in patients who live in areas of high sun exposure [13]. The most common types of cutaneous malignancy are basal cell cancer (BCC) and squamous cell cancer (SCC) with BCC outnumbering SCC by a factor of 4:1. Less common lesions include malignant melanoma and Merkel cell carcinoma. There is a fivefold increase in developing melanoma in post-transplant patient when compared to the general population. In patients with a pretransplantation history of melanoma, there is a 20% recurrence rate after transplantation and a waiting period of at least 5 years before considering transplantation is recommended [14]. Merkel cell carcinoma or neuroendocrine carcinoma is a rare entity with 55 cases reported in transplant population [15]. Merkel cell carcinoma has a much more aggressive clinical course with higher incidence of lymphatic involvement and spread. Risk factors for development of skin cancer include increase age at time of transplant, duration of immunosuppression, smoking, and prior infection by human papilloma virus [16].

Treatment of skin cancer is primarily with surgical excision and treatment of the neck lymphatics. Reduction of immunosuppression may improve prognosis, as well as conversion to a non-potentiating immunosuppressive agent such as rapamycin or everolimus. Education of skin exposure protection from the sun is mandatory. Close clinical follow-up is necessary and early intervention remains critical to preventing metastatic disease and death.

## Malignancies of Aerodigestive Tract

Cancers of the aerodigestive tract have a high morbidity and effect on quality of life. These patients suffer functional impairments related to speaking, swallowing, breathing, tasting, and smelling as well as facial disfigurement. Patients with these functional impairments are at higher risk of emotional disorder compared any other form of cancer [17]. More than 25% of patients develop anxiety with around 15% developing depression [18]. This high emotional burden makes proper treatment and management of head and neck cancers critical.

Recent shifts in epidemiology and management have changed the landscape of cancers of the upper aerodigestive tract. The incidence of head and neck squamous cell carcinoma (HNSCC) has declined over the past 30 years; however, the incidence of oropharyngeal cancer as a subset of HNSCC continues to rise. This is driven by the increasing number of HPV-related malignancies. 70–90% of newly diagnosed cases of oropharyngeal cancer are related to HPV. The majority are caused by the HPV-16 subtype with a smaller amount caused by HPV-18, HPV-33, and HPV-35. Clinical presentation of HPV-related malignancy is characterized by smaller primary tumors with more advanced nodal disease.

Management of HPV-related tumors depends on the treating institution. Current trends reflect the improved survival for HPV-associated disease with a focus on treatment de-escalation compared to non-HPV-associated disease. There are ongoing clinical trials focusing on radiotherapy dose reduction and defining the role of chemotherapy. The smaller size of the primary tumor allows these masses to be more amenable to surgical resection.

Surgical resection is one of the key pillars of management of head and neck cancers. Key concepts include margin control, management of regional metastasis, and reconstruction. Resection often results in large defects. Microsurgical reconstructive have been used extensively after tumor ablation. This allows for restoration of function and cosmetic improvement of areas that could not be reconstructed previously. Patients with liver cirrhosis are at a much higher risk from complications during surgical resection and reconstruction. Patients with Child's class B or C liver failure, low albumin level, increased total bilirubin, prolonged PT, intraoperative blood transfusion of 2 units or more, or ascites have a statistically significant higher chance of postoperative complications [19]. These complications include pulmonary edema, gastrointestinal bleed, myocardial infarction, acute renal failure, and sepsis. Mortality in patients with Child's class A, B, and C cirrhosis are 4.8%, 23.5%, and 66.7% respectively [19]. In these higher risk patients, it is recommended to consider correction of reversible clinical or biological factors prior to surgery when possible.

## Salivary Neoplasms

Salivary gland masses are comprised of a diverse group of malignant and benign tumors with varying behaviors. Salivary glands can be divided into major and minor salivary glands. The major salivary glands are comprised of the parotid glands, submandibular glands, and sublingual glands. Approximately 80% of salivary gland tumors originate in the parotid glands while 10–15% originate in the submandibular glands. The rest originate in sublingual or minor salivary glands. Masses in smaller salivary glands are more likely to be malignant. The primary modality of treatment for salivary neoplasm is through complete surgical resection. Radiation therapy, in combination with surgery, has been shown to improve locoregional control and survival. Adjuvant radiation is recommended in patients with high-grade malignancy. Chemotherapy has not been shown to improve locoregional control or survival and its primary role is for palliation, although the addition of chemotherapy to radiation is currently under investigation. Tumor size is a major prognostic indicator with decreased survival in larger masses. Skin involvement and facial nerve involvement are indicative of advanced malignancy requiring excision of involved structures. Free tissue reconstruction is often used for reconstruction of large defects. There is no current association between cirrhosis and salivary gland neoplasms, and the aforementioned preoperative precautions and postoperative interventions apply equally for these patients, as described earlier to other cancer types of the head and neck region.

## References

1. Camus M, Jensen DM, Matthews JD, Ohning GV, Kovacs TO, Jutabha R, Ghassemi KA, Machicado GA, Dulai GS. Epistaxis in end stage liver disease masquerading as severe upper gastrointestinal hemorrhage. World J Gastroenterol. 2014;20(38):13993–8.
2. Traboulsi H, Alam E, Hadi U. Changing trends in the management of epistaxis. Int J Otolaryngol. 2015;2015:1–7. . Article ID 263987
3. Rustemeyer J, Bremerich A. Necessity of surgical dental foci treatment prior to organ transplantation and heart valve replacement. Clin Oral Investig. 2007;11(2):171–4.

4. Niederhagen B, Wolff M, Appel T. Location and sanitation of dental foci in liver transplantation. Transpl Int. 2003;16(3):173–8.
5. Cheung NH, Napolitano LM. Tracheostomy: epidemiology, indications, timing, technique, and outcomes. Respir Care. 2014;59(6):895–919.
6. De Leyn P, Bedert L, Delcroix M, Depuydt P, Lauwers G, Sokolov Y, van Meerhaeghe A, van Schil P. Tracheotomy: clinical review and guidelines. Eur Assoc Cardiothorac Surg. 2007;32:412–21.
7. Andriolo BNG, Andriolo RB, Saconato H, Atallah AN, Valente O. Early versus late tracheostomy for critically ill patients. Cochrane Database Syst Rev. 2015. [Cited 1 June 2016]. Available from: http://onlinelibrary.wiley.com/doi/10.1002/14651858.CD007271.pub3/full.
8. Young D, Harrison DA, Cuthbertson BH, Rowan K. Effect of early vs late tracheostomy placement on survival in patients receiving mechanical ventilation: the TracMan randomized trial. JAMA. 2013;309(20):2121–9.
9. Halum SL, Ting JY, Plowman EK, Belafsky PC, Harbarger CF, Ostma GN, Pitman MJ, Lamonica D, Moscatello A, Khosla S, Cauley CE, Maronian NC, Melki S, Wick C, Sinacori JT, White Z, Younes A, Ekbom EC, Sardesai MG, Merati AL. A multi-Institutional analysis of tracheotomy complications. Laryngoscope. 2011;122(1):38–45.
10. Epstein SK. Late complications of tracheostomy. Respir Care. 2005;50(4):542–9.
11. Mitchell RB, Hussey HM, Setzen G, Jacobs IN, Nussenbaum B, Dawson C, Brown CA, Brandt C, Deakins K, Hartnick C, Merati A. Clinical consensus statement: tracheostomy care. Otolaryngol Head Neck Surg. 2013;148(1):6–20.
12. Nure E, Frongillo F, Lirosi MC, Grossi U, Sganga G, Avolio AW, Siciliano M, Addolorato G, Mariano G, Agnes S. Incidence of upper aerodigestive tract cancer after liver transplantation for alcoholic cirrhosis: a 10-year experience in an Italian center. Transplant Proc. 2013;45(7):2733–5.
13. Ramsay HM, Fryer AA, Hawley CM, Smith AG, Harden PN. Non-melanoma skin cancer risk in the Queensland renal transplant population. Br J Dermatol. 2002;147(5):950–6.
14. Penn I. Malignant melanoma in organ allograft recipients. Transplantation. 1996;61(2):274–8.
15. Euvrard S, Kanitakis J, Claudy A. Skin cancers after organ transplantation. N Engl J Med. 2003;348:1681–91.
16. Gourin CG, Terris DJ. Head and neck cancer in transplant recipients. Curr Opin Otolaryngol Head Neck Surg. 2004;12(2):122–6.
17. Ahn MH, Park S, Lee HB. Suicide in cancer patients within the first year of diagnosis. Psychooncology. 2015;24(5):601–7.
18. Wu YS, Lin PY, Chien CY, Fang FM, Chiu NM, Hung CF, Lee Y, Chong MY. Anxiety and depression in patients with head and neck cancer: 6-month follow-up study. Neuropsychiatr Dis Treat. 2016;12:1029–36.
19. Kao HK, Chang KP, Ching WC, Tsao CK, Cheng MH, Wei FC. Postoperative morbidity and mortality of head and neck cancers in patients with liver cirrhosis undergoing surgical resection followed by microsurgical free tissue transfer. Ann Surg Oncol. 2010;17(2):536–43.

# Chapter 24
# Oral Surgery on the Patient with Cirrhosis

James Guggenheimer

## Cirrhosis and Dental Disease

Definitive treatment of end-stage liver disease with liver transplantation became an accepted treatment modality in 1983 [1].Subsequently, it was recommended that candidates for liver transplantation undergo a dental examination and treatment of all potential sources of infection [2, 3]. As of 2002–2003, 80% of the respondents to a survey of U.S. organ transplant centers indicted that they "routinely requested" a dental evaluation prior to an organ transplant [4].

Dental evaluations will be able to assess patients' current dental health status, but should also determine if they had regular dental care and have the ability and motivation to maintain their oral health. Unfortunately, a majority of the risk factors for cirrhosis are more likely to be associated with neglect of dental health, lack of dental care, and having untreated dental disease. This can be extrapolated from data from the 2012 liver transplant wait list, which indicated that 61% of the 15,308 adult patients had primary end-stage liver disease as consequences of hepatitis C, alcoholic liver disease, or consequent hepatocellular carcinoma [5]. Since a majority of these causes of liver failure are related to substance abuse, these patients are at greater risk for untreated dental disease. This is based on the likelihood that these patients did not apply the requisite efforts to maintain good oral health and suggests that they may best be served by extraction of their remaining teeth [3, 6].

Consistent alcohol use or abuse has been associated with dental neglect and poor dental health [7, 8]. Patients with alcoholic end-stage liver disease have been shown to have higher rates of dental caries and periodontal disease [8–10]. A subset of 27 patients from Finland with end-stage alcoholic liver disease were found to have higher MELD scores and required a greater number of dental extractions prior to

J. Guggenheimer, DDS
Department of Diagnostic Sciences, University of Pittsburgh School of Dental Medicine, G-137 Salk, 3501 Terrace Street, Pittsburgh, PA 15261, USA
e-mail: guggen@pitt.edu

© Springer International Publishing AG 2017     309
B. Eghtesad, J. Fung (eds.), *Surgical Procedures on the Cirrhotic Patient*,
DOI 10.1007/978-3-319-52396-5_24

liver transplantation when compared with other liver diseases [10]. It is also likely that patients with alcoholic liver disease have abused more than one substance [11, 12]. This includes cigarette smoking [11, 12] that contributes to the development and progression of periodontal disease [8, 13]. Many years of substance abuse are associated with behavioral and sociodemographic attributes that also contribute to a lack of regular dental care and maintenance of good dental health [14, 15].

Irrespective of the cause of cirrhosis and end-stage liver disease, chronic liver failure can be an insidious process with its attendant complications and subsequent involvement of other organs including the heart and kidneys, as well as hepatic encephalopathy [16]. With progressive disability, further deterioration of dental health is likely. Patients become increasingly focused on the need for ongoing medical care that may require multiple hospitalizations, as shown by data from Medicare expenditures [5]. Symptoms of liver failure, including weakness, fatigability, malaise, muscle cramps, diarrhea, anorexia with nausea and vomiting, and anemia with dyspnea [16] are likely to compromise the patients' ability to maintain adequate oral health and to be able to undergo dental care in an ambulatory setting. A study of 300 patients who were evaluated for liver transplantation found that they were significantly more likely not to have had a dental visit during the previous 12 months, were more likely to have evidence of a lack of oral hygiene, and had two or more teeth that were carious and had periodontal disease [9]. Time constraints associated with higher MELD scores and matching liver donor and recipient have also been shown to affect dental care. A study of liver transplant candidates in Finland found that patients with higher MELD scores did not receive a pretransplant dental evaluation and were less likely to have dental treatment prior to the transplant surgery [17].

The medical management of the complications that accompany end-stage liver disease entails the use of medication regimens that may include diuretics and mood modifiers that have xerostomic side effects [11, 18]. A reduction or loss of saliva over an extended period of time will also contribute to the increased development and progression of dental caries [11, 18].

The debilitating manifestations of end-stage liver disease may result in loss of employment in conjunction with dental insurance causing economic stresses that may also preclude obtaining dental care [11]. Although the costs of medical care pre- and post-transplantation may largely be covered by Medicare [5], it does not provide benefits for dental care, and Medicaid has continuously reduced its reimbursement for dental services [19].

Among patients who have had a liver transplant for alcoholic cirrhosis, the risk for recidivism has been reported to range from 10% to 50% [20]. Heavy smoking is also more likely among abusers of alcohol [11, 12] and cessation is often a prerequisite for transplantation [21], but heavier smoking has resulted in an approximate 40% rate of relapse after liver transplantation [20]. The combined effects of these behaviors are likely to contribute to a continuum of dental neglect among these patients with further progression of their dental disease.

The older age of liver transplant candidates, in conjunction with their increased life expectancy post-transplantation [5], and the attendant commitments required for good dental health, suggest that patients' quality of life may be enhanced if they had fewer concerns with the maintenance of their natural dentition and their ability to access dental care on a regular basis. Furthermore, patients from rural or underserved areas may only have access to a general dental practitioner. This may have potential consequences if an acute dental infection should develop and the practitioner is reluctant to perform oral surgery on a patient who is significantly medically compromised [11].

As a consequence of the interactions among all of the foregoing issues and concerns, in conjunction with the compounding risks for an acute dental infection and sepsis from untreated dental disease, a majority of patients with cirrhosis may best be served by extraction of their remaining teeth and fabrication of dentures [3, 6]. Conversely, patients with end-stage liver disease that is not a consequence of substance abuse, who are in good dental health with a history of regular dental care, have attendant resources and support systems, and can be relied upon to comply with optimal health behaviors, should be encouraged to retain their natural dentition [6].

# Dental Infection and Bacteremia

An acute dental infection most frequently results from dental decay that encroaches the dental pulp, allowing bacteria to invade this normally sterile structure. Consequently, there is irreversible inflammation of the neurovascular tissues within the dental pulp and root canals, followed by necrosis. This process is estimated to involve more than 100 million bacteria [22], and if the infection is not contained within the root canal(s), it can extend into the adjacent periapical tissues and cause an abscess. The bacteria will then have access to blood vessels and lymphatics for dissemination that can put the immunocompromised patient at risk for sepsis.

An intraoperative bacteremia that is most likely to occur while a tooth is being luxated during the extraction procedure has resulted in recommendations that patients be premedicated after transplantation [4]. There is, however, no evidence to support the efficacy of this practice either in patients with end-stage liver disease or post-transplantation.

Patients with cirrhosis are at risk for spontaneous bacterial peritonitis [23], and it has been suggested that a bacteremia from dental surgery is another invasive procedure that could increase the risk for this complication [6, 24]. There is also no evidence to support the use of prophylactic antibiotics for this complication [6, 24]. Furthermore, spontaneous bacterial peritonitis has primarily been attributed to Gram-negative intestinal flora [23].

Concerns with the risk of a bacteremia can be minimized by preoperative oral rinses with 0.12% chlorhexidine gluconate mouthwash (Peridex® or PerioGard®). This can be resumed 1 day post-operatively for several days until the extraction site has healed.

## Coagulopathies and Bleeding

Cirrhosis can be accompanied by a number of complex coagulopathies that involve the coagulation proteins and blood platelets [25]. This is described in Chap.2 Hemostasis following tooth extraction does not appear to be a significant management problem based on reports of outcomes after dental surgery, although it may unpredictably occur (Fig. 24.1), even in healthy individuals. The extent of postoperative bleeding has been evaluated in two studies of 157 patients who were candidates for liver transplantation [26, 27]. The first study used absorbable hemostatic sponges for all 23 patients who had 84 extractions [26]. There was one case of bleeding (2.9%) that was readily controlled. In a larger study of 134 liver transplant candidates in Finland, the protocol used topical tranexamic acid that was applied to the extraction sites [27]. In addition, patients whose international normalized ratio (INR) was >2.0 received preoperative fresh frozen plasma, and those whose platelet counts were <100,000 × $10^9$/l were given a platelet transfusion. Despite these measures, postoperative bleeding developed in 12 patients (9%). Bleeding occurred significantly more frequently among the patients with higher INR values and lower platelet counts despite the preoperative replacement regimens.

The results of these two studies are consistent with other reports that have determined that the INR and platelet count may not be predictive of hypocoagulability and postoperative bleeding in patients with end-stage liver disease [25, 28]. To address the risk of bleeding, patients who require dental extractions should initiate oral rinses with 0.12% chlorhexidine gluconate mouthwash at least twice daily for several days prior to surgery. This rinse is bacteriocidal and its antimicrobial

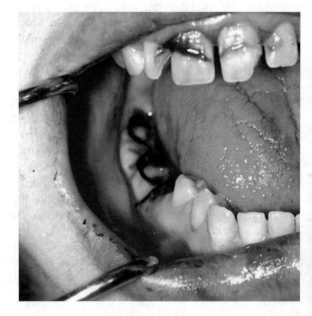

**Fig. 24.1** Postoperative bleeding 2 days after three teeth were extracted on a patient who was on the waiting for a liver transplant for hepatitis C. The area was reopened, curetted, packed with topical hemostatic agents, and resutured

properties will not only diminish the bacteremia associated with dental extractions, but will also reduce gingival inflammation that can contribute to intra- and postoperative bleeding. Dental surgical procedures should be kept as short as possible, with minimal tissue trauma. Topical, absorbable hemostatic agents should be placed over the extraction site(s) and the alveolar mucosa reapproximated with tight sutures. Absorbable hemostatic agents have been used since the 1940s [29]. These products have different textures and constituents, such as cellulose, porcine gelatin, or bovine collagen or thrombin that, on contact, activate blood clotting or platelet aggregation [29].

Any postoperative bleeding can initially be controlled with pressure by biting on a moistened gauze pad or tea bag. Delayed bleeding will entail re-exposing the surgical site, curettage to remove clots and granulation tissue, replacement of the absorbable hemostatic agents, and re-suturing (Fig. 24.1).

## Use of Anesthesia and Analgesics

A toothache has been described as one of the most severe forms of acute pain that has been ranked as 8.5/10 [30]. It results when bacteria cause irreversible inflammation of the neurovascular bundle within the dental pulp and root canals (acute pulpitis). Analgesia for acute dental pain may require an opioid or opioid-acetaminophen combination, but definitive treatment entails either an endodontic (root canal) procedure or extraction of the tooth. Postoperative pain can usually be managed with acetaminophen in conjunction with a nonsteroidal anti-inflammatory drug, preferably ibuprofen [31, 32]. For the patient with cirrhosis, however, these analgesics can have adverse effects since most are metabolized in the liver and excreted by the kidneys [33]. Opioids may also be contraindicated due to the risk for developing or exacerbating concurrent encephalopathy and constipation [33]. In addition, concerns with the use of nonsteroidal anti-inflammatory drugs include impaired renal function and gastrointestinal bleeding [33]. Consequently, acetaminophen that does not exceed 3–4 grams per day may be the drug of choice [33] but may not provide adequate relief of pain if it cannot be augmented with other analgesics.

The need for analgesics following dental surgery can, however, be minimized by use of a long-acting local anesthetic such as 0.5% bupivacaine HCl.(Marcaine™) This anesthetic has been available since 1963 and was approved for dental procedures in 1984 [34]. Bupivacaine, in combination with 1:200,000 epinephrine can provide anesthesia, followed by analgesia for seven or more hours [35]. A single dental cartridge of 1.8 ml contains 9.0 mg. of the anesthetic, and, as a guideline, the maximum safe dose for a healthy adult is 10 cartridges or 90.0 mg. per procedure [35]. Bupivacaine is primarily metabolized in the liver and excreted by the kidneys [35], but with accurate injection techniques, local infiltration with one cartridge can anesthetize several adjacent sites. Furthermore, epinephrine slows absorption of the drug. The injection procedure requires slow administration with frequent, intermittent aspiration. Each quadrant in a mouth with an intact dentition would normally contain eight teeth including the wisdom teeth. In the maxilla, anesthesia would require infiltration of anesthetic for each tooth that could be accomplished with less than the maximum recommended dose. The mandible can be anesthetized with regional blocks that require only two cartridges.

If necessary, surgical sites can be reinjected after several hours. Postoperative pain and swelling can also be limited by the application of ice packs for 20-min on/ off intervals on the day of and 1 day following surgery. Similar to the prevention of bleeding, tissue manipulation and trauma should be kept to a minimum. On the day of surgery and 1 day postoperatively, the diet should be limited to liquids or soft foods. Saline and 0.12% chlorhexidine gluconate mouth rinses can be started 1 day after surgery to maintain cleanliness of the extraction sites.

## Conclusions

Assessment of the dental health status of patients with cirrhosis should be an integral component of their management, particularly if the disease is a consequence of substance abuse and is progressing to liver failure. It is likely that these patients will require dental extractions but studies of outcomes following surgery are limited. Dental extractions performed prior to liver transplantation found no adverse sequelae other than minor bleeding. Surgery can be undertaken using standard practice procedures. Primary concerns appear to be limited to management of postoperative bleeding and pain. Providing interceptive dental care may be an inconvenience but offers far greater benefits than the risks of an acute dental infection and sepsis.

## References

1. National Institutes of Health Consensus Development Conference Statement. Liver transplantation-June 20-23, 1983. Hepatology. 1984;4:107S–10S.
2. Svirsky JA, Saravia ME. Dental management of patients after liver transplantation. Oral Surg Oral Med Oral Pathol. 1989;67:541–6.
3. Little JW, Rhodus NL. Dental treatment of the liver transplant patient. Oral Surg Oral Med Oral Pathol. 1992;73:419–26.
4. Guggenheimer J, Mayher D, Eghtesad B. A survey of dental care protocols among U.S. transplant centers. Clin Transplant. 2005;19:15–8.
5. Kim WR, Smith JM, Skeans MA, Schladt DP, Schnitzler MA, Edwards EB, et al. OPTN/SRTR 2012 annual data report: liver. Am J Transplant. 2014;14:69–96.
6. Douglas LR, Douglass JB, Sieck JO, Smith PJ. Oral management of the patient with end-stage liver disease and the liver transplant patient. Oral Surg Oral Med Oral Pathol Oral Radiol Endod. 1998;86:55–64.
7. Bloom B, Simile CA, Adams PF, Cohen RA. Oral health status and access to oral health care for U.S. adults aged 18–64: National Health Interview Survey, 2008. Vital & Health Statistics – Series 10: data from the National Health Survey. 2012; July 253:1–22.

8. Novacek G, Plachetzky U, Pötzi R, Lentner S, Slavicek R, Gangl A, et al. Dental and periodontal disease in patients with cirrhosis-role of etiology of liver disease. J Hepatol. 1995;22:576–82.
9. Guggenheimer J, Eghtesad B, Close JM, Shay C, Fung JJ. Dental health status of liver transplant candidates. Liver Transpl. 2007;13:280–6.
10. Helenius-Hietala J, Meurman JH, Höckerstedt K, Lindqvist C, Isoniemi H. Effect of the aetiology and severity of liver disease on oral health and dental treatment prior to transplantation. Transpl Int. 2012;25:158–65.
11. Guggenheimer J, Eghtesad B, Stock DJ. Dental management of the (solid) organ transplant patient. Oral Surg Oral Med Oral Pathol Oral Radiol Endod. 2003;95:383–9.
12. Burling TA, Ziff DC. Tobacco smoking: a comparison between alcohol and drug abuse inpatients. Addict Behav. 1988;13:185–90.
13. Ojima M, Hanioka T. Destructive effects of smoking on molecular and genetic factors of periodontal disease. Tob Induc Dis. 2010;8:4–8.
14. Metsch LR, Crandall L, Wohler-Torres B, Miles CC, Chitwood DD, McCoy CB. Met and unmet need for dental services among active drug users in Miami, Florida. J Behav Health Serv Res. 2002;29:176–88.
15. D'Amore MM, Cheng DM, Kressin NR, Jones J, Samet JH, Winter M, et al. Oral health of substance-dependent individuals: impact of specific substances. J Subst Abuse Treat. 2011;41:179–85.
16. Cheney CP, Goldberg EM, Chopra S. Cirrhosis and portal hypertension. In: Friedman LS, Keefe EB, editors. Handbook of liver disease. 3rd ed. Philadelphia: Saunders; 2012. https://www.clinicalkey.com/#!/browse/book/3-s2.0-C20100692406. Accessed 24 Aug 2016.
17. Helenius-Hietala J, Åberg F, Meurman JH, Isoniemi H. Increased infection risk postliver transplant without pretransplant dental treatment. Oral Dis. 2013;19:271–8.
18. Guggenheimer J, Close JM, Eghtesad B, Shay C. Characteristics of oral abnormalities in liver transplant candidates. Int J Organ Transpl Med. 2010;1:107–13.
19. Lee HH, Lewis CW, Saltzman B, Starks H. Visiting the emergency department for dental problems: trends in utilization, 2001 to 2008. Am J Public Health. 2012;102:e77–83.
20. Iruzubieta P, Crespo J, Fábrega E. Long-term survival after liver transplantation for alcoholic liver disease. World J Gastroenterol. 2013;19:9198–208.
21. Fleetwood VA, Hertl M, Chan EY. Liver transplantation to the active smoker: transplant provider opinions and how they have changed: transplantation in smokers: a survey. J Gastrointest Surg. 2015;19:2223–7.
22. Siqueira JF, Rôças IN. Microbiology of endodontic infections. In: Hargreaves KM, Berman LH, Rotstein I, editors. Cohen's pathways of the pulp. 11th ed. St Louis: Elsevier; 2016. https://www-clinicalkey-com.pitt.idm.oclc.org/#!/content/book/3-s2.0-B9780323096355000336. Accessed 8 Sept 2016.
23. Fiorello FJ. Dental management of patients with end-stage liver disease. Dent Clin N Am. 2006;50(4):563–90.
24. Dever JB, Sheikh MY. Review article: spontaneous bacterial peritonitis - bacteriology, diagnosis, treatment, risk factors and prevention. Aliment Pharmacol Ther. 2015;41:1116–31.
25. Tripodi A, Mannucci PM. The coagulopathy of chronic liver disease. N Engl J Med. 2011;365:147–56.
26. Perdigao JP, de Almeida PC, Mota MR, Soares EC, Alves AP, Sousa FP. Postoperative bleeding after dental extraction in liver pretransplant patients. J Oral Maxillofac Surg. 2012;70:e177–84.
27. Helenius-Hietala J, Åberg F, Meurman JH, Nordin A, Isoniemi H. Oral surgery in liver transplant candidates: a retrospective study on the delayed bleeding and other complications. Oral Surg Oral Med Oral Pathol Oral Radiol. 2016;121:490–5.
28. Segal JB, Dzik WH. Paucity of studies to support that abnormal coagulation test results predict bleeding in the setting of invasive procedures: an evidence-based review. Transfusion. 2005;45:1413–25.

29. Gaby M. Absorbable hemostatic agents. Am J Health Syst Pharm. 2006;63:1244–53.
30. Marco CA, Nagel J, Klink E, Baehren D. Factors associated with self-reported pain scores among ED patients. Am J Emerg Med. 2012;30:331–7.
31. Moore PA, Hersh EV. Combining ibuprofen and acetaminophen for acute pain management after third-molar extractions. Translating clinical research to dental practice. J Am Dent Assoc. 2013;144:898–908.
32. Drugs for pain. Med Lett Drugs Ther. 2013;11:31–42.
33. Dwyer JP, Jayasekera C, Nicoli A. Analgesia for the cirrhotic patient: a literature review and recommendations. J Gastroenterol Hepatol. 2014;29:1356–60.
34. Moore PA. Bupivacaine: a long-acting local anesthetic for dentistry. Oral Surg Oral Med Oral Pathol. 1984;58:369–74.
35. Marcaine. FDA prescribing information. https://www.accessdata.fda.gov/drugsatfda_docs/label/2012/018692s015lbl.pdf. Accessed 8 Dec 2015.

# Chapter 25
# Ophthalmic Surgery in Cirrhosis

Jila Noori and Andrew W. Eller

## Introduction

Amongst all surgeries, cataract surgery is the most commonly performed operation in the United States and perhaps in the world. The introduction of modern technology, including the insertion of implant lenses for the restoration of vision, has made it one of the most successful and satisfying of all surgeries with an extremely low complication rate. Therefore, it would not be surprising if many patients with cirrhosis were found to be candidates for this ophthalmic procedure. Particularly if they happen to also have diabetes mellitus or have been treated with corticosteroids, both are risk factors for cataract formation.

As with all surgeries in patients with cirrhosis, there is the increased risk of bleeding due to a reduction in procoagulant factors. A review of the literature revealed a paucity of reports regarding spontaneous ocular hemorrhage in cirrhotic patients with decompensated liver function [1, 2]. There are no published studies that specifically evaluated the propensity for bleeding during or following routine ophthalmic surgeries in cirrhotic patients with coagulopathy. For the purposes of this chapter, studies documenting the risk of hemorrhagic events in systemic hypocoagulable states such as anticoagulant and antiplatelet medications as well as thrombocytopenia were reviewed for their relationship with ophthalmic surgery.

J. Noori, MD
The Retina Service, Department of Ophthalmology, University of Pittsburgh Medical Center, Pittsburgh, PA, USA
e-mail: jilanoori82@gmail.com

A.W. Eller, MD (✉)
The Retina Service, UPMC Eye Center, Department of Ophthalmology, University of Pittsburgh School of Medicine, The Eye and Ear Institute, 203 Lothrop Street, Pittsburgh, PA 15213, USA
e-mail: elleraw@upmc.edu

© Springer International Publishing AG 2017                                    317
B. Eghtesad, J. Fung (eds.), *Surgical Procedures on the Cirrhotic Patient*,
DOI 10.1007/978-3-319-52396-5_25

# Preoperative Considerations

Two major factors must be taken into consideration when evaluating a patient with cirrhosis for ocular surgery. As the majority of eye surgeries are performed under local anesthesia with intravenous sedation, it is very important to assess the cirrhotic patient for their ability to lie comfortably in a supine position for the duration of the operation. Depending on the nature of the surgery, it may take minutes to hours to perform. If the cirrhosis is advanced and the patient has significant ascites, it may be very difficult if not impossible for them to be placed in a supine position. General anesthesia may be an option in this case, but it is accompanied with increased risk. The other major factor of importance, when planning surgery for patients with cirrhosis, is to assess their propensity for abnormal bleeding. This factor should also be considered when selecting the type of anesthesia and the surgical technique.

# Ophthalmic Anesthesia

The anesthetic techniques for ophthalmic surgical procedures have changed dramatically in recent decades. There are two options for local anesthesia of the eye: topical or an injection into the retrobulbar or peribulbar space. Local anesthesia was used in 46% of ophthalmic surgical procedures in 1993, increased to more than 95% in 2003 [3, 4]. In part, this is due to advances in eye surgery that have allowed for increased efficiency and safety and shorter operating times. There have also been advances in the medications used for intravenous sedation as well. Cataract surgery is now more commonly performed with topical anesthesia (tetracaine 0.5%) alone or topical combined with an intracameral injection (nonpreserved lidocaine 1%) for which there is no risk of bleeding [4]. In one study, patients experienced similar total pain and intraoperative discomfort for procedures under topical compared to retrobulbar/peribulbar anesthesia [5].

Retrobulbar anesthesia is typically delivered via a hypodermic needle into the muscle cone behind the eye. There are a number of potential complications with this technique including perforation of the globe and possibly the optic nerve. In addition, there is the risk of a retrobulbar hemorrhage that is increased in a patient with a hypocoagulopathy. A retrobulbar hemorrhage after retrobulbar or peribulbar anesthesia secondary to an arterial perforation can have overwhelming outcomes such as optic nerve and retinal ischemia and subsequently severe visual loss. In cases with a hypocoagulopathy, whenever possible, alternative anesthesia techniques including subconjunctival [6, 7] sub-Tenon [8], topical [9–11], and intracameral [12] should be considered. One study reported a reduced risk of hemorrhagic complications with topical anesthesia when compared with retrobulbar or peribulbar anesthesia, especially in individuals with preexisting systemic conditions [13]. Longer ophthalmic procedures that require more manipulation of the eye, such as retinal detachment repair cannot be performed under topical and require retrobulbar anesthesia.

To reduce the risk of a retrobulbar hemorrhage, rather than the use of a sharp needle, a blunt-tipped catheter can be inserted into the muscle cone through a conjunctival incision. This technique is preferred for patients with any type of bleeding diathesis. General anesthesia has its own associated risks but avoids the potential complications of a retrobulbar injection. It is usually reserved for longer surgeries such as pediatric, or ocular trauma procedures, or for patients with anxiety or claustrophobia [14].

## Expulsive Choroidal Hemorrhage

A tragic hemorrhagic complication specific to intraocular surgery is the expulsive choroidal hemorrhage. This rare adverse event usually leads to either loss of vision or even loss of the eye. Although it is commonly associated with cataract surgery, it can occur with any penetrating ocular surgery such as a glaucoma procedure, corneal transplantation, and retinal surgery. A British national survey reported an incidence of 0.04% for suprachoroidal hemorrhage during cataract extraction [15]. The primary risk factors for this devastating hemorrhagic event include systemic parameters causing arterial fragility such as arterial hypertension, arteriosclerosis, advanced age, and diabetes [16, 17]. Ocular factors associated with an increased risk for the development of a suprachoroidal hemorrhage include choroidal sclerosis, glaucoma, myopia, prolonged intraocular surgery, and hypotony [17].

## Cataract Surgery

In the past few decades, there has been a dramatic technological leap for cataract surgery. Phacoemulsification (ultrasound energy) has become the most commonly applied technique in developed countries, allowing for smaller incisions within a closed more stable eye and shorter operating time. In a series of 51 eyes corresponding to 40 patients at high risk for thromboembolic complications, phacoemulsification surgery with IOL implantation using a clear corneal incision under topical needle-free anesthesia was safely performed without discontinuing anticoagulation or antiplatelet therapy [18]. Cataract extraction with modern techniques can safely and effectively be performed in patients who are warfarinized with an INR of approximately 2.0 [19]. The incidence of suprachoroidal hemorrhage during cataract surgery has markedly decreased from 0.13% in extracapsular extractions (large incision) to 0.03% in phacoemulsification [20]. Studies have failed to show an increased risk of hemorrhagic complications in the perioperative period for cataract surgery when patients were treated with antiplatelet (aspirin or clopidogrel) or anticoagulant therapy [18, 21–24]. Phacoemulsification techniques with the insertion of foldable intraocular lenses (IOLs) through avascular clear corneal incisions under topical anesthesia have elevated cataract extraction surgery into a lower-risk procedure [25]. Therefore, one should expect similar results for a cirrhotic patient with a hypocoagulopathy.

## Vitreoretinal Surgery

There are a number of indications for vitreoretinal surgery including the repair of retinal detachments, treatment of advanced diabetic retinopathy, and surgery for some macular conditions. Unlike cataract surgery that can be performed through an avascular cornea, vitreoretinal procedures require conjunctival and scleral incisions. In addition, occasionally, an incision may be necessary in the highly vascularized retina and choroid. In recent years, a number of studies have evaluated the risk of bleeding in patients undergoing vitreoretinal surgery while on anticoagulant therapy [26–30]. A review of 57 vitreoretinal surgical procedures performed on patients treated with warfarin, there were no cases of anesthesia-related or intraoperative hemorrhage [28]. In another series evaluating the risk of bleeding in vitrectomy surgery, 60 patients treated with warfarin had a median INR of 2.3 ranging up to 4.6, without an increase in perioperative complications [30]. Fu et al. reported on 25 scleral buckle surgeries treated with warfarin anticoagulation. Retrobulbar or peribulbar anesthesia was administered and only one intraoperative subretinal hemorrhage was observed during external drainage of subretinal fluid [29]. Nonetheless, it is prudent to avoid external drainage of subretinal fluid whenever possible in anticoagulated patients. Antiplatelet usage has also been studied in this setting, and it is not considered a risk factor for bleeding [31–34]. Advances in vitreoretinal surgery include a shift from 20-gauge incisions to smaller entrance ports (23, 25, and 27gauge). Consequently, there is decreased risk of bleeding with shorter surgical time, and in select cases, it is feasible to use alternative methods of anesthesia such as subconjunctival or sub-Tenon injections that avoid the risks associated with retrobulbar injections [35].

Intravitreal injections of various medications for a variety of indications have been established as a treatment modality for a number of retinal pathologies. The MARINA and ANCHOR clinical trials for macular degeneration have shown that the anti-VEGF inhibitor ranibizumab can be safely injected into eyes of patients on warfarin anticoagulation and ASA antiplatelet therapy [36, 37].

## Glaucoma Surgery

A rather sudden, marked reduction in intraocular pressure from glaucoma surgery predisposes the eyes to an intra- or postoperative suprachoroidal hemorrhage. Anticoagulation can only exacerbate the extent of a suprachoroidal hemorrhage, making a difficult complication even worse. In a retrospective study reviewing 367 trabeculectomies, none of the 55 patients on aspirin experienced a significant intra-operative or postoperative hemorrhage. Aspirin was associated with a significantly higher risk of hyphema but without significant influence on intraocular pressure at 2 years. In this study, all of the five patients on warfarin suffered hemorrhagic complications (two required reoperation for hyphema evacuation) and four had trabeculectomy failure [38]. These results were confirmed by another retrospective study on eyes undergoing glaucoma surgery [39].

## Oculoplastic Surgery

Overall, the incidence of severe hemorrhagic complications is low in oculoplastic procedures. In a survey the incidence of orbital hemorrhage associated with cosmetic eyelid surgery was 0.055% (1/2000), and orbital hemorrhage with permanent visual loss was 0.0045% (1/10,000) [40].

In a prospective study, serious bleeding with the potential to affect surgical outcome, occurred in 0.4% of oculoplastic surgeries, but neither hepatic cirrhosis nor consumption of anticoagulants and antiplatelet agents were reported as risk factors for bleeding or bruising [41]. In a series of 150 dacryocystorhinostomy procedures, two patients with preexisting clotting abnormalities were found to have significant postoperative bleeding [42].

## Dry Eye Syndrome

In patients with cirrhosis, dry eye syndrome is a particularly common problem [43, 44]. Seventy-eight percent of patients with primary biliary cirrhosis were shown to have ocular surface dryness confirmed by tear-film breakup time and Rose Bengal staining [45]. The dry eye syndrome is a multifactorial disease of the tear film and ocular surface. It can result in symptoms of discomfort, visual disturbance, and tear-film instability with potential damage to the ocular surface, and possible ulceration. Advanced stages of hepatic fibrosis have been correlated with subjective and objective signs of dry eye. It has been hypothesized that as hepatic fibrosis progresses, there is a decrease in the synthesis of essential factors such as vitamin A and growth factors that are necessary for healthy tear film and ocular surface [46]. Tear production is decreased in HCV infection, possibly as a result of lymphocytic infiltration of the lacrimal gland [47]. An impairment of tear dynamics and squamous metaplasia in the ocular surface has been reported in patients with chronic hepatitis C treated with interferon alpha-2b and ribavirin. Moreover, it is emphasized that these abnormalities may persist even 6 months after discontinuation of treatment [48].

Ocular surgery, including cataract and refractive surgery, is known to be associated with an exacerbation of dry eye symptoms. It has been suggested that this may be a result of intraoperative evaporation of the tear film, vigorous intraoperative irrigation of the tear film, elevation of inflammatory factors due to manipulation of ocular surface, intraoperative use of topical anesthesia, and postoperative use of topical eye drops [49]. It is important for the ophthalmic surgeon to be cognizant of potential tear-film deficiencies while planning surgery, as these patients are at a greater risk for postoperative ocular surface disease.

## Summary

Many factors must be assessed while planning an ophthalmic surgery for patients with cirrhosis. These include the patient's coagulation profile, their ability to lie still in a supine position for the length of the operation, and the condition of the ocular surface. Also, surgeons must consider using those surgical techniques associated with a decreased risk of bleeding and shorter duration of surgical time. There is a dearth of information in the literature regarding the risk of bleeding when performing ophthalmic surgeries in cirrhotic patients with coagulopathy. However, a review of published studies evaluating hemorrhagic events in systemic hypocoagulable states demonstrates that there is a low risk for hemorrhagic complications while performing most ophthalmic surgeries.

## References

1. Nemiroff J, Baharestani S, Juthani VV, Klein KS, Zoumalan C. Cirrhosis-related coagulopathy resulting in disseminated intravascular coagulation and spontaneous orbital hemorrhages. Orbit. 2014;33(5):372–4.
2. Sirkanth K, Kumar MA. Spontaneous expulsive suprachoroidal hemorrhage caused by decompensated liver disease. Indian J Ophthalmol. 2013;61920:78–9.
3. Leaming DV. Practice styles and preferences of ASCRS members: 2003 survey. J Cataract Refract Surg. 2004;30:892–900.
4. El-Hindy N, Johnston RL, Jaycock P, et al. The Cataract National Dataset Electronic Multicentre Audit of 55 567 operations: anesthetic techniques and complications. Eye. 2009;23:50–5.
5. Virtanen P, Huha T. Pain in scleral pocket incision cataract surgery using topical and peribulbar anesthesia. J Cataract Refract Surg. 1998;24:1609–13.
6. Petersen WC, Yanoff M. Subconjunctival anesthesia: an alternative to retrobulbar and peribulbar techniques. Ophthalmic Surg. 1991;22:199–201.
7. Vicary D, McLennan S, Sun XY. Topical plus subconjunctival anesthesia for phacotrabeculectomy: one year follow-up. J Cataract Refract Surg. 1998;24:1247–51.
8. Guise PA. Sub-Tenon anesthesia: a prospective study of 6,000 blocks. Anesthesiology. 2003;98:964–8.
9. Kershner RM. Topical anesthesia for small incision self-sealing cataract surgery. A prospective evaluation of the first 100 patients. J Cataract Refract Surg. 1993;19:290–2.
10. Yepez J, Cedeno de Yepez J, Arevalo JF. Topical anesthesia for phacoemulsification, intraocular lens implantation, and posterior vitrectomy. J Cataract Refract Surg. 1999;25:1161–4.
11. Yepez J, Cedeno de Yepez J, Arevalo JF. Topical anesthesia in posterior vitrectomy. Retina. 2000;20:41–5.

12. Karp CL, Cox TA, Wagoner MD, et al. Intracameral anesthesia: a report by the American Academy of Ophthalmology. Ophthalmology. 2001;108:1704–10.
13. Stupp T, Hassouna I, Soppart K, et al. Systemic adverse events: a comparison between topical and peribulbar anaesthesia in cataract surgery. Ophthalmologica. 2007;221:320–5.
14. Holloway KB. Control of the eye during general anaesthesia for intraocular surgery. Br J Anaesth. 1980;52:671–9.
15. Ling R, Cole M, James C, et al. Suprachoroidal haemorrhage complicating cataract surgery in the UK: epidemiology, clinical features, management, and outcomes. Br J Ophthalmol. 2004;88:478–80.
16. Nouvellon E, Cuvillon P, Ripart J. Regional anesthesia and eye surgery. Anesthesiology. 2010;113:1236–42.
17. Ling R, Kamalarajah S, Cole M, et al. Suprachoroidal haemorrhage complicating cataract surgery in the UK: a case control study of risk factors. Br J Ophthalmol. 2004;88:474–7.
18. Barequet IS, Sachs D, Shenkman B, et al. Risk assessment of simple phacoemulsification in patients on combined anticoagulant and antiplatelet therapy. J Cataract Refract Surg. 2011;37:1434–8.
19. Grzybowski A, Ascaso FJ, Kupidura-Majewski K, Packer M. Continuation of anticoagulant and antiplatelet therapy during phacoemulsification cataract surgery. Curr Opin Ophthalmol. 2015;26:28–33.
20. Eriksson A, Koranyi G, Seregard S, Philipson B. Risk of acute suprachoroidal hemorrhage with phacoemulsification. J Cataract Refract Surg. 1998;24:793–800.
21. Katz J, Feldman MA, Bass EB, et al. Risks and benefits of anticoagulant and antiplatelet medication use before cataract surgery. Ophthalmology. 2003;110:1784–8.
22. Kobayashi H. Evaluation of the need to discontinue antiplatelet and anticoagulant medications before cataract surgery. J Cataract Refract Surg. 2010;36:1115–9.
23. Kumar N, Jivan S, Thomas P, McLure H. Sub-Tenon's anesthesia with aspirin, warfarin, and clopidogrel. J Cataract Refract Surg. 2006;32:1022–5.
24. Bonhomme F, Hafezi F, Boehlen F, Habre W. Management of antithrombotic therapies in patients scheduled for eye surgery. Eur J Anaesthesiol. 2013;30:449–54.
25. Barequet IS, Sachs D, Priel A, et al. Phacoemulsification of cataract in patients receiving Coumadin therapy: ocular and hematologic risk assessment. Am J Ophthalmol. 2007;144:719–23.
26. McCormack C, Simcock P, Tullo A. Management of the anticoagulated patient for ophthalmic surgery. Eye. 1993;7:749–50.
27. Gainey SP, Robertson DM, Fay W, Ilstrup D. Ocular surgery on patients receiving long-term warfarin therapy. Am J Ophthalmol. 1989;108:142–6.
28. Dayani PN, Grand MG. Maintenance of warfarin anticoagulation for patients undergoing vitreoretinal surgery. Arch Ophthalmol. 2006;124:1558–65.
29. Fu AD, McDonald HR, Williams DF, et al. Anticoagulation with warfarin in vitreoretinal surgery. Retina. 2007;27:290–5.
30. Chandra A, Jazayeri F, Williamson TH. Warfarin in vitreoretinal surgery: a case controlled series. Br J Ophthalmol. 2011;95:976–8.
31. McMahan L. Anticoagulants and cataract surgery. J Cataract Refract Surg. 1988;14:569–70.
32. Tabandeh H, Sullivan PM, Smahliuk P, et al. Suprachoroidal hemorrhage during pars plana vitrectomy. Risk factors and outcomes. Ophthalmology. 1999;106:236–42.
33. Oh J, Smiddy WE, Kim SS. Antiplatelet and anticoagulation therapy in vitreoretinal surgery. Am J Ophthalmol. 2011;151:934–9.
34. Brown JS, Mahmoud TH. Anticoagulation and clinically significant postoperative vitreous hemorrhage in diabetic vitrectomy. Retina. 2011;31:1983–7.
35. Malik AI, Foster RE, Correa ZM, Peterson MR, Miller DM, et al. Anatomical and visual results of transconjunctival sutureless vitrectomy using sobconjunctival anesthesia performed on select patients taking anticoagulant and antiplatelet agents. Retina. 2012;32:905–11.

36. Rosenfeld PJ, Brown DM, Heier JS, MARINA Study Group. Ranibizumab for neovascular age-related macular degeneration. N Engl J Med. 2006;355:1419–31.
37. Brown DM, Kaiser PK, Michels M, ANCHOR Study Group. Ranibizumab versus verteporfin for neovascular age-related macular degeneration. N Engl J Med. 2006;355:1432–44.
38. Cobb CJ, Chakrabarti S, Chadha V, Sanders R. The effect of aspirin and warfarin therapy in trabeculectomy. Eye. 2007;21:598–603.
39. Law SK, Song BJ, Yu F, et al. Hemorrhagic complications from glaucoma surgery in patients on anticoagulation therapy or antiplatelet therapy. Am J Ophthalmol. 2008;145:736–46.
40. Hass AN, Penne RB, Stefanyszyn MA, Flanagan JC. Incidence of post blepharoplasty orbital hemorrhage and associated visual loss. Ophthal Plast Reconstr Surg. 2004;20:426–32.
41. Custer PL, Trinkaus KM. Hemorrhagic complications of oculoplastic surgery. Ophthal Plast Reconstr Surg. 2002;18:409–15.
42. Bartley GB, Nichols WL. Hemorrhage associated with dacryocystorhinostomy and the adjunctive use of desmopressin in selected patients. Ophthalmology. 1991;98:1864–6.
43. Kedhar SR, Belair ML, Jun AS, et al. Scleritis and peripheral ulcerative keratitis with hepatitis C virus-related cryoglobulinemia. Arch Ophthalmol. 2007;125:852–3.
44. Jacobi C, Wenkel H, Jacobi A, et al. Hepatitis C and ocular surface disease. Am J Ophthalmol. 2007;144:705–11.
45. Giovannini A, Ballardini G, Amatetti S, Bonazzoli P, Bianchi FB. Patterns of lacrimal dysfunction in primary biliary cirrhosis. Br J Ophthalmol. 1985;69:832–5.
46. Gumus K, Yurci A, Mirza E, et al. Evaluation of ocular surface damage and dry eye status in chronic hepatitis C at different stages of hepatic fibrosis. Cornea. 2009;28:997–1002.
47. Haddad J, Deny P, Munz-Gotheil C, et al. Lymphocytic sialadenitis of Sjogren's syndrome associated with chronic hepatitis C virus liver disease. Lancet. 1992;339:321–3.
48. Huang FC, Shih MH, Tseng SH, et al. Tear function changes during interferon and ribavirin treatment in patients with chronic hepatitis C. Cornea. 2005;24:561–6.
49. Li XM, Hu L, Hu J, Wang W. Investigation of dry eye disease and analysis of the pathogenic factors in patients after cataract surgery. Cornea. 2007;26(9 Suppl 1):S16–20.

# Chapter 26
# Non-transplant Management of Portal Hypertension in Children

Jorge D. Reyes

## Introduction

The introduction and development of liver transplantation (Ltx) for previously untreatable end-stage liver disease dramatically changed the care of children with portal hypertension (PH) [1]; indeed, most clinical series attributed extrahepatic portal venous obstruction rather than intrinsic liver disease as the most common entity precipitating PH in children, perhaps because these were the only patients amenable to portosystemic shunt surgery. Over the past five decades experience with the broad clinical spectrum of pediatric diseases producing PH and its outcomes with and without liver transplantation has evolved according to the management strategies used to treat the complications of this disease and has impacted our understanding of its associated pathophysiology [2]. Another important consideration is that though the clinical manifestations and management strategies for PH are similar to those seen in adults, they are not the same. Liver disease is comparatively rare in children and are congenital or hereditary in nature (generally not acquired); also, clinically significant PH is late in most children with cirrhosis succumbing to jaundice, ascites, malnutrition, and infection. Similarly, the frequency and nature of extrahepatic portal obstruction is different in children than in adults [3].

The last 30 years has seen improved results with endoscopic sclerotherapy, and the success of liver transplantation has allowed for pretransplant temporizing approaches such as transcutaneous intrahepatic portosystemic shunts (TIPS). Portosystemic shunt surgery has thus been minimized due to the success of the other approaches mentioned but also because of the concern for shunt thrombosis in the small babies and postshunt encephalopathy. Unfortunately, most of these strategies have not been rigorously studied in children, and they are used almost under the

J.D. Reyes, MD
Roger K. Giesecke Distinguished Chair, Professor and Chief, Division of Transplant Surgery, Department of Surgery, University of Washington, Director of Transplant Services, Seattle Children's Hospital, 1959 NE Pacific Street, Box 356195, Seattle, WA 98195, USA
e-mail: reyesjd@uw.edu

© Springer International Publishing AG 2017
B. Eghtesad, J. Fung (eds.), *Surgical Procedures on the Cirrhotic Patient*,
DOI 10.1007/978-3-319-52396-5_26

mindset of "translational treatment" for what works with adults. This chapter will describe the clinical spectrum of PH in children and review the medical and surgical strategies available to manage it.

## Portal Hypertension

The portal system receives the drainage of the mesenteric and splenic venous beds, with normal pressure that remains between 5 and 10 mmHg. Portal hypertension is an abnormally high blood pressure in this system (>10 mmHg) and can be a consequence to increased resistance and/or increase in blood flow. By measuring pressures via a catheter (using a transjugular approach), a wedged hepatic vein pressure (WHVP), free hepatic vein pressure (FHVP), and a hepatic vein pressure gradient (HVPG) can be determined which will suggest the potential etiologies causing PH, by location of disease – either liver disease/cirrhosis (intrahepatic cause or sinusoidal), extrahepatic thrombosis of the portal vein (extrahepatic cause, presinusoidal), or hepatic venous outflow and beyond (posthepatic, postsinusoidal); a pressure gradient of >4 mmHg is abnormal and portal pressures of >12 mmHg with gradients >10 mmHg are associated with complications of PH (varices and ascites) (Fig. 26.1).

Diseases causing PH in children can be classified according to the aforementioned pressure-gradient table, which places patients into two principle groups – those with

| HPVG (WHVP-FHVP)>12mmHg | |
|---|---|
| Pre-hepatic ⟶ Normal HVPG | Portal or splenic vein thrombosis |
| | AV fistules in the splanchnic bed or spleen |
| Intra-hepatic | Pre-sinusoidal ⟶ Normal HVPG<br>*Sarcoid, Schistosomiasis* |
| | Sinusoidal ⟶ High HVPG (WHVP>FHVP)<br>*Cirrhosis- any cause* |
| | Post-sinusoidal ⟶ Budd Chiari- can't get into hepatic veins (clot in veins) |
| Post-hepatic ⟶ Normal HVPG (High WHVP and FHVP) | Webs in IVC |
| | Cardiac Disease ⟶ constrictive pericarditis, right heart failure |

Fig. 26.1 Hepatic vein measurements and gradients

associated significant liver disease and those associated with no significant liver disease. The performance of these pressure-gradient measurements is feasible and safe in children; however, it may not be necessary in the routine clinical care of these patients if the determination of in one of these groups is evident using other modalities.

Children with liver disease are usually cirrhotic, biliary atresia being the most common disease (60% of childhood cirrhosis, of which 70% may have varices); nonetheless, only in a minority are the complications of PH a dominant feature of their disease. Also, in those patients with early decompensation any evidence of PH will prompt liver transplantation. Late decompensation (with preserved liver function in successfully treated children with the Kasai operation) may manifest complications of PH in adolescence and be amenable to therapy other than transplant. Some patients present persistence of a small caliber portal vein with this disease, which may be a consequence to decreases in flow as cirrhosis develops and can make the reconstruction of the portal vein at transplant difficult. Alpha-1-antitrypsin deficiency is the other notable cirrhotic disease in children, occurring only in the PIZZ phenotype (18% of children affected) with the risk of developing jaundice, hepatomegaly, cirrhosis, and possibly hepatocellular carcinoma at various time points of the disease. The manifestations of PH are usually in concert with other evidence of cirrhosis, because the evolution can span from the neonate to the elderly careful follow up for the development and management of PH is necessary. Postnecrotic cirrhosis (viral or toxic) is rare in children; familial cholestatic syndromes, biliary cirrhosis, and cystic fibrosis (only 2% of whom develop clinically significant PH) account for the other causes of PH. Congenital hepatic fibrosis is an intrahepatic disorder which behaves like an extra-hepatic/pre-sinusoidal disease (as in with no associated liver disease) and is a consequence to the deposition of fibrous bands of dense connective tissue in portal and peri-portal areas; complications of PH can occur in 30–70% patients, which prompts aggressive management. Also of consideration is the associated ductal disease of the kidneys which may lead to renal failure and need for Kidney transplantation, at which time consideration for PH management may be required (including transplantation) (Table 26.1).

Rarely will posthepatic disease cause PH in children, the most notable being constrictive pericarditis particularly tuberculous in origin, and generally in areas of significant endemic disease. Other notable causes for reference are included in Table 26.2.

Given the success of Liver transplantation for patients with Liver disease, many patients presenting with bleeding complications of PH at this time are in association with no significant Liver disease, which has important management and outcome implications. Common diseases for this form of presinusoidal cause of PH are noted in Table 26.3.

These noncirrhotic diseases comprise what is termed extrahepatic portal vein obstruction (EHPVO), bleeding mostly occurring early in life, can be idiopathic (neonatal sepsis), or secondary to malignancy, trauma, hypercoagulable states, intraperitoneal inflammatory processes (portal vein phlebitis), and umbilical vein catheterization. It can also present in the setting of Liver transplantation, Budd Chiari, and cirrhosis. Over 50% of children with EHPVO develop severe bleeding episodes, however, the mortality rate is low (0–2%, vs. the mortality rate in the setting of

**Table 26.1** Intrahepatic
causes of portal hypertension

| Intrahepatic | |
| --- | --- |
| Postsinusoidal | Veno-occlusive disease |
| Sinusoidal | Cirrhosis (BA, A1A) |
| | Nodular regenerative hyperplasia |
| | Hypervitaminosis A |
| | Postnecrotic |
| Presinusoisal | Schistosomiasis |
| | Congenital hepatic fibrosis |
| | Sarcoidosis |
| | Portosclerosis |
| | Hepatic artery-portal vein fistula |

**Table 26.2** Posthepatic
causes of portal hypertension

| Posthepatic |
| --- |
| Heart failure |
| Cardiomyopathy |
| Congenital heart disease |
| Constrictive pericarditis |
| Inferior vena cava thrombosis |
| Congenital web in inferior vena cava |
| Budd-Chiari syndrome |
| Tumor |

**Table 26.3** Prehepatic
causes of portal hypertension

| Prehepatic |
| --- |
| Portal vein thrombosis |
| Portal vein stenosis |
| Cavernous transformation of portal vein |
| Congenital anomalies of portal vein |
| Tumor |

cirrhosis which ranges from 2.5% to 20%). This low mortality rate from bleeding is likely due to the absence of other complications seen in patients with cirrhosis, however, these patients do suffer from massive splenomegaly and hypersplenism, growth retardation, neurocognitive impairment, and encephalopathy. The disease is indolent, the age at presentation is quite variable (from infancy to adolescence), and the frequency and intensity of bleeding is similarly varied and unpredictable.

## Diagnosis and Management

Irrespective of the cause of PH the clinical consequences are the same: bleeding from gastro-esophageal varices, splenomegaly with hypersplenism, hepatopulmonary syndrome, portopulmonary hypertension, neurocognitive impairment, growth retardation, and encephalopathy; depending on the etiology and Liver reserve, ascites may be a component. The principle emphasis which has guided management has been the control of bleeding.

Portal Hypertension should be suspected in children who present with unexplained gastrointestinal bleeding, evidence of porto-systemic collateral circulation, cyanosis, splenomegaly, hypersplenism, or abdominal distention with ascites. Some patients may be referred by a pediatric hematologist/oncologist after an extensive work up for the non-bleeding complications of PH. Generally, the initial history and physical examination will determine the likelihood of the presence or absence of chronic Liver disease; such a determination will then focus the evaluation and severity of the Liver disease, specifically cirrhosis. In the absence of evidence to support cirrhosis, consideration of EHVO as a cause for the PH is quickly assessed by Doppler ultrasonography of the Liver visualizing the Liver (for parenchymal texture, bile ductular dilations, cysts, vascular anomalies, and surface irregularities), portal vein patency and flow changes (reversal of flow), hepatic vein patency (venous outflow), the presence of splenomegaly, renal abnormalities, and visceral rotations. Upper gastrointestinal endoscopy is the second investigative modality for the assessment and potential management of varices and is specifically performed after a bleeding presentation; there are no evidenced based recommendations regarding screening endoscopy, since therapeutic recommendations used in adults have not been studied in children regarding safety or efficacy in the prevention of the first variceal bleed. Computerized tomography or magnetic resonance imaging, and selective angiography with their various arterial and venous phase imaging are used when no lesion can be detected in the portal vein or there is no evidence of Liver disease. Hepatic vein pressure and gradients can be measured as well and determine other pre and post Liver diseases as the cause of PH; this transjugular vein route may also allow for retrograde visualization of the intrahepatic portal venous anatomy, the presence of angiodysplasias, and the performance of a liver biopsy (if indicated). The use of splenoportograms (through the transcutaneous puncture of the Spleen) has been in disuse for many years due to the risk of splenic bleeding or rupture. All of these diagnostic modalities may assist in the planning of a therapeutic strategy [4].

The management of PH in children has, up until recently, focused on the initial control of established bleeding; longer-term strategies are guided by the determination of the presence or absence of Liver disease. Management of the asymptomatic child with PH is highly variable, with endoscopy for monitoring or therapy being the controversial due to the lack of controlled pediatric trials. Endoscopic evaluations of "low" vs. "high" risk varices and algorithms indicating prophylactic variceal obliteration or Beta blockers lack safety data and should be used with caution; the experience with endoscopic variceal ligation (EVL) suggest it to be safer than endoscopic sclerotherapy (EST) in children (Fig. 26.2). However, because the mortality of cirrhotic children at the time of the first bleed can be as high as 15%, screening endoscopy in all children with advanced liver disease and complications of PH may be justified [5].

**Fig. 26.2** Esophago
gastric varices

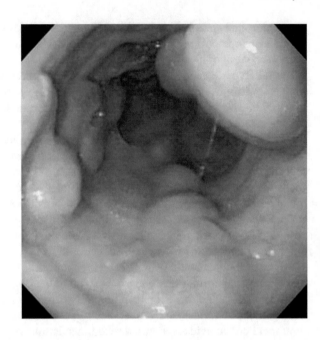

The presence of gastrointestinal bleeding can result in dramatic clinical scenarios, which mandate aggressive resuscitative management to achieve stabilization. Achieving stability, endoscopy can determine a nonvariceal source (with its appropriate management to follow) or a variceal source. In cases of variceal bleeding, endoscopic sclerotherapy or banding with or without pharmacologic therapy is instituted with follow-up EST or EVL as indicated; this therapy is successful in the majority of patients, with recurrence of bleeding in the order of 10–15%. Patients who fail to achieve stability may benefit from pharmacologic support using splanchnic vasoconstrictors such as octreotide or vasopressin; if attempts at control of bleeding with EST or EVL fail, the use of balloon tamponade with a Sengstaken Blakemore tube (SBT) may allow for stabilization and determination of the need for more invasive therapies such as a TIPS or a surgical shunt. The need to consider a SBT insertion is ominous and a provider "should know where this tube is stored"; algorithms for insuflation of esophageal and gastric components vary, as does strategies for removal [6] (Fig. 26.3).

Gastric varices tend to be more common in patients with EHVO; in patients with cirrhosis they should be a consideration for TIPS, shunt surgery (if there is well preserved liver function), or Liver transplantation. Some cirrhotic children with compensated long-standing noncholestatic Liver disease may be considered for shunt surgery, however, it is important to consider procedures which avoid the hepatic hilus (in the expectation of a need for transplantation). A TIPS procedure can control the acute complications of PH and stabilize the child while awaiting transplantation, the most common drawback being the development of encephalopathy. Because the definitive therapy in children with liver disease (or other intrahepatic cause for PH) is liver transplantation, these latter therapies are geared

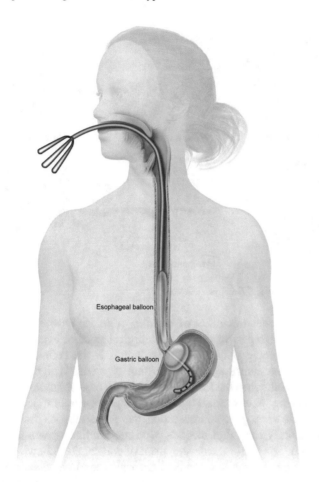

**Fig. 26.3** Sengstaken-Blakemore

toward temporary management and should not risk or complicate the chances for transplantation [7].

In patients without associated liver disease, there is no hepatic dysfunction and therefore the focus is entirely on the bleeding varices. As noted before, approaches that include watchful waiting or prophylactic EVL/EST are common, though not studied as to efficacy. Endoscopic control has been the cornerstone of management for many years and resulted in a decline of shunt surgery; it is believed that the risk of rebleeding will diminish progressively over time given the tendency to develop spontaneous shunts. This approach has been the standard of care for many years given the risk of postshunt complications such as occlusion, rebleeding and encephalopathy. However, it is critical to recognize the limitations of these temporizing measures and their potential for complications.

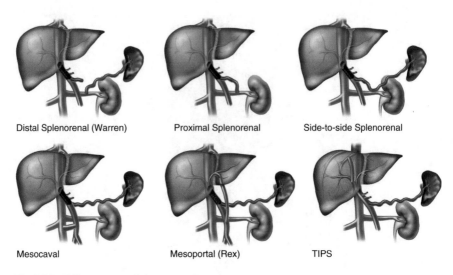

Distal Splenorenal (Warren)        Proximal Splenorenal        Side-to-side Splenorenal

Mesocaval                          Mesoportal (Rex)            TIPS

**Fig. 26.4** Different types of shunt procedures

Surgical approaches to control of bleeding from PH have the goal of decompressing the esophago-gastric varices by a surgical shunt or bypass procedure; this indicated if endoscopic obliteration fails, and it is the definitive treatment for PH. Indeed, because shunt surgery in this group of patients is highly successful, it is of significant benefit when the local therapy fails. In case of failure of a shunt, other procedures such as direct variceal ligation (through a gastrotomy), gastric devascularization, gastric or esophageal transection, and porto-azygous disconnection may allow for temporary control of bleeding with reinstitution of endoscopic management, while time allows for the development of collaterals. Following are the most common shunt procedures in consideration, which are in essence porto-systemic shunts (with or without removal of the spleen) except for the mesoportal or Rex shunt which is a bypass procedure [8] (Fig. 26.4). The surgical strategy should take into account the extent of EHVO and the pattern [9] of collateral flow (to the right or left of the stomach, right-sided vs. left-sided PH). Previously the mesocaval and then the distal splenorenal shunts were the most popular procedures since it did not require removal of the spleen; however, in cases where there is a predominance of right-sided flow a better option may be a proximal splenorenal shunt. The mesenterico-left portal bypass or Rex shunt was introduced by Jean de Ville de Goyet in 1992 for postliver transplant EHVO, and since been extended to all children with PH without associated liver disease; it has the advantage of not placing the patient at risk for long-term complications such as encephalopathy from hyperammonemia or hepatopulmonary syndrome [10–13].

Given the physiologic nature of the reestablishment of flow to the liver with this procedure (creating a shunt between the superior mesenteric vein and the portal venous system at the recess of Rex), important positive physiologic observations have been made in patients thus managed. These include the cure of portal hypertension, reversal of the commonly observed coagulopathy, correction of portal biliopathy, improvement in the not so uncommon evidence of liver atrophy, normalization of hyperammonemia, improvement in neurocognitive ability, improvement in somatic growth, and reversal of hepatopulmonary syndrome. It has been known that chronic diversion of portal blood flow significantly affects the size and function of the liver that has a dependency on hepatotrophic factors such as insulin. Restoration of normal portal inflow may prevent long-term functional deterioration of the liver and its effects on the child. Indeed, for some time it has been debated whether in light of the success of shunt surgery and other therapies, the benefits now outweigh the risk; thus, are we entering into a phase of preemptive/primary procedures before the occurrence of a major bleed to manage children with PH? [14–17].

In summary, it is critically important to assess the nature of disease resulting in PH; the goal of managing the bleeding complication hinges on resuscitation and stabilization, with endoscopic control remaining the cornerstone of therapy. Liver transplantation remains the definitive treatment in patients with cirrhosis and PH; select patients with normal hepatic reserve may benefit from temporizing measures such as TIPS or surgical shunts. Significant progress has been made through the introduction and development of the Rex Shunt, such that it may be introduced as the primary therapy in patients with EHVO, even in the absence of a bleeding episode [18, 19].

# Bibliography

1. Starzl TE. Experience in hepatic transplantation. Philadelphia: WB Saunders Co; 1969. p. 45–8.
2. Reyes J, Iwatsuki S. Current management of portal hypertension with liver transplantation. In: Camaron JL, editor. Advances in surgery, vol. 25. St. Louis: Mosby-Year Book, Inc.; 1992. p. 189–208.
3. Alonso EM, Hackworth C, Whitington PF. Portal hypertension in children. Clin Liver Dis. 1997;1(1):201–22. xiii. Review. PubMed PMID: 15562677.
4. Ling SC. Advances in the evaluation and management of children with portal hypertension. Semin Liver Dis. 2012;32(4):288–97. doi:10.1055/s-0032-1329897. Epub 2013 Feb 8. Review. PubMed PMID: 23397529.
5. Ng NB, Karthik SV, Aw MM, Quak SH. Endoscopic evaluation in children with end-stage liver disease-associated portal hypertension awaiting liver transplant. J Pediatr Gastroenterol Nutr. 2016;63(3):365–9. doi:10.1097/MPG.0000000000001160. PubMed PMID: 26863384.
6. D'Antiga L. Medical management of esophageal varices and portal hypertension in children. Semin Pediatr Surg. 2012;21(3):211–8. doi:10.1053/j.sempedsurg.2012.05.004. Review. PubMed PMID: 22800974.
7. Shneider BL, Bosch J, de Franchis R, Emre SH, Groszmann RJ, Ling SC, Lorenz JM, Squires RH, Superina RA, Thompson AE, Mazariegos GV. Expert panel of the Children's Hospital of Pittsburgh of UPMC. Portal hypertension in children: expert pediatric opinion on the report of the Baveno v Consensus Workshop on Methodology of Diagnosis and Therapy in Portal Hypertension. Pediatr Transplant. 2012;16(5):426–37. doi:10.1111/j.1399-3046.2012.01652.x. Epub 2012 Mar 13. PubMed PMID: 22409296.

8. Millar AJW. Portal hypertension. In: Paediatric surgery, Global Help: Seattle, WA. vol. 1. p. 503–7. 010. *Fig 87.1.*
9. de Ville de Goyet J, Alberti D, Falchetti D, Rigamonti W, Matricardi L, Clapuyt P, Sokal EM, Otte JB, Caccia G. Treatment of extrahepatic portal hypertension in children by mesenteric-to-left portal vein bypass: a new physiological procedure. Eur J Surg. 1999;165(8):777–81. PubMed PMID: 10494645.
10. de Ville de Goyet J, Gibbs P, Clapuyt P, Reding R, Sokal EM, Otte JB. Original extrahilar approach for hepatic portal revascularization and relief of extrahepatic portal hypertension related to later portal vein thrombosis after pediatric liver transplantation. Long term results. Transplantation. 1996;62(1):71–5. PubMed PMID: 8693549.
11. Reyes J, Mazariegos G, Bueno J, Cerda J, Towbin RB, Kocoshis S. The role of portosystemic shunting in children in the transplant era. J Pediatr Surg. 1999;34(1):117–23.
12. Superina R, Bambini DA, Lokar J, Rigsby C, Whitington PF. Correction of extrahepatic portal vein thrombosis by the mesenteric to left portal vein bypass. Ann Surg. 2006;243(4):515–21. PubMed PMID: 16552203; PubMed Central PMCID: PMC1448975.
13. Dasgupta R, Roberts E, Superina RA, Kim PC. Effectiveness of Rex shunt in the treatment of portal hypertension. J Pediatr Surg. 2006;41(1):108–12; discussion 108-12. PubMed PMID: 16410118.
14. Chiu B, Superina R. Extrahepatic portal vein thrombosis is associated with an increased incidence of cholelithiasis. J Pediatr Surg. 2004;39(7):1059–61. PubMed PMID: 15213899.
15. Rangari M, Gupta R, Jain M, Malhotra V, Sarin SK. Hepatic dysfunction in patients with extrahepatic portal venous obstruction. Liver Int. 2003;23(6):434–9. PubMed PMID: 14986818.
16. Starzl TE, Terblanche J. Hepatotrophic substances. In: Popper H, Schaffner F, editors. Progress in liver disease, vol. 6. New York: Grune & Stratton; 1979. p. 135–52.
17. Starzl TE, Porter KA. Francavilla A: the Eck fistula in animals and humans. Curr Prob Surg. 1983;20:687–752.
18. Starzl TE, Porter KA, Kashiwagi N, Putnam CW. Portal hepatotrophic factors, diabetes mellitus and acute liver atrophy, hypertrophy and regeneration. Surg Gynecol Obstet. 1975;141:843–58.
19. Thompson EN, Williams R, Sherlock S. Liver function in extrahepatic portal hypertension. Lancet. 1964;ii:1352.

# Chapter 27
# Trauma in the Patient with Cirrhosis

**Andrew B. Peitzman**

Trauma remains the leading cause of death in patients younger than 45 years in the United States. Globally, five million people die of trauma every year from injury, more deaths than HIV, TB, and malaria combined. The major causes of death are closed-head injury and bleeding in the blunt trauma victim. Exsanguination is the most common cause of death in penetrating injury. The injured patient requires a rapid, systematic, and thorough evaluation guided by the Advanced Trauma Life Support [1]. The steps of the initial resuscitation are: (1) primary survey, (2) resuscitation, (3) secondary survey, and (4) definitive care. The goal of the primary survey is to detect and treat immediately life-threatening injuries guided by the patient's hemodynamic status and injury pattern. Concurrently, venous access is obtained and fluid resuscitation is initiated. Only after stabilization of the patient, the secondary survey, a head-to-toe examination defining all injuries, is commenced. If a trauma patient deteriorates or does not respond as expected, the primary survey is repeated prior to proceeding with the secondary survey.

For patients who present in shock after airway control, support of ventilation, and control of external hemorrhage, attention should be directed to find and treat hemorrhage as the next most frequent early threat to life. Sources of bleeding can be external, thoracic, intra-abdominal, retroperitoneal (most often pelvic fracture), or long-bone fractures. Major hemorrhages from penetrating injury are generally from vascular injuries in the torso or extremity. The most common sources for blood loss in blunt injury are the liver, spleen, mesentery, lung/chest wall, and pelvis. Tension pneumothorax, pericardial tamponade, spinal cord injury, and medical causes of shock are less common etiologies for hypotension. Hard signs or positive diagnostic tests (focused assessment with sonography in trauma [FAST] or diagnostic peritoneal lavage [DPL]) mandate laparotomy [2, 3]. In the patient who presents in extremis, empiric chest tube placement is both diagnostic and therapeutic; the hemothorax

A.B. Peitzman, MD
Trauma and Surgical Services, F-1281,UPMC-Presbyterian, Pittsburgh, PA 15213, USA
e-mail: peitzmanab@upmc.edu

© Springer International Publishing AG 2017                                              335
B. Eghtesad, J. Fung (eds.), *Surgical Procedures on the Cirrhotic Patient*,
DOI 10.1007/978-3-319-52396-5_27

is found and the tension pneumothorax is both diagnosed and treated. Send a blood specimen for type and cross match. Biochemical indices, either base deficit or lactate levels, should be measured to assess global perfusion. Hypotension, tachycardia, and oliguria are obvious signs of hypoperfusion. On the other hand, even with normal vital signs, as many as 75% of trauma patients in the ICU have compensated shock with tissue hypoperfusion [4–7]. In the trauma patient, on-going blood loss is the most common etiology for persistent hypoperfusion.

The abdomen is particularly challenging to evaluate in the trauma patient. Except in cases of evisceration or obvious peritonitis, the history and physical exam findings, which suggest intra-abdominal injury, are often subtle; physical examination alone will miss 45% of intra-abdominal injuries. Severely injured patients often have altered mental status from associated brain injury, shock, or intoxicating agents that mask signs and symptoms of abdominal injury. More obvious injuries, such as complex open extremity fractures, distract both physicians and patients, focusing attention away from occult torso injuries. Delay in diagnosis and treatment of intra-abdominal injury is a common cause of preventable morbidity and mortality in the trauma patient [8, 9]. Furthermore, the majority of blunt solid organ injuries, most frequently spleen and liver, can be managed nonoperatively. The key criterion for observation of a patient with blunt injury to the spleen or liver is hemodynamic stability.

To understand outcomes in the trauma patient, we need to discuss scoring systems for trauma. The burden of anatomic injury in the trauma patient is quantified by the injury severity score (ISS) [10]. The ISS is calculated by the sum of the squares of the AIS (abbreviated injury score) of the most severe injuries from three of six body regions. The AIS reflects the severity/grade of an organ injury. Predicted outcome in a trauma patient is then calculated as the probability of survival using the ISS as the measurement of anatomic burden and the revised trauma score as quantification of the physiologic status of the trauma patient, adjusting for patient age and blunt versus penetrating mechanism of injury (TRISS) [11].

A relationship between cirrhosis and poor outcomes in trauma patients has been demonstrated—both for patients managed nonoperatively and those undergoing operative management [12–45]. Patients with cirrhosis who undergo emergency operation have mortality which is 2–4 times greater than the noncirrhotic patient. Although these observations are well documented, the precise mechanism of this inferior outcome is not elucidated. The effect of anesthesia and hypoperfusion on the liver may further compromise a cirrhotic liver. Cirrhotic patients are often coagulopathic. Add the multiple abnormalities of the *coagulopathy of trauma* [12–14], and this further compounds the ability to secure hemostasis in the cirrhotic trauma patient.

Cirrhosis is a relatively uncommon comorbidity in trauma patients, only 1% of total trauma admissions [26–38]. Several summary observations can be gleaned from the literature: (1) Trauma patients with cirrhosis have higher than predicted mortality. (2) Mortality increases with increasing MELD or Child-Pugh classification. (3) Early deaths after injury in cirrhotic patients are from hemorrhage. Late deaths are a consequence of infection, most commonly pneumonia or sepsis. (4)

The common scoring systems (TRISS) to predict mortality in trauma patients are unreliable in the cirrhotic patient. (5) Operative mortality is dramatically higher in the cirrhotic patient undergoing laparotomy for trauma as compared to the noncirrhotic patient.

In one of the earliest reports on the impact of cirrhosis on survival after injury, Tinkoff et al. [38] reported mortality of 30% for 40 trauma patients with cirrhosis. They had no control group for comparison. The authors reported that the predicted survival using TRISS for the cirrhotic trauma patients was 93%, but only 70% survived.

Talving et al. prospectively studied the impact of cirrhosis on the outcome in trauma patients, based on the Child-Pugh classification [31]. Of 12,102 trauma admissions, 0.08% had cirrhosis. Cirrhotic patients were matched with noncirrhotic cohorts in a 1:2 ratio. The overall complication rate in cirrhotics was 31.5% vs 7.1% in controls ($p < 0.001$). Renal failure and sepsis were the most common complications. Others have reported increased infectious complications in the cirrhotic patient [30]. ICU length of stay was significantly longer in the patient with cirrhosis, 2.7 vs 0.8 days ($p < 0.007$). The in-hospital mortality was 20.7% vs 6.5%, comparing cirrhotics to noncirrhotic, respectively ($p = 0.001$). Within the cirrhotic patient group, mortality increased significantly with Child-Pugh classification: 8.0% in Class A, 32.2% in Class B and 45.5% in Class C ($p = 0.003$). Similarly, mortality for patients with a MELD of 10 or greater had 30.0% mortality vs 9.5% for controls, odds ratio 4.07 ($p = 0.016$).

From the same center, the authors queried the effect on outcome of the cirrhotic patient undergoing trauma laparotomy; 46 patients were reported over 12 years at a busy urban trauma center (4771 trauma patients underwent laparotomy) [41]. Each cirrhotic patient was matched with two noncirrhotic patients. The overall mortality comparing the cirrhotic to the noncirrhotic trauma patient undergoing laparotomy was 45% vs 25% with an odds ratio of 7.60 ($p = 0.021$). Stratifying by Injury Severity Score (ISS), cirrhotic patients with an ISS≤15 incurred mortality of 29% vs 5% in the noncirrhotic group ($p = 0.013$) (Table 27.1). For cirrhotic patients with more severe injury, ISS 16–25, mortality was 56% vs 11% for noncirrhotic trauma patients ($p = 0.024$). Differences in mortality for the most severely injured patients, ISS >25, were not significant (70% in cirrhotic, 75% in noncirrhotic trauma patients). The authors emphasized that mortality for emergency operation in general surgery patients has been reported from 46% to 86%. In elective setting, intensive preoperative and perioperative optimization can achieve a mortality rate less than

**Table 27.1** Comparison of mortality of trauma patients undergoing laparotomy based on Injury Severity Score (From Demetriades et al. [41])

| Injury severity score | Cirrhotic pts | Noncirrhotic pts | Odds ratio |
|---|---|---|---|
| ≤15 | 29% | 5% | 8.00* |
| 16–25 | 56% | 11% | 10.00* |
| >25 | 70% | 75% | NS |

*$p < 0.05$

10% for elective abdominal procedures. With laparotomy for trauma or emergency general surgery, we have little opportunity to correct existing organ dysfunction, thus the high operative mortality. Lin et al. [36] reported an operative mortality rate of 43% for blunt trauma victims undergoing laparotomy. Multiple logistic analysis revealed significant predictors of operative mortality to be shock on admission ($p = 0.021$) and MELD score ($p = 0.012$). Using receiver-operating characteristic (ROC) curve analysis, a MELD score greater than or equal to 17 predicted high risk of mortality. On the other hand, Peetz et al. demonstrated that improvement in MELD score with 72 h of ICU admission for the cirrhotic trauma patient was associated with improved mortality [27] (Fig. 27.1).

A review of the National Trauma Data Bank [26] reported 956 trauma patients with cirrhosis (0.11% of 885,000 trauma admissions). The overall mortality for patients with cirrhosis was four times greater than those without (17.7% vs 4.4%, $p < 0.001$). Mortality remained much higher in cirrhotic trauma patients, even when accounting for age, preexisting comorbidities, ISS and TRISS. Cirrhotic patients undergoing laparotomy had a significantly higher mortality than cirrhotics who did not (44.2% vs 16.8%). In addition, cirrhotic patients undergoing laparotomy had mortality of 44.2% vs 17.3% in noncirrhotic patients who underwent laparotomy. Trauma patients with cirrhosis were also more likely to develop complications (27.4% vs 5.2%). The authors concluded that cirrhosis is a strong predictor of poor outcome in trauma patients, especially if undergoing laparotomy.

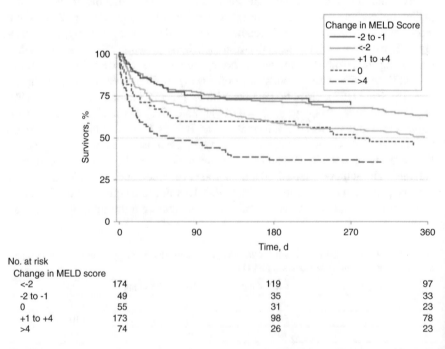

**Fig. 27.1** Survival in cirrhotic trauma patients by changes in MELD score (From Peetz et al. [27])

Christmas et al. appropriately describe trauma and cirrhosis as the deadly duo [32]. Sixty-one trauma patients with cirrhosis were compared to a matched group of control patients (1:2); with no difference in age, ISS or GCS between the groups. Intensive care unit stay, hospital length of stay, transfusion requirements in the first 24 h postinjury and mortality (33% vs 1%) were significantly higher in the trauma patients with cirrhosis. Fifty-five percent of the deaths in the cirrhotic group were due to sepsis. Mortality rose as Child's class increased: Child's A (15%), Child's B (37%) and Child's C (63%) (Fig. 27.2). Mortality in cirrhotics undergoing laparotomy incurred a 55% mortality vs 21% mortality in cirrhotics who did not require an exploratory laparotomy. The authors concluded that, regardless of the severity of injury, cirrhosis carries a poor prognosis in the trauma patient. In this study, splenectomy was the most common abdominal operation in the trauma patient with cirrhosis. As hemodynamic instability remains the primary indication for operation on the trauma patient with splenic injury, this management is compounded in the cirrhotic patient. Fang et al. [43] reported a significantly higher failure rate for nonoperative management of splenic injuries in the patient with cirrhosis (92 vs 19%). In fact, the cirrhotic patients who failed nonoperative management of blunt splenic injury had lower ISS, lower grade splenic injury, greater need for blood transfusion and higher mortality compared to noncirrhotic patients with splenic injury. The authors concluded that high-grade splenic injury, multiple injuries and elevated PT should prompt early laparotomy in the cirrhotic patient.

In a multicenter study of 77 cirrhotic patients with blunt splenic injury (case control matched with noncirrhotic trauma patients), Cook et al. [45] report an inpatient mortality of 27% for cirrhotics with blunt splenic injury, correlating with higher MELD scores, higher ISS, lower platelet count, and higher incidence of splenectomy. All patients with a MELD >19 died. Multivariable analysis demonstrated that the presence of cirrhosis was a significant risk factor for mortality in blunt splenic injury (OR 10.9).

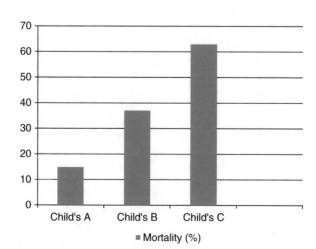

**Fig. 27.2** Mortality by Child's classification in trauma patients with cirrhosis [32]

In the largest and more recent series of blunt splenic injury in cirrhotics, Bugaev et al. [44] queried the National Trauma Data Bank for 2002–2010. Of 77,752 adult patients with blunt splenic injury, 289 had cirrhosis (0.37%). Initial nonoperative management of the splenic injury was attempted in 86% of cirrhotics and 90% of noncirrhotics. Patients with cirrhosis were more likely to fail nonoperative management (17% vs 10%, $p = 0.004$), despite more frequent use of angioembolization (13% vs 8%, $p = 0.001$). The patients with cirrhosis incurred more complications, had longer length of hospital and intensive care unit stay and higher mortality (22% vs 6%, $p = 0.001$) which was independent of mode of treatment. Mortality in patients with cirrhosis was 14% with successful nonoperative management of the splenic injury, 30% for patients undergoing immediate laparotomy, and 46% with failed nonoperative management ($p < 0.05$). Failure of observation was predicted by high-grade splenic injury (OR 11.6) and preexisting coagulopathy (OR 3.28). Mortality correlated with male sex (OR 4.34), hypotension (OR 3.15), preexisting coagulopathy (OR 3.06) and GCS less than 13 (OR 6.33). The authors suggest that patients with high-grade splenic injury (grade 4 or 5) or coagulopathy may benefit from prompt surgery (Table 27.2).

On the other hand, Barmparas et al. [42] reported no difference in success of nonoperative management of liver injury in cirrhotic trauma patients in a report from the National Trauma Data Bank (14% failure rate). However, cirrhotic patients had a higher mortality (28% vs 7%, $p < 0.01$), particularly if they required a laparotomy (58% vs 17%, $p < 0.01$) or if they failed nonoperative management (50% vs 4%, $p < 0.01$). The authors concluded that a trial of nonoperative management with blunt liver injury in the stable patient with cirrhosis was reasonable, acknowledging a higher risk of mortality of the patients required laparotomy.

The impact of cirrhosis on outcome after brain injury was addressed by Cheng et al. [28]. One year after traumatic brain injury, cirrhotic patients had higher mor-

**Table 27.2** Spleen organ injury scale [21]

| Grade[a] | Injury type | Description of injury |
|---|---|---|
| I | Hematoma | Subcapsular, <10% surface area |
| | Laceration | Capsular tear, <1 cm parenchymal depth |
| II | Hematoma | Subcapsular, 10–50% surface area |
| | | Intraparenchymal, <5 cm in diameter |
| | Laceration | Capsular tear, 1–3 cm parenchyma depth that does not involve a trabecular vessel |
| III | Hematoma | Subcapsular, >50% surface area or expanding; ruptured subcapsular or parenchymal hematoma; intraparenchymal hematoma ≥5 cm or expanding |
| | Laceration | >3 cm parenchymal depth or involving trabecular vessels |
| IV | Laceration | Laceration involving segmental or hilar vessels producing major devascularization (>25% of spleen) |
| V | Laceration | Completely shattered spleen |
| | Vascular | Hilar vascular injury which devascularizes spleen |

[a]Advance one grade for multiple injuries up to grade III

tality (52.2%) compared to noncirrhotic patients (30.6%) with increased risk of mortality of 1.75 ($p$, 0.001). Similarly, cirrhosis has a profound negative effect on outcome in burn patients [40]. The overall mortality rate in the burn patients was 50% in cirrhotics and 14.8% in noncirrhotics. With logistic regression, age (OR 1.08), total body surface area burned (OR 1.08), inhalation injury (OR 3.17), and cirrhosis (OR 8.78) had independent effects on mortality.

How can we summarize the literature on the trauma patient with cirrhosis? The injured patient with cirrhosis should be aggressively monitored and promptly treated. Blunt splenic injury is the most common indication for trauma laparotomy. The conundrum we have in management of the trauma patient with blunt injury to the spleen is the high mortality for the patient who fails nonoperative management of the splenic injury versus the high mortality for emergency laparotomy in the cirrhotic patient. The risk is greater with higher admission MELD, baseline coagulopathy or high-grade splenic injury. With no optimal answer, the balance may be monitoring of the cirrhotic patient who meets criteria for nonoperative management, understanding the high risk of failure and operating early with high-grade splenic injury or when failure of nonoperative management is apparent.

# References

1. Advanced Trauma Life Support Student Manual. Chicago: American College of Surgeons; 2012.
2. Rozycki GS, Ballard RB, Feliciano DV, Schmidt JA, Pennington SD. Surgeon-performed ultrasound for the assessment of truncal injuries: lessons learned from 1540 patients. Ann Surg. 1998;228:557–67.
3. Soffer D, Schulman CI, McKenney MG, et al. What does ultrasonography miss in blunt trauma patients with a low Glasgow Coma Score (GCS)? J Trauma. 2006;60:1184–8.
4. Rixen D, Raum M, Bouillon B, Lefering R, Neugebauer E. Base deficit development and its prognostic significance in posttrauma critical illness: an analysis by the trauma registry of the Deutsche Gesellschaft fur unfallchirurgie. Shock. 2001;15:83–9.
5. Davis JW, Parks SN, Kaups KL, Gladen HE, O'Donnell-Nicol S. Admission base deficit predicts transfusion requirements and risk of complications. J Trauma. 1996;41:769–74.
6. Claridge JA, Crabtree TD, Pelletier SJ, Butler K, Sawyer RG, Young JS. Persistent occult hypoperfusion is associated with a significant increase in infection rate and mortality in major trauma patients. J Trauma 2000;48:8–14; discussion −5.
7. Abramson D, Scalea TM, Hitchcock R, Trooskin SZ, Henry SM, Greenspan J. Lactate clearance and survival following injury. J Trauma. 1993;35:584–8; discussion 8-9.
8. Enderson BL, Maull KI. Missed injuries. The trauma surgeon' s nemesis. Surg Clin North Am. 1991;71:399–418.
9. Choi KC, Peek-Asa C, Lovell M, Torner JC, Zwerling C, Kealey GP. Complications after therapeutic trauma laparotomy. J Am Coll Surg. 2005;201:546–53.
10. Baker SP, O'Neill B, Haddon Jr W, et al. The injury severity score: a method for describing patients with multiple injuries and evaluating emergency care. J Trauma. 1974;14:187–96.
11. Champion HR, Copes WS, Sacco WJ, et al. The major trauma outcome study: establishing national norms for trauma care. J Trauma Acute Care Surg. 1990;30:1356–65.
12. Hess JR, Brohi K, Dutton RP, et al. The coagulopathy of trauma: a review of mechanisms. J Trauma Acute Care Surg. 2008;65:748–54.

13. Maegele M, Schochl H, Mitch C. An update on the coagulopathy of trauma. Shock. 2014;41:21–5.
14. Mitra B, Cameron PA, Mori A, et al. Acute coagulopathy and early deaths post major trauma. Injury. 2012;43:22–5.
15. Ochsner MG. Factors of failure for nonoperative management of blunt liver and splenic injuries. World J Surg. 2001;25:1393–6.
16. Velmahos GC, Toutouzas K, Radin R, et al. High success with nonoperative management of blunt hepatic trauma: the liver is a sturdy organ. Arch Surg. 2003;138:475–80; discussion 480-1.
17. van der Wilden GM, Velmahos GC, Emhoff T, et al. Successful nonoperative management of the most severe blunt liver injuries: a multicenter study of the research consortium of new England centers for trauma. Arch Surg. 2012;147:423–8.
18. Velmahos GC, Toutouzas KG, Radin R, Chan L, Demetriades D. Nonoperative treatment of blunt injury to solid abdominal organs: a prospective study. Arch Surg. 2003;138:844–51.
19. Malhotra AK, Fabian TC, Croce MA, et al. Blunt hepatic injury: a paradigm shift from operative to nonoperative management in the 1990s. Ann Surg. 2000;231:804–13.
20. Watson GA, Rosengart MR, Zenati MS, et al. Nonoperative management of severe blunt splenic injury: are we getting better? J Trauma. 2006;61:1113–8. discussion 8-9
21. Moore FA, Davis JW, Moore Jr EE, Cocanour CS, West MA, McIntyre Jr RC. Western Trauma Association (WTA) critical decisions in trauma: management of adult blunt splenic trauma. J Trauma. 2008;65:1007–11.
22. Peitzman AB, Harbrecht BG, Rivera L, Heil B. Failure of observation of blunt splenic injury in adults: variability in practice and adverse consequences. J Am Coll Surg. 2005;201:179–87.
23. Peitzman AB, Heil B, Rivera L, et al. Blunt splenic injury in adults: multi-institutional Study of the Eastern Association for the Surgery of Trauma. J Trauma. 2000;49:177–87. discussion 187-9
24. Gaarder C, Dormagen JB, Eken T, et al. Nonoperative management of splenic injuries: improved results with angioembolization. J Trauma. 2006;61:192–8.
25. Skattum J, Naess PA, Eken T, Gaarder C. Refining the role of splenic angiographic embolization in high-grade splenic injuries. J Trauma Acute Care Surg. 2013;74:100–3; discussion 103-4.
26. Morrison CA, Wyatt MM, Carrick MM. The effects of cirrhosis on trauma outcomes: an analysis of the National Trauma Data Bank. J Surg Res. 2008; doi.org/10.1016/j.jss.2008.04.034
27. Peetz A, Salim A, Askari R, et al. Association of model for end-stage liver disease score and mortality in trauma patients with chronic liver disease. JAMA Surg. 2016;15:41–8.
28. Cheng C-Y, Ho C-H, Wang C-C, et al. One-year mortality after traumatic brain injury in liver cirrhosis patients-- a ten-year population-based study. Medicine. 2015;94:1–9.
29. Nau C, Wutzler S, Dorr H, et al. Liver cirrhosis but not alcohol abuse is associated with impaired outcome in trauma patients--- a retrospective, multicentre study. Injury. 2012;44:661–6.
30. Patel MS, Malinoski DJ, Nguyen X-MT, et al. The impact of select chronic diseases on outcomes after trauma: a study from the National Trauma Data Bank. J Am Coll Surg. 2011;212:96–104.
31. Talving P, Lustenberger T, Okoye OT, et al. The impact of liver cirrhosis on outcomes in trauma patients: a prospective study. J Trauma Acute Care Surg. 2013;75:699–703.
32. Christmas AB, Wilson AK, Franklin GA, et al. Cirrhosis and trauma: a deadly duo. Am Surg. 2005;71:996–1000.
33. Georgiou C, Inaba K, Teixeira PGR, et al. Cirrhosis and trauma are a lethal combination. World J Surg. 2009;33:1087–92.
34. Dangleben DA, Jazaeri O, Wasser T, et al. Impact of cirrhosis on outcomes in trauma. J Amer Coll Surg. 2006;203:908–13.
35. Wutzler S, Maegele M, Marzi I, et al. Association of preexisting medical conditions with in-hospital mortality in trauma patients. J Amer Coll Surg. 2009;209:75–81.

36. Lin B-C, Fang J-F, Wong Y-C, et al. Management of cirrhotic patients with blunt abdominal trauma: analysis of risk factor of postoperative death with model for end-stage liver disease score. Injury. 2011;43:1457–61.
37. Shoko T, Shiraishi A, Kaki M, et al. Effect of pre-existing medical conditions on in-hospital mortality: analysis of 20,257 trauma patients in Japan. J Amer Coll Surg. 2010;211:338–46.
38. Tinkoff G, Rhodes M, Diamond D, et al. Cirrhosis in the trauma victim. Effect on mortality rates. Ann Surg. 1990;211:172–7.
39. Gacouin A, Locufier M, Uhel F, et al. Liver cirrhosis is independently associated with 90-day mortality in ARDS patients. Shock. 2016;45:16–21.
40. Burns CJ, Chung KK, Aden JK, et al. High risk but not always lethal: the effect of cirrhosis on thermally injured patients. J Burn Care Res. 2013;34:115–9.
41. Demetriades D, Constantinou C, Salim A, et al. Liver cirrhosis in patients undergoing laparotomy for trauma: effect on outcomes. J Amer Coll Surg. 2004;199:538–42.
42. Barmparas J, Cooper Z, Ley EJ, et al. The effect of cirrhosis on the risk for failure of nonoperative management of blunt liver injuries. Surgery. 2015;158:1676–85.
43. Fang J-F, Chen R-J, Lin B-C, et al. Liver cirrhosis: an unfavorable factor for nonoperative management of blunt splenic injury. J Trauma Acute Care Surg. 2003;54:1131–6.
44. Bugaev N, Breeze JL, Daoud V, et al. Management and outcome of patients with blunt splenic injury and preexisting liver cirrhosis. J Trauma Acute Care Surg. 2014;76:1354–61.
45. Cook MR, Fair KA, Burg J, et al. Cirrhosis increases mortality and splenectomy rates following splenic injury. Am J Surg. 2015;209:841–7.

# Index

Printed in the United States
By Bookmasters